Hemovigilance

Hemovigilance

An Effective Tool for Improving Transfusion Safety

EDITED BY

René R.P. De Vries MD

Past President of the International Haemovigilance Network (IHN) and Head of the Blood Transfusion Service, Department of Immunohematology and Blood Transfusion, Leiden University Medical Center, Leiden, The Netherlands

Jean-Claude Faber MD

President of the International Haemovigilance Network (IHN) and retired as Medical Director, Blood Transfusion Service of the Luxembourg Red Cross, Luxembourg

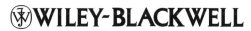

A John Wiley & Sons, Ltd., Publication

This edition first published 2012, © 2012 by John Wiley & Sons, Ltd

Copyright is not claimed for chapters 19 and 27, which are in the public domain.

Wiley-Blackwell is an imprint of John Wiley & Sons, formed by the merger of Wiley's global Scientific, Technical and Medical business with Blackwell Publishing.

Registered office: John Wiley & Sons, Ltd, The Atrium, Southern Gate, Chichester, West Sussex, PO19 8SQ, UK

Editorial offices: 9600 Garsington Road, Oxford, OX4 2DQ, UK
          The Atrium, Southern Gate, Chichester, West Sussex, PO19 8SQ, UK
          111 River Street, Hoboken, NJ 07030-5774, USA

For details of our global editorial offices, for customer services and for information about how to apply for permission to reuse the copyright material in this book please see our website at www.wiley.com/wiley-blackwell

Library of Congress Cataloging-in-Publication Data
Hemovigilance : an effective tool for improving transfusion safety / edited by René R.P. De Vries, Jean-Claude Faber, Pierre Robillard.
    p. ; cm.
  Includes bibliographical references and index.
  ISBN 978-0-470-65527-6 (hardcover : alk. paper)
  I. Vries, René R. P. de.   II. Faber, Jean-Claude.   III. Robillard, Pierre.
  [DNLM: 1. Blood Safety.   2. Blood Banks–standards.   3. Blood Transfusion–standards. WH 460]
  615.3'90289–dc23

                                                          2012002552

A catalogue record for this book is available from the British Library.

Wiley also publishes its books in a variety of electronic formats. Some content that appears in print may not be available in electronic books.

Set in 9/12pt Meridien by Aptara Inc., New Delhi, India

1   2012

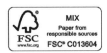

Contents

Part 6 Developments

Appendices

List of Contributors

Ramir Alcantara MD
Registrar
Blood Services Group
Health Sciences Authority
Singapore

Ai Leen Ang MD, FRCPath
Consultant
Blood Services Group
Health Sciences Authority
Singapore;
Department of Haematology
Singapore General Hospital
Singapore

Simon A. Brown MBBS, MD, FRCP, FRCPath, FRACP, FRCPA
Clinical Advisor and Consultant Haematologist
Queensland Blood Management Program & Pathology
Queensland
Brisbane, Australia

Hannah Cohen MD, FRCP, FRPath
Consultant Haematologist and Honorary Senior Lecturer
University College London Hospitals and University College
    London
Department of Haematology
London, UK

Magdy Elekiaby MSc, MD
Head of Blood Transfusion Center
Shabrawishi Hospital
Giza, Egypt

Madhav Erraguntla PhD
Senior Research Scientist
Knowledge Based Systems Inc
College Station, TX, USA

Katherine Forrester PhD
Transfusion Researcher
Scottish National Blood Transfusion Service
Edinburgh, UK

Gamal Gabra MD
Transfusion Medicine Consultant
Birmingham Blood Transfusion Center
Birmingham, UK

Peter R. Ganz PhD
Director, Centre for Biologics Evaluation
Health Canada
Ottawa, ON, Canada;
Adjunct Professor
Faculty of Medicine
University of Ottawa
Ottawa, ON, Canada

Naoko Goto MS
Deputy Director
Safety Vigilance Division
Blood Service Headquarters
Japanese Red Cross Society
Tokyo, Japan

Giuliano Grazzini MD, PhD
Director, National Blood Centre
Istituto Superiore di Sanità
Rome, Italy

Mark Grumbridge RGN BSc Dip N
Transfusion Practitioner
Department of Haematology
St George's Hospital and Medical School
London, UK

Reinhard Henschler MD
Head, Department of Production
Institute for Transfusion Medicine and
    Immunohaematology
Clinics of the Johann Wolfgang Goethe University
    Frankfurt/Main
German Red Cross Blood Donor Services
    Baden-Wuerttemberg-Hessen
Frankfurt/Main, Germany

Salwa Hindawi MD, FRCPath, CTM
President of Saudi Society of Transfusion Medicine
ISBT Eastern Mediterranean Regional Director
Member of WHO Advisory Panel on Blood Safety
Director of Blood Transfusion Services
King Abdalaziz University, Jeddah
Saudi Arabia

Satoru Hino MPharm
Deputy Director General
(General Manufacturing/Distribution Supervisor)
Blood Service Headquarters
Japanese Red Cross Society
Tokyo, Japan

Christopher J. Hogan MBBS, BSc (Hons), FRCPA
Principal Medical Officer
National Blood Authority, Canberra;
Chair, Australian Haemovigilance Advisory Committee
Canberra, Australia

Jerry A. Holmberg PhD
Director, Scientific Affairs
Novartis Vaccines and Diagnostics Inc.
Emeryville, CA, USA

Hany Kamel MD
Corporate Medical Director
Blood Systems Inc.
Scottsdale, AZ, USA

Mickey B.C. Koh MD, PhD, FRCPath
Consultant Haematologist
Director, Stem Cell Transplant Programme
St George's Hospital and Medical School
London, UK;
Medical Director, Cell Therapy Facility
Health Sciences Authority
Singapore;
Division Director
Blood Services Group
Health Sciences Authority
Singapore

Wim de Kort MD, PhD
Director, Donor Services
Sanquin Blood Supply Foundation
Nijmegen, The Netherlands

Matthew J. Kuehnert MD
Director, Office of Blood, Organ, and other Tissue Safety
Division of Healthcare Quality Promotion
Centers for Disease Control and Prevention (CDC)
Atlanta, GA, USA

Juergen Luhm PhD
Quality Manager
Institute for Transfusion Medicine and Immunohaematology
Clinics of the Johann Wolfgang Goethe University
    Frankfurt/Main
German Red Cross Blood Donor Services
    Baden-Wuerttemberg-Hessen
Frankfurt/Main, Germany

Tanneke Marijt-van der Kreek MD
Chief Donor Physician in Southwestern Region
Sanquin Blood Supply Foundation
Rotterdam, The Netherlands

Brian McClelland MD
Scottish National Blood Transfusion Service
Edinburgh, UK

Shun-ya Momose BPharm
Director
Safety Vigilance Division
(Safety Management Supervisor)
Blood Service Headquarters
Japanese Red Cross Society
Tokyo, Japan

Markus M. Mueller
Consultant in Transfusion Medicine
Department Head of Blood Donation
Institute for Transfusion Medicine and Immunohaematology
Clinics of the Johann Wolfgang Goethe University
    Frankfurt/Main
German Red Cross Blood Donor Services
    Baden-Wuerttemberg-Hessen
Frankfurt/Main, Germany

Thea Mueller-Kuller PhD
Quality Manager
Institute for Transfusion Medicine and Immunohaematology
Clinics of the Johann Wolfgang Goethe University
    Frankfurt/Main
German Red Cross Blood Donor Services
    Baden-Wuerttemberg-Hessen
Frankfurt/Main, Germany

Fátima Nascimento MD
Senior Consultant in Transfusion Medicine
General Directorate of Health
Lisbon, Portugal

Hitoshi Okazaki MD, PhD
Senior Director
Research and Development Department
Central Blood Institute
Blood Service Headquarters
Japanese Red Cross Society
Tokyo, Japan

Hans-Ulrich Pfeiffer Dipl Biol
Production Manager
Institute for Transfusion Medicine and
    Immunohaematology
Clinics of the Johann Wolfgang Goethe University
    Frankfurt/Main
German Red Cross Blood Donor Services
    Baden-Wuerttemberg-Hessen
Frankfurt/Main, Germany

Constantina Politis MD
Associate Professor of Medicine
Athens University;
Head of the Hellenic Coordinating Haemovigilance Centre
    (SKAE)
Athens, Greece

Simonetta Pupella MD
Responsible Medical Area, National Blood Centre
Istituto Superiore di Sanità
Rome, Italy

Philippe Renaudier MD, MS
French Society of Vigilance and Transfusion Therapeutics
    (SFVTT)
Regional Coordination of Hemovigilance
Agence Régionale de Santé Lorraine
Nancy, France

Martin R Schipperus MD, PhD
Hematologist
Head, Department of Hematology
Haga Teaching Hospital;
President, TRIP Dutch National Hemovigilance Office
The Hague, The Netherlands

Erhard Seifried MD, PhD
Professor of Transfusion Medicine
Chair for Transfusion Medicine and Immunohaematology
Medical Director and CEO
German Red Cross Blood Transfusion Service
    Baden-Wuerttemberg—Hessen
Institute for Transfusion Medicine and
    Immunohaematology
JW Goethe University Frankfurt/Main
Frankfurt/Main, Germany

Walid Sireis MUDr
Head, Quality Management
Institute for Transfusion Medicine and Immunohaematology
Clinics of the Johann Wolfgang Goethe University
    Frankfurt/Main
German Red Cross Blood Donor Services
    Baden-Wuerttemberg-Hessen
Frankfurt/Main, Germany

**Lisa J. Stevenson RN, Grad Dip Health Med Law,
Cert Transfus Practice, Cert Crit Care**
Transfusion Nurse Consultant
Blood Matters Program
Department of Health and Australian Red Cross Blood
    Service
Melbourne, Victoria, Australia

Paul F.W. Strengers MD, FFPM
Director, Medical Affairs and Product Development
Division of Plasma Products
Sanquin Blood Supply Foundation
Amsterdam, The Netherlands

D. Michael Strong PhD
Affiliate Professor
Department of Orthopaedics and Sports Medicine
University of Washington School of Medicine
Seattle, WA, USA

Kenji Tadokoro MD, PhD
Executive Officer
Blood Service Board of Management;
Director General
Central Blood Institute
Blood Service Headquarters
Japanese Red Cross Society
Tokyo, Japan

Clare Taylor PhD FRCP FRCPath
Consultant in Haematology and Transfusion Medicine
Former Medical Director of SHOT
c/o SHOT Office, Manchester Blood Centre
Manchester, UK

Dafydd Thomas MBChB, FRCA
Consultant in Intensive Care Medicine
Morriston Hospital
Swansea, Wales

Anita van Tilborgh-de Jong MD
Senior Hemovigilance Physician
TRIP Dutch National Hemovigilance Office
The Hague, The Netherlands

Peter Tomasulo MD
Chief Medical and Scientific Officer
Blood Systems Inc.
Scottsdale, AZ, USA

Tomislav Vuk MD
Specialist in Transfusion Medicine
Head of Quality Control and Quality Assurance Department
Croatian Institute of Transfusion Medicine
Zagreb, Croatia

Barbara I. Whitaker PhD
Director, Data and Special Programs
AABB
Bethesda, MD, USA

Johanna Wiersum-Osselton MD
National Coordinator
TRIP Dutch National Hemovigilance Office
The Hague, The Netherlands
and
Senior Donor Physician
Sanquin Blood Supply Foundation
Rotterdam, The Netherlands

Lorna M. Williamson BSc, MD, FRCP, FRCPath
Medical and Research Director
NHS Blood and Transplant
Watford, UK

Jeroen de Wit PharmD
Vice Chair, Executive Board
Sanquin Blood Supply Foundation
Amsterdam, The Netherlands

Erica M. Wood MBBS, FRACP, FRCPA
Consultant Haematologist
Chair, Serious Transfusion Incident Reporting (STIR)
    Expert Group
Blood Matters Program
Department of Health and Australian Red Cross Blood
    Service
and
Department of Clinical Haematology, Monash University
Melbourne, Victoria, Australia

Jun Wu MD, PhD
Blood Safety Surveillance and Health Care Acquired
    Infection Division
Public Health Agency of Canada
Ottawa, ON, Canada

Pauline Y. Zijlker-Jansen MD
Hemovigilance and Tissue Vigilance Physician
TRIP Dutch National Hemovigilance Office
The Hague, The Netherlands

Foreword

Hemovigilance is one of the most important activities for those of us who are active in the field of blood transfusion. Irrespective of your profession, whether blood banker, quality manager, donor physician, nurse, phlebotomist, laboratory technician, transfusing physician or hospital nurse, the safety of blood products from their "origin" in the blood donor until their use in the recipient is of utmost importance. The phrase "safety from vein to vein" was coined to illustrate the breadth of the field. Today, the field of hemovigilance is even more wide-ranging, covering blood components, tissues and cell preparations including donor vigilance, materiovigilance and safety of the patient.

While hemovigilance is well known to those who work in the field of transfusion medicine, there are important differences between countries when it comes to the implementation of national hemovigilance programs.

The International Hemovigilance Network (IHN) has done an excellent job in establishing common definitions and in bringing together the different national activities. Today in Europe, EU directives define our common standards in blood transfusion and similar approaches are taken in other regions of the world.

In June 2009, René de Vries, then President of the International Hemovigilance Network, was asked by Maria Khan, responsible for transfusion publications at Wiley-Blackwell, about the need for a handbook on hemovigilance that would outline and guide the reader on procedures of the transfusion chain. Maria asked René whether he believed such a book would be beneficial and, if so, who might make suitable editors and authors for the project.

The request from Wiley-Blackwell fell on fertile soil. After consultation with the IHN Board, René confirmed the need for such a book and moreover advised that the IHN Board had recently been discussing a similar idea. They were therefore willing to embark on the project. Finally, two IHN Board members agreed to take on the editorship of this book: René de Vries and Jean-Claude Faber.

Hemovigilance: An Effective Tool for Improving Transfusion Safety is the first book on this subject and its aim is to become *the* textbook on hemovigilance. This may well be the case since all the ingredients to achieve this aim are present: the editors developed a master plan and communicated this to all the authors, gathering the best experts from all over the world. Contributors demonstrated their commitment, writing their chapters according to the uniform instructions and definitions set out by the editors. The book is as comprehensive as is possible for such a big subject and many diverse examples from different settings are given.

It not only provides clear-cut answers to the 'Whats?' and 'Whys?', but also to the 'How do Is?' Examples of national and international hemovigilance systems and a summary of past achievements as well as new developments and future challenges will help readers to integrate their local or national experience into the global scheme.

We are very pleased with the new hemovigilance book and we hope that many readers from both within the field of transfusion medicine and from other fields such as quality and safety management, and regulatory affairs, will enjoy it. We are confident that *Hemovigilance: An Effective Tool for Improving Transfusion Safety* will contribute to the improvement of safety and quality of blood transfusion.

Erhard Seifried* and Markus M. Mueller
Frankfurt/Main, Germany
March 2012

---

*past president of the International Society for Blood Transfusion (ISBT).

PART 1
General Introduction

CHAPTER 1

Introduction

René R.P. de Vries

Department of Immunohematology and Blood Transfusion, Leiden University Medical Center, Leiden, The Netherlands

Why did we produce this book?

Hemovigilance deals with the safety of blood transfusion. Although such safety has been a major concern ever since blood transfusions started being given, both the concept and the name "hemovigilance" were born less than 20 years ago. Today hemovigilance is an established but also quickly developing field in transfusion medicine, for which a comprehensive text has thus far been lacking.

This book is the first book on hemovigilance. The only other book that comes somewhat near is *Blood Safety and Surveillance*,[1] which mainly deals with product safety and has a quite different scope. Apart from that, there are only less detailed and less complete chapters on hemovigilance in books on transfusion medicine, such as in *Rossi's Principles of Transfusion Medicine*[2] and reviews in journals.[3–5]

Our aim is that this book becomes *the* book on hemovigilance.

Who would want to read or consult this book?

Professionals may want to consult this book so that they can easily find practical information on the different aspects of this new and quickly developing field. We aim this book specifically at the following categories of professionals:
• staff and quality management officers of blood establishments;

• hospital Transfusion Committees, hemovigilance officers, and all personnel involved in the transfusion process in the hospital (medical doctors, nurses, logistic people, quality officers);
• staff of regional and national hemovigilance offices.

This book will also be valuable as a teaching aid, both for teachers and students of hemovigilance. Finally, relevant parts are easily assessable for non-medical personnel (hospital managers, health and regulatory authorities).

What can you expect to find in this book?

This book is an introduction to and a manual for the subject of hemovigilance.

You will find both "the how" examples of the actual information derived, and what is done with it. Of course, a book like this cannot be comprehensive with regard to all information, and so we include references to the most pertinent papers on the subject and links to websites with more details.

One thing we don't include is detailed descriptions of different types of transfusion reactions in patients and how to deal with them. For this type of information, please consult general textbooks on transfusion medicine or, for example, the monograph on transfusion reactions written by Popovsky.[6] The same advice applies to information on complications in donors.

Hemovigilance: An Effective Tool for Improving Transfusion Safety, First Edition. Edited by René R.P. De Vries and Jean-Claude Faber.
© 2012 John Wiley & Sons, Ltd. Published 2012 by John Wiley & Sons, Ltd.

How to use this book?

After reading the General Introduction (Part 1), you can go straight to one or more of the next parts depending on your area of interest. The content of each part is briefly summarized below:

• Part 1, a general introduction, contains (in addition to this introduction to the book), an introduction to hemovigilance (Chapter 2) and to its concepts and models (Chapter 3).

• Part 2, Surveillance of the Blood Transfusion Chain, is split into two sections. If you want to know how to establish a hemovigilance system in your hospital or blood establishment, go to Section 2.1 where the different parts of the transfusion chain are discussed: Setting up or consolidating a system (Chapter 4); preparation of blood components (Chapter 5); testing, issuing, and transport (Chapter 6); and clinical activities (Chapter 7). Section 2.2 (Chapters 8 to 11) describes how established hemovigilance systems work at the level of a blood establishment and a hospital.

• Part 3 deals with national and regional hemovigilance systems. The nine chapters provide examples of how different national hemovigilance systems function and what data they generate. The results of one of the best functioning hemovigilance systems (SHOT) are also presented and discussed in Part 5, Chapter 24.

• Part 4 covers hemovigilance at the international level. The European system is discussed as an example of international frameworks in Chapter 21. Chapter 22 deals with international collaboration, specifically the International Hemovigilance Network (IHN). Hemovigilance is still mainly confined to developed countries (as reflected by the membership of the IHN) and so the objectives and obstacles encountered in developing countries may be quite different. Therefore, we include a separate chapter on hemovigilance in developing countries (Chapter 23).

• Part 5 summarizes the most important achievements of more than 15 years of hemovigilance activities.

• Part 6 discusses three important new developments in hemovigilance: Vigilance of alternatives for blood components (Chapter 25); Surveillance of clinical effectiveness of transfusion (Chapter 26); and Biovigilance (Chapter 27).

• The three appendices include a Glossary with the main terms peculiar to the field of hemovigilance, and lists of definitions of adverse reactions in patients and donors.

For a more detailed guide to the book's various parts and sections, please take a look at Chapter 2.

References

1 Linden JV, and Bianco C (eds), 2001, *Blood Safety and Surveillance*. Marcel Dekker, New York.

2 Simon TL, Synder EL, Solheim BG, Stowell CP, Strauss RG, and Petrides M (eds), 2009, *Rossi's Principles of Transfusion Medicine*, 4th edition, Wiley-Blackwell, Oxford, UK.

3 Faber JC, 2002, Haemovigilance around the world. *Vox Sang* **83**(Suppl 1): 71–6.

4 Robillard P, Chan P, and Kleinman S, 2004, Hemovigilance for improvement of blood safety. *Transfus Apher Sci* **31**(2): 95–8.

5 De Vries RRP, Faber JC, and Strengers PFW, 2011, Haemovigilance: An effective tool for improving transfusion practice. *Vox Sang* **100**: 60–7.

6 Popovsky MA, 2007, *Transfusion Reactions*, second edition. AABB Press, Bethesda, MD, USA.

CHAPTER 2

Hemovigilance: A Quality Tool for the Blood Transfusion Chain

René R.P. de Vries

Department of Immunohematology and Blood Transfusion, Leiden University Medical Center, Leiden, The Netherlands

This chapter is an introduction to hemovigilance, starting with a brief historical overview of the safety of blood transfusion as background.

History of blood transfusions

The first blood transfusions were attempts to transfuse humans with animal blood (lambs were the favorite creatures) to "treat" all kinds of illnesses in the 17th century. In the 18th century, however, the French king Louis XIV forbade the transfusion of animal blood to people by law because it was considered too dangerous.[1] In the 19th century, Henri Leacock and James Blundell pioneered interhuman transfusion as a life-saving therapy for severe blood loss.[2] Blundell warned others, however, to apply this therapy only as *ultimum refugium* because it was, again, considered dangerous.[3] Particularly after the discovery of the ABO blood groups by Landsteiner,[4] blood transfusion became less dangerous but certainly still not without risk.

There is only scattered documentation of the surveillance of the safety of blood transfusion and blood components in the literature (for example, see Reference 5) although this situation is improving.

Introducing hemovigilance

The word "hemovigilance" comes from the French *hémovigilance* and is derived from the Greek *haema* meaning "blood" and the Latin *vigilans* meaning "watchful." It was coined in France in 1994 to function in the same way as the term "pharmacovigilance" does for drugs. Figure 2.1 shows a beautiful picture of a lion, already the symbol of vigilance in the 17th century.

Pharmacovigilance started in France in the 1970s in order to prevent a repeat of anything along the lines of the thalidomide/Softenon drama (also known as the Contergan scandal), in which more than 10,000 children were born with severe congenital deformities due to the use of thalidomide by their mothers during pregnancy. Similarly, as a reaction to the HIV/AIDS scandal in the 1980s and early 1990s, a complete surveillance system for blood transfusion was initiated in France in 1994, and was the start of hemovigilance.

Several definitions exist for hemovigilance and you will encounter several of them throughout this book. The International Hemovigilance Network (IHN) has formulated the following definition:

> *A set of surveillance procedures covering the whole transfusion chain (from the collection of blood and its components to the follow-up of recipients), intended to collect and assess*

Hemovigilance: An Effective Tool for Improving Transfusion Safety, First Edition. Edited by René R.P. De Vries and Jean-Claude Faber.
© 2012 John Wiley & Sons, Ltd. Published 2012 by John Wiley & Sons, Ltd.

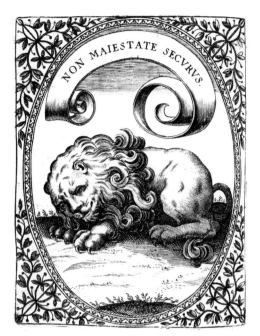

Figure 2.1 This picture, from an edition printed in Brussels in 1649 and kept in the library of Leiden University, the Netherlands, is from Saavedra's *Idea de un Príncipe Político Christiano (Idea of a Political-Christian Prince)* (http://www.emblematica.com/en/cd01-saavedra.htm). The lion was a symbol of vigilance because he needs little sleep. If he does sleep, it was believed that he was doing so with his eyes open because he knows that he is not safe in his majesty *(non majestate securus)*. Reproduced from Biblitotheca Thysiana with permission from Leiden University Library.

information on unexpected or undesirable effects resulting from the therapeutic use of labile blood products, and to prevent their occurrence or recurrence.[6]

A simpler and yet perhaps more complete definition is: "A set of surveillance procedures of the whole transfusion chain intended to minimize adverse events or reactions in donors and recipients and to promote safe and effective use of blood components".

Blood components

There are three kinds of labile blood components: erythrocytes (red blood cells), platelets, and fresh-frozen plasma.

Plasma derivatives such as clotting factor concentrates, immunoglobulins, and albumin are called *blood products*. In Europe, these products are considered to be pharmaceuticals, and the manufacturers have to comply with regulations different to usual hemovigilance ones. The same applies to drugs that are used as alternatives for, or to minimize the use of, blood components, such as Erythropoietin, Tranexamic acid, and Clopidogrel.

Quality system

Hemovigilance is an important part of the quality system for blood transfusion (see Figure 2.2). Other methods for identifying errors, adverse events, and reactions include audits of practice and the investigation of complaints.

Like any discipline, hemovigilance involves the use of specific terms with precise meanings as follows:

• An *adverse event* is an undesirable and unintended occurrence in the blood transfusion chain (which consists of the collection, testing, preparation, storage, distribution, ordering, issuing, and administration of blood and blood components). It may or may not be the result of an error or an incident (see below) and it may or may not result in an adverse reaction in a donor or recipient.

• An *incident* is a case in which the patient is transfused with a blood component that did not meet all the requirements for a suitable transfusion for that patient, or that was intended for another patient. Incidents thus comprise transfusion errors and deviations from standard operating procedures (SOPs) or hospital policies that have lead to

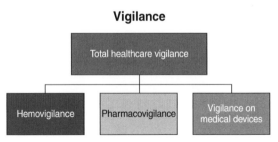

Figure 2.2 Hemovigilance as part of a quality management system for healthcare.

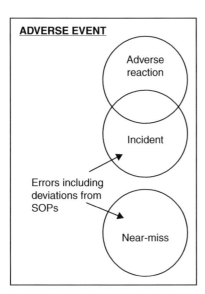

Figure 2.3 Adverse events: Relationship between adverse reactions, incidents, and near-misses (*source:* ISBT proposed standard definitions for surveillance of non-infectious adverse transfusion reactions, July 2011; developed by the ISBT working party on hemovigilance in collaboration with the International Hemovigilance Network; reproduced by permission www.isbtweb.org/working-parties/haemovigilance/definitions).

mistransfusions. It may or may not lead to an adverse reaction (see below).

• A *near-miss* is an error or deviation from standard procedures or policies that is discovered before the start of the transfusion and that could have led to a wrongful transfusion or to a reaction in a recipient.

• An *adverse reaction* is an undesirable response or effect in a patient or donor temporally associated with the collection or administration of blood or blood component. It may, but need not, be the result of an incident.

Figure 2.3 shows the interrelationship of these terms.

Adverse reactions in recipients

An adverse reaction to the transfusion of a blood component is synonymous with a *transfusion reaction*. The severity of an adverse reaction in a recipient is graded according to an internationally accepted scale (see Appendix B).[7]

Another aspect in this regards is the *imputability*, which is the likelihood that an adverse reaction in a recipient can be attributed to the blood component transfused.

There are many different types of transfusion reactions (see Table 2.1 on page 9), which can be subdivided in several ways according to their pathogenesis. A common subdivision is into infectious and noninfectious transfusion or adverse reactions. We also use some internationally accepted definitions throughout this book (see Appendix B).[7]

Adverse reactions or complications in donors

Because the etiology of adverse reactions in a donor is quite different from those in a recipient, they are also known as *complications*. For several reasons, the severity of donor complications are graded according to a different scale to adverse reactions in recipients, although the two scales are similar. This donor scaling is also internationally accepted and evaluated (see Appendix C and/or www.isbt-web.org/members_only/files/society/StandardSurveillanceDOCO.pdf).

Legal framework

In the European Union (EU), certain aspects of hemovigilance (mainly product-related adverse events) are legal requirements that are governed by Directives. One important distinction made in the EU Directives concerning blood products is between Blood Establishments (BEs) and Hospital Blood Banks (hBBs):

• A *Blood Establishment* is any structure or body that is responsible for any aspect of the collection and testing of human blood or blood components, whatever their intended purpose, and their processing, storage, and distribution when intended for transfusion. This does not include hBBs.[8]

• A *Hospital Blood Bank* is a hospital unit that stores, distributes, and may perform compatibility tests on blood and blood components exclusively for use within hospital facilities, including hospital-based transfusion activities.[8]

Summary

Hemovigilance is a system for

• observing, recording, reporting, and analyzing when something goes wrong in the blood transfusion chain (see the next section);

• using the lessons learned to take action to avoid that problem going wrong again.[9]

Hemovigilance systems exist at three levels:

• blood establishment and the hospital level (the blood transfusion chain);

• regional or national level;

• international level.

Hemovigilance in the blood establishment and the hospital: The blood transfusion chain (Part 2)

Soon after the establishment of hemovigilance programs, it was recognized that blood products were actually extremely safe in the developed countries where these programs were functioning, but that transfusion safety consists of more than blood component safety. Notably the UK Serious Hazards of Transfusion (SHOT) scheme draws attention to the fact that transfusion errors are serious and unacceptably common (see Chapter 14). Later it also became clear that many adverse reactions are unavoidable and therefore they are a calculated risk of blood transfusion, as can be seen from Table 2.1.[9]

More recently the donor has received due attention in hemovigilance programs. Because the safety of the donor (rather than of the donated blood) is also the subject of vigilance, this part of hemovigilance is also called *donor vigilance.*

A donor can also be seen as the start of the *blood transfusion chain* (see Figure 2.4). We use this scheme of the blood transfusion chain throughout the book.

Establishing a hemovigilance system (Part 2, Section 2.1)

Hemovigilance systems exist at three levels: (i) the hospital and BE from which that hospital obtains the blood components for transfusion (the basic unit of hemovigilance); (ii) regional and national; and (iii) international.

The basic unit of hemovigilance is the blood transfusion chain shown in Figure 2.4. In order to establish a functioning hemovigilance system in this unit, one needs to follow general principles of a quality system and adapt these to the local situation. Section 2.1 provides a framework and guidance and gives practical tips and examples illustrating the do's and don'ts.

Although there are certainly many similarities with hemovigilance in one transfusion chain, the establishment of a regional or national hemovigilance system faces some quite different challenges, such as confidentiality issues, governance, contact with media, and so on. These are discussed in Part 3. The establishment of an international hemovigilance system is discussed in Part 4.

Hemovigilance systems at three levels (Parts 3 and 4)

Regional and preferably national hemovigilance programs have added value compared to local systems as regards improving the safety of transfusion.

The first hemovigilance system was established in 1993 in Japan (see Chapter 13).

As a reaction to the HIV scandal, the first national hemovigilance system in Europe was initiated in France in 1994. Soon after, other European countries followed this initiative, starting with the UK in 1996. Today almost all EU countries have established a hemovigilance system and the number of hemovigilance systems outside Europe is also steadily increasing.

The functioning of a European hemovigilance system meant to stimulate the development of a coordinated approach to the safety of blood and blood products is described in Chapter 21.

In 1997, the initiative was taken to found the European Hemovigilance Network with the aim of increasing the safety of clinical blood transfusion medicine in Europe. Members of the network are (national) hemovigilance systems. The network started with five members and grew to over 25 members, including some from outside Europe. As a result of this growth, the scope and the name

Table 2.1 Preventable and nonpreventable adverse events.[9]

Type of adverse reaction	Related to the quality of blood component?	Related to failure in clinical transfusion process?	Preventable by
Transfusion-transmitted bacterial infection	Yes	Possibly due to failure to inspect component before transfusion	Donor skin cleansing Diversion pouch on donation line Pathogen reduction Correct storage conditions
Transfusion-transmitted viral infection (HBV, HCV, HIV-1/2, other)	Yes	No	Donor selection Donation testing Pathogen reduction
Transfusion-transmitted parasitic infection (malaria, other)	Yes	No	Donor selection Donation testing Pathogen reduction
Hemolysis due to incorrect storage	No	Yes	Quality assured clinical transfusion process
Immunological hemolysis due to ABO incompatibility	No	Yes	–
Immunological hemolysis due to other alloantibody	No	Yes	–
Anaphylaxis or hypersensitivity	No	No	Unpredictable and unavoidable
Post-transfusion purpura	No	No	Unpredictable and unavoidable
Transfusion Related Acute Lung Injury (TRALI)	Yes	No	TRALI risk may be reduced with Fresh Frozen Plasma (FFP) from male donors
Graft-Versus-Host Disease	Yes	Yes, due to failure to select component or failure to recognize patient at risk	Use of irradiated components for at-risk patients; use of amotosalen treated platelets
Transfusion Associated Circulatory Overload (TACO)	No	Yes, due to failure to recognize patient at risk	Avoid over-infusion
Febrile non-hemolytic TR	Yes	No	Incidence may be reduced by leucodepletion

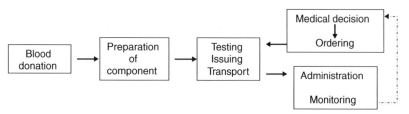

Figure 2.4 The blood transfusion chain.

was changed to the International Hemovigilance Network (IHN). See Chapter 3 for more on the IHN.

Results and achievements (Part 5)

Probably the most important result of hemovigilance has been that it has shown that since the mid-1990s, blood transfusion in Europe is quite safe and notably that blood products are extremely safe compared with other activities and products in healthcare.

The majority of the serious adverse reactions and events that nevertheless do occur happen in the hospital part of the blood transfusion chain. Particularly, the data from the UK hemovigilance system Serious Hazards of Transfusion (SHOT, see Chapter 14) have drawn attention to the fact that about 50% of these are due to administrative errors. The measures installed subsequently resulted in a further increase of the safety of clinical blood transfusion in the hospital.

Well-functioning hemovigilance systems, such as AFSSAPS in France (Chapter 12), Serious Hazards of Transfusion (SHOT) in the UK (Chapter 14), and TRIP in the Netherlands (Chapter 15), have documented the success of various measures to even further improve the safety of blood products. Two examples—(i) the deviation pouch applied during blood drawing from a blood donor in order to minimize the risk on contaminating skin bacteria and (ii) the decision to use only plasma from male donors—have been demonstrated to result in significant decreases of serious adverse reactions due, respectively, to bacterial contamination of blood products (particularly platelets) and TRALI reactions.

The results of many activities of the EHN/IHN, such as the contribution to the high quality of hemovigilance in Europe through digital information exchange, meetings, and seminars, are difficult to measure but are certainly important. Concrete results include: (i) the standardization of definitions and reporting of serious adverse events and reactions in collaboration with the International Society of Blood Transfusion (ISBT) Working Party for Hemovigilance (see Appendix B); (ii) the stimulation and structuring of donor vigilance also in collaboration with the Working Party for Hemovigilance (see Appendix C).

These definitions (see www.isbt-web.org/docu mentation and www.ihn-org.com) are being used by the European Commission for the reporting according to the EU Directives requirements.

After completing the standardization of the definitions, IHN decided to embark on an ambitious project to establish an international hemovigilance database. The compliance with the international definitions was not yet optimal and the database project will contribute to improving that situation. With these results, it will be possible to make comparisons between data generated by different systems.

New developments: Vigilance of alternatives for and appropriateness of transfusion and tissue-/bio-vigilance (see Part 6)

Data from an anesthesiology survey in France indicated that many more perioperative deaths are due to under-transfusion or delayed transfusion than to adverse reactions of transfusions given in time.[10] Also the safety of measures that are often proposed to stimulate blood saving strategies (e.g., cell savers) and medicinal products (e.g., anti-fibrinolytics) have to be taken into account. Presently, not enough is known about the safety of these alternatives to be sure whether they can be recommended.

Another issue is optimal blood usage. The awareness that apart from vital indications the efficacy of blood transfusions is often unknown, not established, or even negative has resulted in a significant reduction of the use of blood products as documented by many hemovigilance systems. One step further would be the surveillance of appropriate or optimal blood use in a more detailed way, for example, through the collection of a set of indicators, which may be provided easily by most hospital information systems. In a still broader framework, there is also a need for data on the benefit of transfusion of a blood component in different clinical situations in order to be able to make risk-benefit calculations.[11]

Audit methods may sometimes be more appropriate to measure and analyze critical parameters for optimal blood use, such as compliance with guidelines (see www.optimalblooduse.eu). Nevertheless, it is expected that existing hemovigilance systems, including the hemovigilance officials in hospitals, may in the near future also contribute to the surveillance of optimal blood use.[12]

Hemovigilance systems will also be exposed to the vigilance and surveillance of other human products that are transplanted: first, cells and tissues, and at a later stage, organs for transplantation. In the USA, the word "biovigilance" has already been coined for this combined activity (www.aabb.org/programs/biovigilance). The European Commission has combined these activities in one directorate. It is clear that there are many similarities with hemovigilance and this will present opportunities for other activities to be shared and based on the expertise obtained in hemovigilance.

Appendices

The appendices of this book contain a Glossary with the main terms peculiar to the field of hemovigilance (Appendix A), definitions for the surveillance of noninfectious adverse transfusion reactions (Appendix B), and complications related to blood donation (Appendix C).

References

1 Bernard J, 1992, *La Légende du Sang*. Flammarion, Paris.

2 Schmidt PJ, and Leacock AG, 2002, Forgotten transfusion history: John Leacock of Barbados. *BMJ* **325**(7378): 1485–7.

3 Blundell J, 1818, Experiments on the transfusion of blood by the syringe. *Lancet* **9**: 57–92.

4 Landsteiner K, 1901, Ueber Agglutinationserscheinungen normalen menschlichen Blutes. *Wien. Klin. Wochenschr.* **14**: 1132–4.

5 AuBuchon JP, and Dzik WS, 2010, Reports on clinical transfusion medicine in the early days of transfusion. *Transfusion* **50**: 963–7.

6 www.ihn-org.com/about/definition-of-haemovigilance [accessed February 21, 2012].

7 ISBT, 2011, Proposed standard definitions for surveillance of non-infectious adverse transfusion reactions. http://www.isbtweb.org/fileadmin/user_upload/WP_on_Haemovigilance/ISBT_definitions_final_2011_4_.pdf [accessed February 22, 2012].

8 European Union, 2004, Commission Directive 2004/33/EC implementing Directive 2002/98/EC of the European Parliament and of the Council as regards certain technical requirements for blood and blood components. *Official Journal of the European Union*, 30.03.2004, L91/25–L91/39.

9 McClelland DBL, Pirie E, Franklin IM, for the EU Optimal Use of Blood Project Partners, 2010, *Manual of optimal blood use*. Scottish National Blood Transfusion Service.

10 Lienhart A, 2006, Les risques de la transfusion et la non transfusion en France. *La Gazette de la Transfusion* **199**: 6–10.

11 McClelland B, and Contreras M, 2005, Appropriateness and safety of blood transfusion. *BMJ* **330**(7483): 104–5.

12 Reesink HW, Panzer S, Gonzalez CA, Lena N, Muntaabski P, *et al.*, 2010, Haemovigilance for the optimal use of blood products in the hospital. *Vox Sang* **99**: 278–93.

CHAPTER 3

Concepts and Models

René R.P. de Vries[1] and Jean-Claude Faber[2]
[1]Department of Immunohematology and Blood Transfusion, Leiden University Medical Center, Leiden, The Netherlands
[2]Blood Transfusion Service, Luxembourg Red Cross, Luxembourg

This chapter introduces you to the concepts and models of hemovigilance.

Introduction

Current hemovigilance systems contain significant conceptual and organizational differences, related to scope and structure. In effect, many roads lead to Rome, and irrespective of the structure of the system hemovigilance can provide valuable data for priority settings and evaluation of corrective strategies.

These system differences, however, may have important implications for the interpretation and comparison of the data from different systems. On the one hand, as shown in Table 3.1, there are more reports per 1000 units in systems where all reactions are reported compared to those where only serious reactions need to be reported. On the other hand, whether the reporting is mandatory (as in France) or voluntary (as in the Netherlands) does not have to affect the reporting rate and differences in reporting rate may be observed in systems using the same concepts and models.

Some systems and methods are more efficient and/or cheaper than others. Certainly, there has been a learning process during the establishment of hemovigilance systems. For instance, lessons were learned from both the early French and UK systems,[1,2] despite them being quite different, and later systems have been developed according to hybrid and novel models.

It is still too early to draw conclusions regarding cost-effectiveness of the different concepts and models.

Scope

Products and processes

The discipline of hemovigilance was triggered by the fact that blood components were unsafe. Therefore, in the beginning activities were mainly focused on product safety, the products in this case being blood components. Soon, however, it became clear that hemovigilance should not be confined only to product safety, because some processes in the blood transfusion chain appeared to be weaker links than the blood components themselves.[3]

In Europe, an international scheme has been operating since 2008, in which each EU member state has to provide the European Commission (EC) annually with blood component-related incidents.[4-8] (See also Chapter 21 on page 244–247.)

Recipients and donors

At first, hemovigilance focused exclusively on the safety of the *recipient* of a blood component. But as the concept of the blood transfusion chain extended "from vein (of the donor) to vein (of the recipient)",[3] *donor* safety also became a subject for hemovigilance. Since 2006, an increasing number of systems have also started to collect data of donor complications data.[9]

Hemovigilance: An Effective Tool for Improving Transfusion Safety, First Edition. Edited by René R.P. De Vries and Jean-Claude Faber.
© 2012 John Wiley & Sons, Ltd. Published 2012 by John Wiley & Sons, Ltd.

Table 3.1 Reporting in different hemovigilance systems.

Country/region	*Reports/ 1000 units	What is reportable	Type of system (at creation)
UK	0.20	Serious reactions + IBCT	Voluntary
Ireland	1.22	Serious reactions + IBCT	Voluntary
France	2.83	All reactions	Mandatory
Netherlands	2.90	All reactions	Voluntary
Québec	7.07	All reactions	Voluntary

*P. Robillard, personal communication; data are from 2006.

"Hot and cold" hemovigilance

"Hot" hemovigilance means the immediate reporting of an incident. This allows immediate corrective measures to be taken, which is very important for product-related incidents and hemovigilance at the level of the hospital or the blood establishment. (See also the Rapid Alert System discussed on page 15.)

Regional, national, and international hemovigilance systems and activities mainly deal with "cold" hemovigilance, for instance the analysis of data and trends on an annual basis and the follow-up of corrective measures proposed on the basis of these data and/or trends.

Report all adverse events/reactions or only the serious ones?

The reporting of *all* adverse events is better for vigilance purposes and for creating awareness, because serious adverse events are rare. It does, of course, require more resources, however.

In most hemovigilance systems, all adverse events (AE) are reported, and in most countries only the reporting of serious adverse reactions (AR) is compulsory. The advantage of also reporting incidents and near-misses, is that these reports offer more and "relatively cheap" (namely, no harm is done) learning opportunities.

Data on more than just blood components?

Safety data of measures that proposed to stimulate blood-saving strategies (e.g., cell savers) and the use of medicinal products (e.g., anti-fibrinolytics or erythrocyte stimulating agents) as compared with blood components are lacking. Some hemovigilance systems (e.g., the Dutch system TRIP) are considering broadening their scope in order to help with providing the data on which an advice on the treatment with blood components or blood alternatives should be based.[10]

Structure

Integration in quality systems

Hemovigilance should be part of a quality system for the blood transfusion chain. In several systems this is indeed the case and some are able to close the Deming quality circle of plan, do, check, act for their system. However, other systems do not go much beyond the reporting of transfusion reactions.

Errors and adverse events occur in many aspects of the process of healthcare. For most patients and clinicians, blood transfusion is only one element of the whole process of clinical care and transfusion risks are a small proportion of the risks to which patients are exposed. Moreover, compared to medicinal drugs, blood components are very safe.[11,12] For these reasons a quality management system for blood transfusion should be part of a hospital's wider quality system in general and an integrated part of the quality system of the patient's safety activities in particular.

Integration in other patient safety activities

Blood safety activity globally is not well integrated into other aspects of patient safety, which are very active in many countries. Efforts need to be made to improve this situation. For instance, in Italy there are plans to integrate the hemovigilance program with the program for clinical risk management for other patient safety movements.

International collaboration

We will briefly introduce here two activities on the field of international collaboration. The first is the International Hemovigilance Network (IHN), which has operated successfully for more than 10 years and grew from the European Hemovigilance Network (EHN).[13,14] The second is the Global Steering Committee on Hemovigilance (GloSCH), a recent initiative with the aim of stimulating hemovigilance particularly in developing countries.

The aim of the IHN is to develop and maintain a worldwide common structure with regards to the safety of blood/blood products and hemovigilance of blood transfusion. The objectives are exchange of valid information between the members of the Network, rapid alert/early warning between the members, joint activities between the members, and educational activities in relation to hemovigilance.

The main activities of the IHN are: a website (www.ihn-org.com) with an open part and a closed part only for official contact persons (OCPs) and participants; an annual general meeting where the Board informs the members of their activities in the past year and important decisions are taken; the organization of an annual Seminar (IHS), which is a scientific two-day meeting; working parties to harmonize definitions and make comparisons on quality indicators, both for safety and appropriate use; and finally the running of an international database on hemovigilance.

The network is briefly structured as follows. Members are (regional or) national hemovigilance systems that are represented by OCPs. Other individuals active in hemovigilance systems may become participants of the network. The OCPs convene yearly to discuss and decide on strategy and budget. Participants may attend these meetings but have no right of vote. The day-to-day running of the network is delegated to a Board consisting of five people.

In 2008, the World Health Organization, the Government of Canada, the ISBT, and the IHN took the initiative for a Global Steering Committee for Hemovigilance (GloSCH). The goal of this initiative is to promote hemovigilance specifically in developing countries. One of the objectives is the production of a guidance document providing Recommendations for Establishing a National Hemovigilance System.

Reporting structure

Safe incident reporting must be blame-free.[15] By creating a failures management culture where physicians and nurses are not afraid of reporting incidents and where reporting is not anonymous but done in an atmosphere of confidence, transfusion practice is improved. In the complex system of healthcare, attention to the safety for the patient therefore also implies attention to the safe functioning of the employer and of the healthcare process.

There are many different reporting structures depending on local situations, legal frameworks, and so on.[16,17] Examples may be found in Chapters 4–21.

Governance

Governance of a hemovigilance system can be organized by a competent authority, a manufacturer, professional organizations, or a Public Health Organization. Combinations are also possible. Examples will be further discussed in Chapters 4–21. Here we briefly summarize the main advantages and disadvantages of each type of governance, by using a particular system as an example:

• *Competent Authority (France: afssaps):* A competent authority (CA) is any person or organization that has the legally delegated or invested authority, capacity, or power to perform a designated function. Advantages are the creation of a centralized system, with sufficient resources and personnel, and that the hemovigilance system is embedded in a multidisciplinary organization including pharmaco- and materio-vigilance. Disadvantages are a top-heavy system, influenced by politics and public opinion, and that reporting to the competent authority may result in under-reporting of errors.

• *Manufacturer (Singapore):* Advantages are the availability of better qualified people, more impetus for change, and less fear for error reporting. The main disadvantage is that the manufacturer may have a conflict of interest.

• *Professional organizations (the Netherlands, TRIP):* Advantages are high qualities of the reports because they are checked by an expert committee, and the whole transfusion chain is covered. Disadvantages are that reporting is on a voluntary basis and therefore is dependent on the willingness of the professionals to report. Also central steering is lacking.

• *Public Health Authority (Canada):* Advantages are the expertise in surveillance methodology and that the handling and analysis of databases can easily be implemented. Disadvantages are no prior knowledge of blood transfusion and therefore confidence of the blood transfusion community was lacking.

Centralized or not

Hemovigilance systems may be organized in a strictly centralized way or be more or less decentralized.

The classical example of a centralized system is the French system (see Chapter 12). Advantages of such a system are that it may guarantee uniformity of data and thus comparability. Disadvantages may be that it is more expensive and that healthcare professionals may be less motivated to report.

An example of a more decentralized system is the UK system SHOT (see Chapter 14), which has certainly provided valuable data and advices (see Chapters 14 and 24) and at much lower costs.

Legal status

Reporting may be on a voluntary or a mandatory basis, and each arrangement has its advantages and disadvantages.

Within the EU, all legal provisions in the Blood Directives have to be transposed into national law by Member States. This has been achieved by most of the Member States within two years time. Member States are free to go beyond what the Directives require: in the context of hemovigilance and traceability several Member States have done so, for example by requiring mandatory notification of all reactions/events to the Competent Authority or by requiring systematic documented feedback of the transfusion of a blood component in a hospital (user) to the blood establishment (producer). This leads to an extensive corps of data available, but whether such extended national requirements in the context of hemovigilance increase safety for the patient and induce change in transfusion practice is not really known. At least it has the potential of raising penalties when cases of infringements to the laws are encountered.

Passive or active

In general, hemovigilance systems deal with passive hemovigilance. Examples of active hemovigilance would be specific transfusion safety research projects and post-marketing surveillance of new components by manufacturers.

Rapid alert system

The rapid alert system (RAS) is an information channel for very quick diffusion of important information in relation to emerging threats, of whatever kind. It allows for quick and safe transmission of precise, correct, and reliable data to competent contact persons in a system. They may decide on possible action in order to maintain or increase safety (through corrective or preventive action) in the case of a proven problem or defect, a potential problem or risk, or even a justified doubt.[13]

In the case of the IHN, the RAS works via fax, e-mail, and website (protected domain). The OCP in one member country of the IHN is informed that a problem has emerged in his or her country, for example through the national hemovigilance system or by other means. This key person analyses the information and decides whether this information should be diffused to the contact persons in the other country members of the IHN. It is the responsibility of the respective contact persons in the other countries to take up the information, evaluate it, and decide upon the actions in their country. In the past, the RAS has been used on different occasions, including the following:

• appearance of clusters of clinical signs after transfusion;

- hidden or apparent defects of disposable material used in transfusion (such as leakages of filter housings, holes in collection bags, defects in apheresis material);
- difficulties with reagents (lack of performance in terms of sensitivity or specificity);
- problems with equipment.

References

1 Noel L, Debeir J, and Cosson A, 1998, The French haemovigilance system. *Vox Sang* **74**(Suppl 2): 441–5.

2 Williamson L, Cohen H, Love E, Jones H, Todd A, and Soldan K, 2000, The Serious Hazards of Transfusion (SHOT) initiative: The UK approach to haemovigilance. *Vox Sang* **78**(Suppl 2): 291–5.

3 Dzik WH, 2003, Emily Cooley Lecture 2002: Transfusion safety in the hospital. *Transfusion* **43**(9): 1190–9.

4 European Union, 2003, Directive 2002/98/EC of the European Parliament and of the Council of January 2003 setting standards of quality and safety for the collection, testing, processing, storage and distribution of human blood and blood components and amending Directive 2001/83/EC. *Official Journal of the European Union* 8.2.2003: L33/30. http://eur-lex .europa.eu/LexUriServ/LexUriServ.do?uri=OJ:L:2003: 033:0030:0040:EN:PDF [accessed February 14, 2012].

5 European Union, 2005, Directive 2005/61/EC of 30 September 2005 implementing Directive 2002/98/EC of the European Parliament and of the Council as regards traceability requirements and notification of serious adverse reactions and events. *Official Journal of the European Union* 1.10.2005: L256/32.

6 European Union, 2005, Directive 2005/62/EC of 30 September 2005 implementing Directive 2002/98/EC of the European Parliament and of the Council as regards Community standards and specifications relating to a quality system for blood establish-ments. *Official Journal of the European Union* 1.10.2005: L256/41.

7 Faber JC, 2004, The European Blood Directive: A new era of blood regulation has begun. *Transfus Med* **14**: 257–73.

8 Watson R, 2005, EU tightens rules on blood safety. *BMJ* **331**: 800.

9 Jorgensen J, and Sorense BS, 2008, Donor vigilance. *ISBT Science Series* **3**(1): 48–53.

10 Strengers PFW, 2010, Adverse effects of alternatives to blood transfusion. *Blood Transfusion* **8**(Suppl 1): 13–6.

11 Hanlon JT, Pieper CF, Hajjar ER, Sloane RJ, Lindblad CI *et al.*, 2006, Incidence and predictors of all and preventable adverse drug reactions in frail elderly persons after hospital stay. *J Gerontol A Biol Sci Med Sci* **61**(5): 511–5.

12 Thomsen LA, Winterstein AG, Søndergaard B, Haugbølle LS, and Melander A, 2007, Systematic review of the incidence and characteristics of preventable adverse drug events in ambulatory care. *Ann Pharmacother* **41**: 1411–26.

13 Faber JC, 2005, Haemovigilance in the European Community. In *Transfusion in Europe: The White Book 2005*, Rouger P and Hossenlopp C (eds). Elsevier Publications SAS.

14 De Vries RRP, Faber JC, and Strengers PFW, 2011, Haemovigilance: An effective tool for improving transfusion practice. *Vox Sang* **100**: 60–7.

15 Strengers, PFW, 2007, Is haemovigilance improving transfusion practice?—The evidence from Europe. In Dax EM, Farrugia A, Vyas G (eds): *Advances in Transfusion Safety; Volume IV*. International Conference Proceedings Developments in Biologicals, vol 127. Karger, Basel; pp. 215–24.

16 Faber JC, 2003, Hemovigilance: Definition and overview of current hemovigilance systems. *Transfusion Alternatives in Transfusion Medicine* **5**: 237–45.

17 Faber JC, 2004, Worldwide overview of existing haemovigilance systems. *Transfus Apher Sci* **31**(2): 99–110.

PART 2

Hemovigilance of the Blood Transfusion Chain (Blood Establishment and Hospital)

SECTION 2.1

Setting up a Hemovigilance System

CHAPTER 4

Setting Up or Consolidating a System for Donor Hemovigilance at the Level of a Blood Establishment

Johanna Wiersum-Osselton[1,2], Wim de Kort[2], Tanneke Marijt-van der Kreek[2], and Jeroen de Wit[2]

[1]Transfusion Reactions in Patients (TRIP), Dutch National Hemovigilance Office, The Hague, The Netherlands
[2]Sanquin Blood Supply Foundation, The Netherlands

Introduction

In a definition adapted from the general meaning of hemovigilance, we see *donor hemovigilance* as "the systematic monitoring of adverse reactions and incidents in the whole chain of blood donor care, with a view to improving quality and safety for blood donors." Here, the term donor *hemo*vigilance is used to make the distinction from donors of tissues, cells, or organs. In this chapter, we use "donor vigilance" in the interests of brevity.

Products and processes

Introduction

In this chapter we review some key points for the (re)designing and implementation of a donor vigi-

lance system at the level of a blood establishment, including blood establishments within hospitals. We give an overview of types of donation complications and define the main processes involved in donor vigilance. This process-based approach will assist in ensuring that all aspects of care are included in assigning responsibilities to staff members of categories and subsequently covered in training.

Processes

Donor vigilance is embedded within the primary blood establishment process, which runs from donor recruitment, health screening, whole blood donation, and apheresis donation procedures to post-donation care and counseling. Figure 4.1 depicts the main aspects of donor vigilance (in the shaded bars) and shows which parts of the donation process they cover.

We consider four aspects of donor vigilance in this chapter:

- Complications related to blood donation (donor adverse reactions).
- Errors (adverse incidents) in donor care.
- Post-donation information: focus on aspects relating to donor safety.
- Counseling and procedures relating to unexpected findings.

This chapter incorporates (chiefly in the sections "Complications related to blood donation (donor adverse reactions)" and "Counseling and procedures relating to unexpected findings") material from Chapter 8, Section 1, of the DOMAINE manual[1] (DOnor MAnagement IN Europe, a European project). This material is included by kind permission of the chapter authors Elze Wagenmans, Crispin Wickenden, Ellen McSweeney, and Wim de Kort as well as the manual's editors Wim de Kort and Ingrid Veldhuizen. Minimal editorial changes have been made.

Hemovigilance: An Effective Tool for Improving Transfusion Safety, First Edition. Edited by René R.P. De Vries and Jean-Claude Faber.
© 2012 John Wiley & Sons, Ltd. Published 2012 by John Wiley & Sons, Ltd.

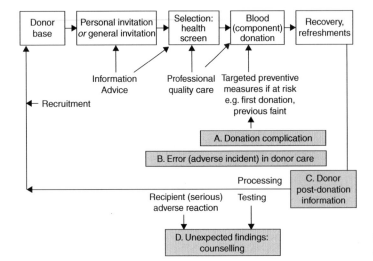

Figure 4.1 The donation process and donor hemovigilance.

Later in the chapter, we return to these processes in donor vigilance and particularly emphasize the need to "close the loop"; that is, to always incorporate steps that review safety and quality of donor care and consider ways to improve.

Note that we do not address aspects of post-donation information relating to recipient safety, nor the study of epidemiological follow-up of donors (seroconverting donors, examining infectious risks, etc.), because these are part of general, product- and recipient-related hemovigilance. Effective use of the donated blood also lies largely outside the scope of this chapter, although the counseling section includes comments about counseling donors whose products are rejected for clinical use.

Complications related to blood donation (donor adverse reactions)

Introduction

Donor safety is of paramount importance during blood sessions and is assured, in so far as it can be, by donor information, donor selection guidelines, adequately trained staff, Standard Operating Procedures (SOPs), and appropriate facilities. Despite these measures, various adverse events and reactions can and do occur during and after blood donation. These complications can be a negative experience for donors and so preventing them must be a priority.

Blood establishments have a duty of care to minimize the risks to donors. This is particularly the case because donating is of no proven health benefit for donors (other than for those who have hemochromatosis). The uneven risk-to-benefit ratio for blood donors also places an ethical responsibility on healthcare givers, the users of blood donations, to avoid wastage and unnecessary use of blood transfusions.

When donor complications do occur, it is essential that they are managed appropriately. It is also essential that blood establishments analyze their complication rates and compare their data with those of other blood services, so as to promote best practice.

This section categorizes types of complications, identifies guidelines for managing and preventing complications, describes the effect of complications on donor motivation, and provides information on hemovigilance, notification, and monitoring.

Definitions and classification of complications of blood donation

A *donor adverse reaction* is any unintended response in a blood donor associated with the collection of blood or blood components.

A *serious adverse reaction* is any unintended response in a blood donor associated with the collection of blood or blood components that is fatal, life-threatening, disabling, incapacitating, or which results in, or prolongs, hospitalization or morbidity.[2]

Donor adverse reactions can manifest themselves in several ways. To facilitate benchmarking, an internationally accepted description and classification of adverse events and reactions was required. The Working Group on Complications Related to Blood Donation, a joint working group of the International Society of Blood Transfusion (ISBT) and the International Hemovigilance Network (IHN), then the European Hemovigilance Network (EHN), was established for this purpose. In the public arena, the group uses the term "complication related to blood donation" in preference to "adverse event or reaction." However, the Working Group defines complications related to blood donations as "adverse reactions or incidents related in time to a blood donation (whole blood or apheresis)."[3] The group classifies complications into two main categories: (i) those with predominantly local symptoms and (ii) those with predominantly generalized symptoms (the categorization is shown in Appendix C on complications related to blood donations. We use the term "complication related to blood donation" in this chapter.

What is known: Complication statistics and risk factors

Complications related to blood donation appear to occur in about 1% of all whole blood donation procedures.[4] However, a higher frequency (3.5%) has been estimated from a donor hemovigilance program on more than 6 million whole blood donations procedures in 2006.[5] The differences in definitions most probably explain these different estimates of donor complication frequencies, but in any case donor reactions are relatively frequent.

It is well recognized that certain categories of donors have higher reaction rates.[6–9] Young age and first-time donor status have been associated with higher reaction rates in many studies. Eder reported a complication rate of 10.7% in 16 and 17 year olds, 8.3% in 18 and 19 year olds, and 2.8% in donors aged 20 years and older.[6] She also found a higher incidence of donation-related injury (particularly physical injury from syncope-related falls) in 16 and 17 year olds compared with older donors.[6] Wiltbank *et al.*, and later Kamel *et al.* in an extended study from the same group, found that compared to donors with no reactions, the strongest predictor of a reaction was a donor's blood volume of less than 3500 ml.[7,9] In addition, Kamel *et al.* showed that 24% of the moderate and severe vasovagal reactions of the study were delayed, that is, occurring more than 15 minutes after the collection. These delayed reactions were significantly associated with females. Off-site delayed reactions (12% of the delayed reactions) were more likely to be associated with a fall, with head trauma, with other injury, and with the use of outside medical care.[9]

Reporting limitations

It is accepted that the reported rate of reactions is much less than the true reaction rate. Newman solicited information from 1000 randomly selected donors three weeks after donation.[10] He found that 36% of donors had had one or more adverse events. The most common systemic adverse events were fatigue (7.8%), vasovagal symptoms (5.3%), and nausea and vomiting (1.1%). The most common arm findings were bruise (22.7%), arm soreness (10%), and hematoma (1.7%). (Note that some groups distinguish between bruising and hematoma, where generally speaking bruising is described as flat discoloration and hematoma is associated with swelling as a result of bleeding into subcutaneous tissue.)

Causes

Jørgensen found that approximately one-third of complications were caused by inserting the needle and two-thirds were vasovagal in nature.[4] He comments that 99% of all complications collated by the EHN/ISBT common working group for 2005 belonged to four common categories: (i) vasovagal reactions (86% of all complications); (ii) hematomas (13%); (iii) nerve injuries (1%); and (iv) arterial punctures (0.4%). The other reported complications together account for 1% of all complications.

Specific complications and long-term complications

Some complications are specific to apheresis donations, for example, citrate reactions, hemolysis, air embolism, allergic reactions to ethylene oxide used in the sterilization of the harness, and thrombocytopenia and protein deficiency from excessive platelet or plasma donations respectively.[11] The majority of apheresis donors experience some mild citrate related side effects, for example a metallic taste in the mouth and/or tingling around the lips. This is an accepted occurrence and is considered to be a physiological effect of the anti-coagulant used in apheresis donations. Most blood establishments only report citrate-related complications if they are moderate or severe or they result in the donation being discontinued.

Potential adverse long-term consequences of donation, such as iron depletion with or without associated anemia[12,13] or increased bone resorption, as has been reported in apheresis donors,[14] are not currently reported as complications of donation. However, this may change, given time.

In some settings, harvesting of peripheral blood stem cells from allogeneic and sometimes also family or autologous donors is performed by the blood establishment. This requires pre-treatment with growth factors (granulocyte colony stimulating factor, G-CSF). Side effects include the near-universal flu-like symptoms, muscle and bone pains, and expected alterations in biochemical and hematological parameters. As well as the frequent occurrence of symptoms of hypocalcemia during the apheresis procedure and the anticipated reduction in platelet counts, complications may arise from the use of central venous catheters. Rare but serious complications have also been described, including splenic rupture, anaphylaxis, and vasculitis.[15] G-CSF is also administered, commonly with steroids, to donors from whom granulocytes are collected, who may also report allergic reactions to the sedimenting agent that is used. The importance of clear information and careful procedures for informed consent and donor clearance cannot be over-stressed. Care of these donors lies beyond the scope of this book. International guidelines exist for follow-up of these donors and appropriate arrangements should be made.[16]

Attention should also be paid to the group of donors who are treated partly or solely for the purposes of hyper-immune plasma donation, with "booster" vaccinations (tetanus, hepatitis B) or Rhesus D positive cells.

If a serious medical event or reaction occurs in a blood donor, it may not always have been caused by the blood donation. This is what is meant by the term *imputability*, which assesses the level of likelihood that an observed reaction can be ascribed to the donation. For instance, if a donor develops myocardial infarction in a blood center but before the health screen, it cannot have been caused by the removal of blood, although a certain level of emotional tension may have played a role. Imputability may be impossible to assess in the case of late events, for example, development of rheumatoid arthritis in long-term follow-up of a stem cell donor.

Serious (severe) and non-serious

Complications range in severity from mild to moderate to severe. The Working Group on Complications Related to Blood Donation has adopted the same generic criteria to define "severe" complications of blood donation as are used for serious adverse reactions in recipients of blood transfusion.[2,3] Non-severe complications may be further classified as either "mild" or "moderate." An overview of the levels of severity is given in Appendix C.

The vast majority of all complications are mild. However, some rare complications are severe, such as accidents related to vasovagal reactions and nerve injuries with long-lasting symptoms.[4] These can have serious consequences for donors and can impact on their daily life. A brief faint, which would be classed as moderate (non-serious), is rated as serious if it leads to a fall necessitating hospitalization: what matters is the outcome for the donor.

Vasovagal reactions that occur after the donor has left the donation site are of particular concern, due to the potential for the donor to come to harm. These are called *delayed reactions*. It is believed that delayed vasovagal reactions account for 10% of all vasovagal reactions.[4] Occasional deaths have occurred as a result of accidents following delayed vasovagal reactions.[4] Sorensen carried out a retrospective analysis of Danish data relating to 2.5 million donations.[17] She found that severe complications occurred with an incidence of 19 per 100,000 procedures; two-thirds of these were due to vasovagal reactions with loss of consciousness and one-third due to needle insertion.

Recognizing and treating complications related to blood donation

The care of donors with complications starts with careful observation of all donors during and after the phlebotomy. The steps in recognition and treatment of the complication are depicted in Box 4.1. These should be covered in training, SOPs, and daily blood service practice.

Box 4.1 Stages in the care of donors with complications related to blood donation

1. Detect
All staff must be alert to signs of complications.

2. Treat promptly
Clear SOPs are required; this should also specify response to (possible) nerve injury.

3. Counsel
Discuss: Were there factors that contributed to the complication?
Provide advice on avoiding a recurrence.

4. Record
Categories suitable for use by donor attendants.
Information should be available next time the donor comes for targeted preventive care.

5. Follow-up
Remain in contact until full recovery.
Counsel: Consider change of donation type or permanent deferral.
Compensate for financial loss.

Recording and vigilance

Reliably recording the occurrence of complications associated with blood donation–even if

minor—forms the backbone of donor vigilance. It serves the following purposes:

- Medical dossier information and compliance with Good Manufacturing Practice (GMP).
- Ethical requirement to give factual account of what happened to the donor.
- Targeted preventive measures next time the donor attends.
- Review of individual (serious) cases.
- Aggregate data for review of quality of care and trends, for benchmarking between organizations, for provision of information to donors, and so on.
- In some countries: mandatory reporting of serious adverse reactions and events.

All staff attending donors should receive instruction in recording complications related to blood donation. The categories of complications, such as those proposed by the Working Group,[3] should not depend on a doctor's medical diagnosis, but be suitable for use by frontline staff. Procedures also apply to late (delayed) complications, hence staff handling telephone calls or other incoming information from donors need to ensure that a donor is put in touch with staff qualified to handle information about late complications.

The later section "Monitoring and assessment" starting on page 30 discusses how recorded information may be validated, evaluated, and used to improve blood establishment practice.

Errors (adverse incidents) in donor care*

Any error or quality incident during the various phases of the donation process should be reported to the blood establishment quality management system. Table 4.1 shows some examples

---

*Note that the European Directive[2] uses the term "adverse event" in the sense of adverse occurrence, i.e., errors and incidents. In international usage an adverse event could be either an adverse reaction or an incident. For the sake of avoiding confusion, we do not use the term adverse event in this chapter.

Table 4.1 Examples of errors or incidents involving defective materials, with possible adverse consequences for the donor.

Problem	Example	Type of risk to donor (note possible risks to recipient as well)
Errors in identification of donor or donation	Donor attends when the computer system is "down." Wrong donor ID assigned when information entered into computer afterwards.	Risk of excessive number of donations, failure of look-back or trace-back procedure.
Errors in donor screening procedures	• Donor reports hospitalization, such as "the cardiologist says I can donate." Donor attendant accepts this although safety requirements require deferral. • Male donor accepted when hemoglobin below threshold for male donors.	Increased risk of adverse reaction or anemia.

Mistakes in collection procedure	• Disposable wrongly placed on automatic weigher.
	 • Wrong IV solution during apheresis:
	   ○ Saline used instead of citrate.
	   ○ Citrate solution instead of saline for volume replacement.
	 • Citrate not running.
	 • Donor still connected when squashing air out of collection bag.
		Too large a volume removed.
		
		 Risk of clotting.
		 Risk of citrate toxicity.
		
		 Risk of clotting.
		 Risk of air embolism.

Defective materials	• Leaky apheresis set (harness): during the procedure plasma trickles to the floor. • Tubing bent. • Spurting reservoir. • Reservoir explodes.	Wasted collection, theoretical risk of infection in donor. Hemolysis Hemolysis Donor blood sprayed all round center

of errors or incidents in donor care, with the resultant risk of harm to donors and in some cases recipients.

Blame-safe reporting

The examples in Table 4.1 illustrate the importance of a non-punitive atmosphere to encourage reporting by all members of staff who discover an anomaly. Incident reports should be seen as valuable signals that can reveal weak areas in the standard operating procedures. If there is a threat of disciplinary measures to staff who have made a mistake, staff members will cover up to protect themselves or their colleagues and opportunities to learn from mistakes will be missed.

All incidents should be discussed within the center team and reported to the quality management system, with enumeration of the corrective measures taken. These should explain actions in relation to the donor, to the collected unit, and to the staff members or process involved. Donors should be informed if there has been an error. Errors or incidents with potentially serious consequences should be systematically reviewed within the quality cycle.

Learning opportunities

A blood establishment is a highly standardized organization in which errors and incidents occur only rarely. Look for opportunities to share incident reports, for instance in team meetings, to prevent complacency among staff and encourage pride in adhering to safety procedures. Illustrative reports of adverse incidents can be used to praise staff who through alertness detect errors and avert harm to donors or recipients. Examples can also be used by staff to respond to donors who react negatively to the repeated checks.

Donor post-donation information

The donor may develop symptoms or be diagnosed with an illness within the days or weeks following the whole blood or apheresis donation. Vigilance requires that donors report relevant information to the blood establishment: this requirement should be included in the standard information that all donors receive. Procedures need to be in place for this information to be recorded, assessed, and appropriately acted upon (if necessary). The information imparted by the donor should be transmitted to staff (for instance, a donor physician) qualified to assess its relevance and take appropriate actions.

Broadly, there are four types of donor post-donation information, as illustrated in Figure 4.2:

• The donor has symptoms or has received a medical diagnosis, and there is a possibility that the recent donation (the *product*) was unsuitable for transfusion (and perhaps also earlier donations). Occasionally donors may contact the blood establishment concerning information that they forgot to mention during the pre-donation screening; the review of this information follows the same principles.

• The donor has a (late) *complication* and needs to receive appropriate care and counseling.

• The donor has symptoms; there is no relation to the recent donation but an assessment should be made about *future donations*. This might be termed "inter-donation information", but the term "post-donation information" is helpful because it reinforces the need to consider whether there is a relation to past donations.

• The information has no consequences for suitability of products or for future donations. Staff should be careful in how they respond so as to stress the importance of communicating relevant information (see Box 4.2).

Box 4.2 Train staff to respond in a way that encourages donors to inform the blood service of medical details

Consider the following two responses to donors. The second donor is more likely to ring up on a future occasion:

• Thank you. We don't need to know about that.
• Thank you for telling us about your sore throat. Your donation was two weeks ago. If it was a shorter time, like one or two days, the bacteria might have been in your blood and we could have stopped your donation from being used for patients.

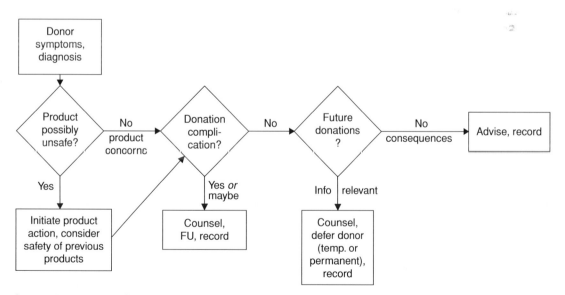

Figure 4.2 Assessing and acting on post-donation information.

There may also be a combination of the first two types in the above list. In the context of donor vigilance, we will not further discuss the steps relating to safety of the donated blood and components manufactured from it. Communication regarding information that is relevant for donor safety should largely follow the pathways that are in place for late-occurring adverse reactions.

A specific case of post-donation information involves information arising at the donor's next attendance. Often this occurs when discussion of a response to a screening question reveals that the donor responded inaccurately on a previous occasion. If it is found that a previous donation may have been unsafe, this should be reported and dealt with through the quality procedures and recall or "look-back" initiated if appropriate. We do not discuss this situation further here because it is part of "general" hemovigilance, relating to recipient safety. Consequences relating to donor safety should be discussed and dealt with directly. Even if there were no concerns about safety of blood components, a report may be made to the quality system because it may be a trigger for review and improvement of screening procedures.

Counseling and procedures relating to unexpected findings

Donor screening and the tests performed by blood establishments are in place for two purposes: (i) to protect the donor from harm (complications) arising from donation and (ii) to protect recipients from receiving a (potentially) unsafe blood component. When abnormal results are found, the donor must be informed and if necessary referral must be made to healthcare providers. Further information on counseling techniques, facilities, and so on may be found in the DOMAINE manual.[1]

Here are some examples of situations where counseling should be provided:
• In the event of a positive (abnormal) result of screening for infectious disease markers. Staff counseling donors with transmissible diseases should receive specific training for this situation.

• After unexpected results: for example, anemia, irregular erythrocyte antibodies, raised blood pressure, a heart murmur (if physical examination is included in donor screening check-up). Any information given to donors in relation to such findings should be uniform and delivered by staff who have been specifically trained in these counseling techniques.
• To donors whose donation is (repeatedly) unsuitable for clinical use: for example, whole blood with filtration problems, lipemic plasma detected in component manufacturing.
• A special category of unexpected results: false-positives.
• After a recipient adverse reaction. The general information given to all donors should explain the existence of traceability procedures and archiving of samples for use in the event of recipient adverse reaction.
• In the event of unexpected laboratory findings by the hospital on testing for crossmatching or in post-transfusion investigations in the patient.

In several of the above situations the donor has no health problem, but is counseled because the blood establishment has a problem using the donated blood. Many donors have difficulty understanding the message that they cannot donate blood and yet it is not because they have an illness. Clear explanations should be given and the information should also be given to the donor in writing.

Prerequisites and requirements

In this section, we assume that the blood establishment is already functioning, with staff qualified to conduct donation procedures and a basic quality system in place. The authors can supply contact addresses for materials, advice, and assistance for reaching the basic standards for blood establishments.

There can be various triggers for wanting to start or improve a donor vigilance system. For example, it can be "top down", perhaps a new regulatory requirement to submit reports on serious adverse incidents associated with blood donation. In other cases a serious complication might have revealed that staff members were not confident in providing treatment and follow-up. Internationally, there is a growing awareness of the importance of vigilance and traceability which is encouraging blood establishments to examine their own systems and make them more effective as a tool for monitoring and improving donor care.

Whatever the trigger, it is crucial that the project is adopted, decided upon, and supervised by those responsible for managing donor care and collection procedures. Consensus should be reached about the scope of the project and possible financial implications should be examined. Box 4.3 lists some points that need to be addressed in the project plan.

Box 4.3 Donor vigilance project plan

- Scope: what are the objectives? What will be the output (reports) and what will they be used for (under whose responsibility)?
- Who will lead the project, how will they consult and communicate progress to the responsible managers?
- Strategy: paper or digital or a combination?
- Integration with existent donor care procedures and the existent quality system.
- Staffing, financial, and training implications.
- IT implications.

If there are several blood establishments in a country, explore the possibility of harmonizing, using common definitions (which should be based on, or mappable to, the international standard), and sharing materials as they are developed.

Preparation

Digital or paper?

In settings where use is made of a computer system for donor and donation data, a digital record should be made in, or linked to, this system in all cases of complications of blood donation. However, the use of separate (additional) reporting forms for donation complications may be considered in the interests of recording additional data, not routinely tracked for uncomplicated donations, which will be transferred to a separate donor vigilance database. Choose a method that fits in with the general working methods in the blood establishment and its quality cycles and is sustainable. For example, a stand-alone database filled from detailed paper complication reports and serviced by a PhD researcher can generate high-quality scientific information but is not suitable for routine surveillance of complications of blood donation. The system should combine optimal recording with controlled but convenient access for analysis once the vigilance procedures become standard practice.

Access to information

Normal blood establishment procedures should guarantee confidentiality of donors' personal identifying and medical information. If complication data is extracted and stored or uploaded into a separate system, the confidentiality of information that is traceable to individual donors must be guaranteed.

What level of confidentiality is required *within* a single blood establishment where there are several departments or collection centers? In most organizations there will be sufficient confidence and a strong enough sense of collaboration between centers for overviews comparing centers to be openly shared and discussed. However, the leadership should consider whether this is appropriate and modify arrangements (for instance, presentation of data that is anonymous as to collection center) if that is felt to be safer.

Another issue is the protection of the identity of a blood establishment, where there is to be voluntary exchange or comparison of data between systems. Each establishment must remain in ownership of its own data, and any publication of information must ensure that individual establishments remain anonymous. The situation regarding anonymity of organizations may be different in the case of mandatory notifications of (serious) complications to competent authorities. While donor and patient identity will generally be protected, these reports enter the public domain and authorities may publish aggregate institutional data.

Implementation timetable

This should be agreed at managerial level, taking staffing and financial issues into consideration. Circumstances may suggest piloting procedures in one part of the establishment (e.g., a region or collection center) and rolling them out progressively:

• DO allow sufficient time for drafting documents and allowing staff from different levels and different departments to review them before they are formalized.

• DO submit request for IT support at an early stage.

• DON'T plan large-scale implementation during another major change within blood establishment (e.g., reorganization); in those circumstances start with small initial steps.

• DO make the written procedures and instructions on caring for donors with complications, if not previously available, an early priority.

Standard Operating Procedures (SOPs)

The management of complications must be clearly documented in the SOPs. The role of different professions, for example, medical doctors, nurses, and donor attendants, must be clearly outlined in these procedures. The SOPs must contain comprehensive information on the sequential steps that must be taken in the initial management of each complication and on the follow-up of donors after they have left the donation session. The indications for referring donors for further medical assessment or treatment, for example, to an Accident and Emergency Department, must be clearly defined. The standard advice that is given to donors who have had complications must be specified. Some donors who have had severe complications may be advised not to donate again: for example, a donor who had lost consciousness and suffered a head injury. The type and severity of complication that will lead to a donor being advised not to donate again must be clearly defined.

Furthermore, the SOPs will give guidance on how to register the complication in the blood bank information system.

It is also advisable to develop a SOP and an induction program for volunteers, because they play a valuable part in the process of collecting blood. Their duties and the limits of their duties must be clear; volunteers must be happy to take on the role that is expected of them and must be deemed competent for it. Even in settings where their main role is limited to the serving of refreshments, volunteers are ideally positioned for observing donors after donation. Informally they can reinforce the advice that has already been given by the trained staff by advising the donor to sit and taking the refreshments to them individually. Volunteers are generally grateful to receive explicit instructions on the initial response to a complication and on how to summon the trained blood bank staff for assistance.

Documentation of jobs: Tasks and responsibilities

Each of the tasks in the processes described in the earlier section "Products and processes" starting on page 21 needs to be clearly assigned to the group (level) of staff who carry responsibility for that task. It is recognized that staffing of blood establishments will vary between countries. Table 4.2 shows suggested tasks and roles for different collection center staff. This is the basis for designing the training program, and will also show which groups need to receive feedback information on their own performance as well as that of the donor vigilance program as a whole. The assigned responsibilities should also be stated in the relevant SOPs so that staff are aware of their own tasks but also know where they should hand over to a more senior member of staff.

More detailed guidance on staff responsibilities and training programs can be found in Chapter 11 of the *Donor Management Manual*.[18]

Monitoring and assessment

We consider two aspects in this section: (i) the validation of recorded data on donor complications; and (ii) the ongoing monitoring (assessment) of what is recorded.

Data validation

Recorded data, particularly if coded, can be subject to a number of errors. It is clear that if the wrong

Table 4.2 Staff responsibilities in caring for donors with complications.

Task	Staff	
Overall responsibility for donor care	Chief donor physician (medical responsibility): Donor care lead manager	
Recognize complication	Donor attendant (phlebotomist)	(DA)
	Registered nurse	(RN)
	Donor physician	(Dr)
	Volunteer serving refreshments	
Treat complication	DA, RN, Dr	
Basic life support (resuscitation), automated external defibrillator (AED) if available	Dr, RN, trained DA	
Counsel	Dr, RN	
Record	DA, RN, Dr	
Verifying recorded information	RN, Dr	
Telephone or walk-in contacts	(Telephone) receptionist connect donor to Dr/RN	
Postal/written contacts including complaint form	Complaints staff, forward to Dr/RN	
Receive information after donor has left center; record info	Dr/RN	
Refer for outside medical attention	Dr/RN	
Follow-up contacts	Dr/RN	

type of complication is entered or there is total failure to record, this will lead to inferior care (for instance, irrelevant advice) and reduced usefulness of the whole activity of registering complication data. For this reason, it is worth investing in procedures to check (validate) recorded data on complications of blood donation. A number of possible pragmatic approaches are listed in Box 4.4.

> **Box 4.4 Validating complication data**
> - Checking of donation forms by session RN or Dr; verifying complication recording in computer system.
> - Use of computer generated session overview list.
> - Download of recorded data:
>   ○ Contact involved staff if code is clearly incorrect, request for correction.
>   ○ Cross-check serious complications with medical notes and reports to quality system.
> - Question in donor screening form: did you suffer a complication last time?

Ongoing complications monitoring

Most adverse event systems focus on severe complications. It is highly recommended that data on non-severe complications is also retained. Both severe and non-severe complications can be investigated, analyzed, and monitored so as to determine

the root cause thereof. The resulting corrective and preventative actions taken will improve processes and procedures.

The use of a system to monitor adverse events in blood donors may be a useful adjunct to monitoring donor deferral rates. Used in conjunction with deferral codes, the information can be used to assess the impact of any changes to procedures or selection criteria. A useful example would be a change in the upper or lower age limit. When assessing the impact of this change, it would be useful to observe adverse event rates to ensure that there was no increase. In addition, the availability of this data is useful to benchmark against the experiences of other organizations that apply different selection criteria. The data can help support the evidence base to change donor selection criteria, obviously within the limits set by the national or supranational regulations (for instance, the EU in Commission Directive 2004/33/EC[19]).

Figure 4.3 illustrates different levels at which recorded data may be used. First, in the opinion of the authors, *all* serious donor reactions should also be reported in the blood establishment quality system with a view to examining critically the quality of care. The director of donor care and senior donor management staff should systematically

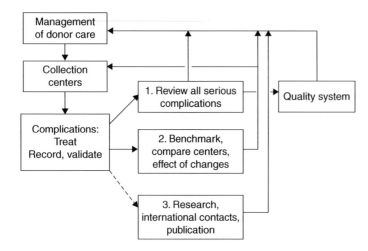

Figure 4.3 Using recorded information on complications associated with blood donation.

review these serious reports and consider whether measures are needed to reduce the likelihood of repetition. In situations where there is a requirement to report to an authority, the data reported to the quality department will generally be the source of the report that is made.

In the European Union, legislation mandates that blood establishments notify the competent authority in their country of any serious adverse events or serious adverse reactions which may have an effect on the quality or safety of blood or blood components.[2] Most donor adverse reactions do not affect the quality or safety of the blood or blood components and are subject to voluntary notification in the European Union. In other parts of the world, the regulations differ. In the United States, the FDA requires notification of a fatality related to blood donation.

Second, aggregate data can be presented in regular (monthly or quarterly) surveillance reports to center supervisors so that they can see whether their rates of recorded complications are higher or lower than those at other centers. As explained above, standardized working procedures, use of self-explanatory descriptive categories, and staff training are the optimal basis for obtaining comparable data. Nevertheless there may be differences between centers in whether they record, for instance, a minor reaction where the donor became pale but rapidly recovered when distracted by staff who also reclined the chair. Staff from the centers should consider and discuss:

• Are "all" complications being recorded? Are rates of faints with loss of consciousness more uniform than rates of vasovagal reactions without loss of consciousness?

• Are changes in figures the result of altered recording or of a true change in incidence?

With these caveats, regular examination of such overviews can enable staff members to benchmark their own experience against that of other centers or review the effect of changes in practice. The recorded data can be regarded as performance indicators for centers to review and improve their blood donor care.

A third level at which recorded donor complication data can be employed is in research, for instance to further elucidate risk factors or prospectively evaluate the effect of specific preventive measures. Through publication and international contacts the work can benefit donor care worldwide.

Denominator

Advance planning is advisable for reports both for internal use and for planned sharing of data with, for instance, the donor association. A count of numbers of donors who fainted or sustained a hematoma should be expressed as a rate in relation to a denominator: complications per 1000 (or 100) donors who attended, or per 1000 venepunctures performed ("needles in arm"), or 1000 successful collections. Although each of these possible denominators has advantages and disadvantages, there will be a fairly constant relation with a few percentage points of difference between them.

Other organizations prefer to express the rate as a ratio: 25 per 1000 becomes 1 in 40. A denominator figure that can be reliably and consistently produced from routinely recorded information should be used.

Where possible, data for whole blood donation and apheresis should, however, be separated in view of the different profile of complications associated with these types of donation. A further breakdown between rates in male and female donors, repeat or first-time donations is scientifically relevant but will not be necessary within an organization that has fairly uniform catchment populations of donors across its centers.

Training and assessment

Based on the staff profiles and responsibilities that we defined in the earlier section "Documentation of jobs: Tasks and responsibilities" (starting on page 30), all staff will have to receive training and be assessed for competency. Particularly in the case of a totally new system or a major change in working method, this can be arranged using a "train the trainer" method. In common with other training programs, documents and confirmation of certification should be archived.

For training, written instructions and group discussion may be sufficient for staff to acquire basic proficiency. Opportunities for enhancing skills in practice should be sought and may be quite simple. For instance, in some settings it is standard practice for the session physician or registered nurse to be called to attend a donor with complications. Typically the donor attendant's and the senior's advice to the donor will be identical in content. The donor attendant will learn from the physician's feedback about how a donor is recovering and what the donor has just said may have contributed to the faint.

When implementing the procedures, the training program for new staff should also be modified to include the donor vigilance processes outlined in "Products and processes" starting on page 21. Staff alertness and skills will be further promoted by routine (e.g., monthly) discussion of figures and case material in team meetings.

Particular consideration is needed for training in basic life support skills and the use of an AED, if available. Accredited trainers and training materials are available and should be used. Ensure that staff members receive updates and refresher training according to national guidelines. For financial reasons, this training may be limited to selected staff. Although this is acceptable, it imposes rota constraints. Each center should hold an up-to-date register of certified staff members and copies of certificates should be archived by the personnel department.

Implementation, evaluation of measures for improvement, and performance indicators

The success of implementing any new practice depends on careful preparation but also on getting collection center staff interested. Is this yet another form-filling exercise for over-stretched staff, or will they appreciate a simple but comprehensive system for logging complications that occur in their donors? Will donor care supervisors make donation complications and donor adverse incidents a regular topic at the regional meetings and create a climate in which center team leaders share their experiences and suggestions for improving the processes? Despite the convenience of circulars, personal contacts between those leading implementation and team leaders in the centers are invaluable in gaining their enthusiasm. Until there is good reporting the data are of little use to guide practice!

The recorded vasovagal reactions and hematomas, expressed as rates per 1000 successful collections, can be adopted as performance indicators for the donation process and regularly reviewed. Once the background vigilance system is in place, it can be used to address questions. For instance, are rates different in mobile drives? Is there an increase in warm weather and can this be prevented? Is there a change when a new type of donation chair, new needle type, or new apheresis machine is introduced? The annual rate of adverse incidents reported to the quality system could be another performance indicator. The same system will allow the effects of measures to be tracked.

Consideration should be given to the wider use of the information captured in the donor vigilance data. Notably, the official donor information should be revised and brought up to date with both local information and relevant findings from published research. This could also be made available on the blood establishment website, along with tips on avoiding adverse reactions.

Concluding remarks

In the light of several studies it is likely that many minor donation complications are not reported by donors and not documented. *Better recording* should be our aim so that data can be used to design improvements in donor care. It is to be applauded that some blood establishments are publishing results of donor vigilance reporting and of research on measures to reduce complication rates. Gradually this will lead to a *safe climate* for sharing data, so that countries will be able to learn from examples of "best practice".

An often-heard comment is that there is considerable *variation of complication rates* between the centers of a single blood establishment with uniform working procedures, definitions, and SOPs. It is possible that the recording performance may play a role. On the other hand, the differences in recorded rates may represent true differences. These may be partly related to the recognized risk factors such as donors' age, sex, and first-time donor status or ambient temperatures. In addition all who work with donors are aware of the effect of the surroundings: if one donor has fainted it is common for others to follow. Unraveling and learning from the causes of variation is an important potential outcome of sharing, comparing, and discussing data both by center staff and between blood establishments.

There are numerous areas for possible future work: research into complications of frequent donation, for example, iron depletion following multiple whole blood donation; the possibility of osteopenia or lower serum albumin level associated with frequent apheresis donation; the possibility of long-term effects such as cytopenia after frequent platelet apheresis; effect of repeated "booster" vaccination for hyperimmune plasma collection; monitoring long-term safety of donors who have been treated with hematopoietic growth factors.

Care should always be taken in publishing data about donation complications. Sensationalist publication could destroy much good work in recruitment and developing a well-informed donor panel. Transparency however can contribute to providing balanced information to donors and enabling progressive improvements to donor care. The presence of a well managed system for donor vigilance can improve donor confidence and contribute towards donor retention, which is essential in donor management and ensuring continuous availability of safe donated blood for transfusion.[20–22]

References

1 Wagenmans E, McSweeney E, Wickenden D, and de Kort W, 2010, Donor Safety Issues. In: de Kort, and W, Veldhuizen I (eds). *Donor Management Manual.* DOMAINE Project, Nijmegen, the Netherlands; pp. 158–78.

2 European Union, 2003, Directive 2002/98/EC of the European Parliament and of the Council of 27 January 2003 setting standards of quality and safety for the collection, testing, processing, storage and distribution of human blood and blood components and amending Directive 2001/83/EC. *Official Journal of the European Union,* L33, 8/02/2003, p. 30.

3 ISBT Working Group on Complications Related to Blood Donation, International Society of Blood Transfusion Working Party on Haemovigilance and European Haemovigilance Network, 2008, *Standard for Surveillance of Complications Related to Blood Donation.* http://www.isbtweb.org/fileadmin/user_upload/WP_on_Haemovigilance/ISBT_StandardSurveillanceDOCO_2008_3_.pdf [accessed February 24, 2012].

4 Jørgensen J, and Sorensen BS, 2008, Donor vigilance. *ISBT Science Series* **3**(1): 48–52.

5 Eder AF, Dy BA, Kennedy JM, Notari EP, Strupp A, *et al.*, 2008, The American Red Cross donor hemovigilance program: complications of blood donation reported in 2006. *Transfusion* **48**(9): 1809–19.

6 Eder AH, Hillyer CD, By BA, Notari EP and Benjamin RJ, 2008, Adverse reactions to allogeneic whole blood donation by 16- and 17-year-olds. *JAMA* **299**(19): 2279–86.

7 Wiltbank TB, Giordano GF, Kamel H, Tomasulo P, and Custer B, 2008, Faint and prefaint reactions in whole-blood donors: an analysis of predonation measurements and their predictive value. *Transfusion* **48**(9): 1799–1808.

8 Trouern-Trend JJ, Cable RG, Badon SJ, Newman BH, and Popovsky MA, 1999, A case-controlled multicentre study of vasovagal reactions in blood donors: influence of sex, age, donation status, weight, blood pressure, and pulse. *Transfusion* **39**(3): 316–20.

9 Kamel H, Tomasulo P, Bravo M, Wiltbank T, Cusick R, *et al.*, 2010, Delayed adverse reactions to blood donation. *Transfusion* **50**(3): 556–65.

10 Newman BH, Pichette S, Pichette D, and Dzaka E, 2003, Adverse effects in blood donors after whole-blood donation: a study of 1,000 blood donors interviewed 3 weeks after whole-blood donation. *Transfusion* **43**(5): 598–603.

11 Winters JL, 2006, Complications of donor apheresis. *Journal of Clinical Apheresis* **21**(2): 132–41.

12 Farrugia A, 2007, Iron and blood donation – an under-recognised safety issue. *Developmental Biology* **127**: 137–46.

13 Page EA, Coppock JE, and Harrison JF, 2010 Study of iron stores in regular plateletpheresis donors. *Transfusion Medicine* **20**(1): 22–9.

14 Dettke M, Buchta C, Bieglmayer C, Kainberger F, Macher M, and Hocker P, 2003, Short and long term effects of citrate on bone metabolism and bone mineral density in healthy plateletpheresis donors. *Journal of Clinical Apheresis* **18**: 87.

15 D'Souza A, Jaiyesimi I, Trainor L, and Venuturumili P, 2008, Granulocyte Colony-Stimulation Factor administration: adverse events. *Transfusion Medicine Reviews* **22**: 280–90.

16 World Marrow Donor Association international standards for unrelated hematopoietic stem cell donor registries, version 1 November 2008, http://www.worldm arrow.org/fileadmin/WorkingGroups_Subcommittees/Accreditation/Documents/standards_history/WMDA_Standards-version_November_2008_01.pdf [accessed 20 October, 2010].

17 Sorensen BS, Johnsen SP, and Jorgensen J, 2008, Complications related to blood donation: a population-based study. *Vox Sang* **94**(2): 132–7.

18 Demetriades M, Pastila S, Domanovic D, and Wagenmans E, 2008, Human Resources Management. In: de Kort, W., Veldhuizen, I. (eds). *Donor Management Manual*. DOMAINE Project, Nijmegen, the Netherlands; pp. 209–20.

19 Commission Directive 2004/33/EC of 22 March 2004 implementing directive 2002/98/EC of the European Parliament and of the Council as regards certain technical requirements for blood and blood components. *Official Journal of the European Union,* L91, 30/03/2004, p. 25.

20 France CR, France JL, Roussos M, and Ditto B, 2004, Mild reactions to blood donations predict a decreased likelihood of donor return. *Transfusion and Apheresis Science* **30**(1): 17–22.

21 Newman BH, Newman DT, Ahmad R, and Roth AJ, 2006, The effect of whole-blood donor adverse events on donor return rates. *Transfusion* **46**(8): 1374–9.

22 France CR, Rader A, and Carlson B, 2005, Donors who react may not come back: Analysis of repeat donation as a function of phlebotomist ratings of vasovagal reactions. *Transfusion and Apheresis Science* **33**(2): 99–106.

CHAPTER 5

Preparation of Blood Components

Tomislav Vuk
Croatian Institute of Transfusion Medicine, Zagreb, Croatia

Introduction

Transfusion treatment has a specific and unique place in clinical practice. Such a role derives from the fact that blood products used in patient treatment are manufactured from human blood, the supplies of which are limited, thus representing an irreplaceable national resource. The biological origin of blood products also implies a series of specific risks, some of which are unpredictable while others are only partially preventable.

In the past few decades, and especially since the emergence of HIV/AIDS, there have been increasing demands for continuous improvement of the safety, quality, and clinical efficacy of transfusion treatment. These demands have first of all entailed the introduction of ever more sensitive laboratory tests (in particular in the detection of blood transmissible disease markers), ever stricter donor selection criteria, introduction of pathogen inactivation methods, reconsideration of the criteria for clinical use of blood/blood products, and many other measures.

In parallel with these interventions, there is growing awareness that full accomplishment of the above requirements is inconceivable without the implementation of an efficient system of quality management in the blood transfusion service. This needs to include systematic surveillance of the overall processes of this complex system in which an array of mutually dependent activities are intermingled and a great number of workers of frequently varying professions and educational levels are involved.

As this chapter describes, the processing of blood components is a key link in the transfusion medicine chain, implying a series of processes and sub-processes that are often crucial for the final product's quality and safety. Therefore, it is no surprise that from early on blood establishments recognized (based on the model of manufacture in the pharmaceutical industry) the need to adopt Good Manufacture Practice (GMP) principles in order to ensure specified quality demands and reduce the rate of input material and final product waste by strict regulations on the premises, equipment, personnel, documentation, and other requirements. With time, these GMP principles have been increasingly adjusted to the needs and specificities of the blood transfusion service. Elements of the ISO 9000 series of standards have also found application in blood transfusion to emphasize the need of continuous quality improvement and adjustment to user requirements through corrective measures. In most industrialized countries, these systems along with accreditation/licensing of blood transfusion institutions have become legal liabilities.

The system of hemovigilance should be integrated into the system of quality management in order to enable efficient management of data

Hemovigilance: An Effective Tool for Improving Transfusion Safety, First Edition. Edited by René R.P. De Vries and Jean-Claude Faber.
© 2012 John Wiley & Sons, Ltd. Published 2012 by John Wiley & Sons, Ltd.

collected by surveillance of the overall chain of blood transfusion, with the ultimate goal of quality improvement, enhanced safety of transfusion therapy, and reduction in the rate of errors. There are considerable differences worldwide in the level of implementation of the hemovigilance system, rate and scope of reporting, definitions, and so on.[1] Many organizations and associations offer great support to the establishment and promotion of this system all over the world, thereby underlining the need of its integration in all segments of the work in blood transfusion. Therefore, it is of utmost importance that the hemovigilance system be considered in a context wider than the initial focusing on the patient (and then on the donor), and be included in all processes of the overall chain of blood transfusion.

The process of blood product manufacture should include a series of surveillance mechanisms to prevent adverse events that may compromise the quality of blood products. In addition, a traceability system should be ensured so as to enable (in the case of undesired adverse events or reactions), the prompt identification of the causes (related to the materials, equipment, or personnel), target testing, the identification of other products from the same donation or manufacturing batch, and the prevention of possible further damage.

Beside the blood product manufacture according to effective working instructions and regulations, the personnel involved in the manufacture process are also responsible for proper assessment of the conformity of input materials and products based on macroscopic inspection, control of package and seal integrity, and of accurate blood product labeling in all steps of the manufacture. They perform surveillance of the manufacture devices and equipment operation, control of computer and other manufacture records, and ensure product traceability and identification throughout the manufacturing process. They also control environmental conditions in the manufacturing and storage premises, and assess their conformity with specified requirements. They have to report nonconformities, errors, and adverse events, in line with valid regulations.

The establishment of a systematic, comprehensive, and efficient system of blood product quality control in accordance with legal provisions is of the utmost importance to assess the stability and quality of the production process. The specific nature of blood products and the fact that each blood product is of a unique composition, thus representing a batch by itself, means that the manufacture process must be monitored by use of measurement results obtained in an acceptable number of samples. This information should then be used to assess the need of implementing proper corrective measures.

Establishment of appropriate quality indicators in this segment of the blood transfusion service is highly relevant for efficient surveillance of the manufacturing process. These should be informative and objective indicators of conformity between measurement results and preset quality objectives.

By its definition and tasks, the system of hemovigilance promotes the upgrading of the quality and safety of transfusion treatment through efficient management of data collected by process surveillance. Analysis and continuous monitoring of data enable the possible defects and problems to identify, the possible causes to investigate, and decisions on the introduction of corrective/preventive measures to make on time.

The introduction of computerization and varying levels of automation in the blood product manufacture has enabled better traceability, comprehensive surveillance of the manufacturing processes, faster data accessibility, and a higher level of the manufacture standardization, eventually resulting in the higher quality and safety of blood products. In addition, an array of procedures and interventions have recently been introduced in the blood product manufacture, aimed at reducing the risk associated with transfusion therapy and the rate of adverse reactions (e.g., exclusive use of plasma obtained from male donors in clinical routine, pathogen inactivation, and so on).

Full achievement of high quality and safety of the products and services is impossible without well-organized, structured, quality education of all those involved in blood transfusion. In addition to professional education, staff should receive continuous education on all aspects of quality management and hemovigilance.

Products and processes: Standards, specifications, and documentation

Products

The term *blood components* refers to various products obtained from human blood and intended for prevention or treatment of disease. The biological origin of these products differentiates them substantially from drugs in the pharmaceutical industry, primarily for their limited resources and a number of specific risks, as follows:

• Every transfusion of a blood product is a transplantation procedure in which the complex biosystems of the donor and the recipient come into close interaction.

• The extremely high number of infective agents that can be transmitted by transfusion means that donor blood cannot be tested for the presence of each of them. The currently available tests for the detection of markers of diseases transmitted by blood are characterized by very high sensitivity but not complete elimination of the window period.

• Every donor blood unit and blood product unit differs according to composition, and so standardization of therapeutic dose is almost impossible. With the exception of the compulsory testing performed on all donations, other quality control testing is done on a limited number of samples. Therefore, the amount of active substances cannot be determined or the sterility tested in every single blood product.

• Even with the provision of optimal conditions of blood product conservation and storage, these products undergo changes that may entail various consequences for the product quality as well as for the safety and efficacy of the transfusion therapy.

In addition to the above risks that are exclusively consequential to biological factors, it should be noted that errors are one of the leading causes of morbidity and mortality associated with transfusion therapy. These errors are frequently of a multifactor nature, reflecting a systemic process flaw.

The ever-growing demands for risk reduction and consequently ever more strict requirements in donor selection have entailed a new risk of decreasing the blood supplies available. Responsible management of the limited supplies of blood products is a common liability of the transfusion service and the clinicians, especially considering the possible side effects of transfusion therapy.

Accordingly, transfusion medicine obviously has a specific and unique position within the healthcare system, which should be recognized and appropriate measures implemented. In the real world, however, the quality and safety of blood products generally depend on the level of a particular country's socioeconomic development. The level of quality system implementation and thus of hemovigilance as one of its components also depends on these factors. In this context, there are valuable World Health Organization (WHO) incentives helping the establishment of national transfusion services on the principles of economic and rational organization, promoting knowledge about blood product quality and safety, emphasizing the role of voluntary blood donation, offering support to the countries that need it, and so.[2] In this way, WHO encourages rational and optimal utilization of the existing resources. Additionally, WHO promotes the introduction of hemovigilance through the Global Steering Committee for Hemovigilance (GloSCH), in developing countries in particular. This incentive has been actively supported by the International Hemovigilance Network (IHN).[3]

Standards and specifications

The standard requirements and specifications that a Department of Blood Product Manufacture has to meet in terms of premises, staff, equipment, and materials to warrant maximal safety and quality of the manufacture process are discussed below, using the Council of Europe Guide for the preparation, use, and quality assurance of blood components[4] and PIC/S: GMP Guide for Blood Establishments[5] as a framework. Although this section of the chapter focuses mainly on quality assurance procedures in the manufacture of blood products, it is a prerequisite for further discussion on hemovigilance in this segment of the transfusion service.

Premises, equipment, and materials

The premises intended for blood product manufacture should be appropriately designed to prevent the occurrence of intersections and errors, while enabling distinct product separation in different stages of processing, appropriate cleaning, and maintenance. Non-authorized personnel should be denied admittance to the processing areas, and these processing areas should be separated from the laboratories. Storage premises need to be regularly surveyed and controlled. Specified conditions required in these premises must be recorded, whereby timely identification of any deviation should be warranted by appropriate alert systems. There must be written instructions on the activities to be performed in case of any deviation of storage conditions from the required ones. In storage premises there should be no mixing of quarantined products and products suitable for release. Nonconforming products and recalled products should be stored in a separate area.

Equipment must be appropriate and qualified for the intended use, calibrated and regularly maintained, with written records on all these steps. On using the equipment, the manufacturer's instructions must be strictly followed. The equipment should imply no risk for the handling staff members. All instruments and accessories suspected or known to result in nonconformity of blood components or that may pose a risk for the operators should be declared inappropriate, properly labeled, and excluded from use until the nonconformity is resolved and correct performance verified. All measuring instruments, the correct operation of which influences product quality, should be calibrated and labeled with the date of calibration expiry. The size, frequency, and range of measurement accuracy of the instruments are to be set in line with the respective legislation.

The materials used in the processing of blood components should be purchased from approved suppliers. On the receipt of the material, proper inspection needs to be performed. Critical materials that may influence the quality of final product

should be clearly defined and released to use under the responsibility of Quality Assurance (QA). On establishing and performing quality control, requirements for incoming materials should be specified, procedures regulated for the inspection and testing of incoming materials, and records taken to prove that all sampling, inspection, and testing procedures have indeed been properly performed. The incoming material passing the quality control should be so labeled as to clearly distinguish it from the unapproved or quarantined materials.

Considering the critical role of the materials used in the transfusion service for the quality and safety of blood products, an efficient system of materiovigilance should be established to the benefit of both the transfusion institution and the manufacturer. Any incoming material nonconformity should be reported and documented and the complaint together with the defective material be forwarded to the supplier/manufacturer. A special system of monitoring the frequency of particular material nonconformities should also be established to identify the trends and to allow for quality comparison of various manufacturers supplying the same type of materials. These data can prove useful in the process of purchase and selection of suppliers.

Personnel: Qualifications

Only personnel with proper education and qualification for these specific activities can be involved in the process of blood product manufacture. Personnel should understand and be familiar with the GMP principles for work in the transfusion service and with all regulations on the activities they perform. They also should have relevant knowledge of microbiology and hygiene. In line with the plan of training, personnel should receive education for work according to the respective Standard Operating Procedures (SOPs) and other documents. Along with initial training, personnel should be included in the program of continuous training. All educational activities and qualifications need to be recorded. It is of utmost importance that the QA manager and Processing Manager are different persons functioning independently of each other.

Documentation

Good documentation is an essential part of a quality management system (QMS). Properly kept documentation ensures standardization of performance, traceability, and control of all procedures. Therefore, quality documentation is a basis of an efficient hemovigilance system. Documents should be written using an unambiguous, clear, intelligible style with short, concise sentences. Wherever possible, documents should also be graphically presented to be readily visually legible. Records can be kept in writing or stored in an electronic medium. Each document should have a unique label and be inspected and approved by an authorized person prior to release. Documents need to be periodically reviewed to ensure that they constantly meet the respective requirements. Obsolete documents should be promptly withdrawn and destroyed, while one (original) copy is properly labeled and stored separately from valid documentation. All SOPs and procedures related to blood product manufacture should be kept at the site of the manufacture process.

All critical points of the manufacture process should be described in detail. Among others, these include the following:
- receipt, control, and storage of the materials used in blood product manufacture;
- incoming control of donated blood/blood components;
- management of nonconformities, errors, and adverse events in blood product manufacture;
- equipment handling and maintenance;
- surveillance of the manufacture conditions;
- product labeling in each step of the process;
- safety and hygiene requirements;
- cleaning and sanitation of premises in the case of spilled content and contamination;
- work in the open system;
- preparation of all blood products;
- macroscopic inspection of products;
- storage of blood products;
- release of blood products;
- use of computer software.

It is advised that SOPs be written by the employees working on the process, and then their accuracy and comprehensiveness be checked by other workers. SOPs should be validated, reviewed, and approved by the responsible professionals, and regularly controlled. Valuable assistance on writing SOPs in the field of transfusion medicine can be found at http://www.eubis-europe.eu/blood_manual_details.php.[6]

Although the manufacture of blood products is generally based on several simple physical procedures, their combinations with or without the use of additional additive solutions and some additional procedures of pathogen inactivation increase the number of blood products that can be obtained. Their characteristics may exert some effects on the recipient and therapeutic outcome. Therefore, every blood product manufacturing institution should have a valid list of approved products and should inform the users on the basic product characteristics, their indications, contraindications, possible side effects, and on storage and administration conditions. Transfusion institutions need to have written regulations on the mode of informing the users on the characteristics of the products released.

Processes

The process of blood product manufacture consists of a number of phases described below, including critical control points and surveillance mechanisms.

Manufacture planning

Quality planning of blood collection and blood product manufacture reduces the risk of excessive and unnecessary disposal of excess stocks of blood products and the risk of patient health threats due to inadequate stocks of blood products for transfusion therapy. Therefore, manufacture planning should be regulated by work instructions as part of the overall management of blood product stocks. Plan development requires close collaboration among all those responsible for blood collection, blood component production, and clinical use. As regards stock management, optimal, minimal, and maximal amounts of blood products according to blood groups should be identified for each blood establishment, thus enabling timely response and introduction of preventive measures.

Receipt of blood units in the processing area

Incoming control of blood units collected can be performed prior to entry in the processing area or by the personnel in the processing department, depending on the work organization in particular blood establishments. The amount of blood units received should be compared with data in the respective documentation; the possible non-conforming material should be separated from blood units entering the production. Inspection of blood units includes macroscopic inspection, package integrity, and appropriate labeling. The time elapsed from blood withdrawal to the component production must be strictly controlled.

Manufacture of blood products

Simultaneous replacement of all blood components is required in a very small proportion of patients. Patient treatment according to the principles of "directed transfusion," that is the replacement of only those blood components that are actually lacking, improves therapeutic efficacy, reduces the rate and severity of side effects, and enables more rational management of donated blood. Furthermore, upon separation of particular blood components, storage conditions such as temperature, anticoagulant solution, and plastics composition can be modified to achieve optimal values for the respective blood component, thus enabling better functional preservation and longer storage of the separated and concentrated blood component. For these reasons, whole blood manufacture has been abandoned or reduced to a negligible proportion for a limited number of indications in industrialized countries.

Separation of a particular blood component as a single product can be achieved by proper selection of the speed and time of centrifugation. What are the critical points for product quality in this step of the manufacturing process? The centrifuges used in the manufacture of blood products should be validated and regularly maintained, and these activities should be properly documented. In addition, placement of blood units in the carriers and tare weight determination are also important parameters to be monitored. An ideal traceability system would enable identification of the centrifuge employed on each blood unit/blood component centrifugation. It is the only way to identify rapidly and efficiently the possible problem in this segment of the manufacturing process in the case of quality deviation.

Upon whole blood centrifugation, separation into blood components follows, with or without red blood cell (RBC) concentrate leukofiltration (some blood collection systems include whole blood filtration). Currently, partially automated methods are generally employed on whole blood separation, although fully automated methods have recently become available. Processing automation enables better standardization of the preparation, thus reducing variation in the product quality. These devices offer the possibility of the storage of all necessary data on the separation of whole blood donations and data analysis with appropriate software.

RBC concentrate, plasma, and platelet concentrate are mostly manufactured from whole blood units. Depending on the blood product type, they can be additionally modified by different procedures such as filtration, washing, irradiation, pathogen inactivation procedures, and so on. Some of the blood product modification procedures are only rarely performed, thus increasing the risk of errors or greater variability in the product final control. These procedures include the washing of RBC and platelet concentrates, plasma volume reduction, and the manufacture of RBC suspension in plasma. As a result, these procedures require frequent personnel training, evaluation of their competences, and strict quality control performance (all units).

In the manufacture of plasma for clinical use, plasma exclusively obtained from male donors has been used in ever more countries due to the risk of the Transfusion Related Acute Lung Injury (TRALI). As TRALI is a serious adverse reaction, efficient mechanisms of surveillance should be established (preferably computer-assisted blocking) to prevent the manufacture of plasma for clinical use from female donor blood. The risk of TRALI development in the recipients is also considerably reduced by the use of additive solutions on RBC and platelet preservation.

Pathogen inactivation in plasma is performed in some countries, whereas in most countries where inactivation is not performed plasma is safeguarded by quarantine. Some methods of pathogen inactivation are available for platelet concentrates; however, their implementation is rarely uniform even within a country, let alone among different countries.

Bacterial contamination of blood products is one of the leading causes of morbidity and mortality associated with transfusion treatment and may occur in any segment of the transfusion chain. The majority of agents isolated from contaminated blood products belong to the physiological flora of the skin and are introduced into the blood container on venepuncture. The *closed* system of manufacture is used as a standard that maximally reduces the risk of bacterial contamination of the blood product. Even when closed system of manufacture is used, those working in the manufacture process should pay due attention on macroscopic inspection of the blood product to the possible presence of damage and control of each seal integrity. When the manufacture is performed in a so-called *open* system, the premises, protective clothes, procedures, and control mechanisms should be described in detail to minimize the possibility of contamination. The manufacture of blood components associated with sterile barrier break should be done within a sterile laminar flow area with regular control of the microbiological air purity, number of air particles, air flow velocity, and filter integrity. Only previously trained and educated personnel are allowed to work in this area.

When 100% bacteriological control of platelet concentrates is performed, the algorithm of their release should be strictly defined. The procedures in the case of positive results of bacteriological screening should also be regulated. The system of traceability should be organized to identify all products from a donation suspected of nonconformity, including their final destination, within the shortest period of time. Such a traceability system is a precondition for an efficient system of product withdrawal, trace-back, and look-back procedures.

Labeling

Labeling is one of the critical points in the chain of blood product safety. The appropriate method of product labeling enables clear product identification in all phases of the production process. Therefore, written instructions on the mode of labeling should be available. Computer-assisted and controlled labeling is preferred because of the reduced risk of errors. Labels should contain all the necessary data on the blood component, and the critical ones need to be in the machine-readable format. Each donation should be labeled by a unique number, so that every blood product manufactured is traceable back to the donor on the one hand and to its final destination on the other hand. This is one of the critical requirements of the hemovigilance system.

Use of computer systems

The introduction of computerization in the blood product manufacture has enabled better traceability, more comprehensive surveillance of the manufacturing process, and faster data availability. In turn this enables faster identification of the causes of nonconformities or deviations in the manufacturing process. The computer program should be validated and properly maintained, and its use described in the SOPs. Computer-stored data must be protected from loss (by data back-up), unauthorized access, and changes. The computer-stored data must be readily and easily transformed to a written document. Computer hardware and software should be regularly controlled, with appropriate records maintained on these controls. Only authorized persons should make changes in the computer program, based on validated and approved procedures, and records kept on these actions. A failure in the computer system should not cause any interruption in the process performance.

In-process control

A series of control measures have to be performed during the processing of blood components. Macroscopic inspection of intermediate and final blood components is of critical importance. On this examination, all nonconforming blood components should be singled out, properly labeled, and stored in line with regulations until disposal. The nonconformity status needs to be entered in the computer software. To prevent the risk of sterile barrier break, the integrity of each seal must be controlled carefully. The personnel in the manufacturing department have to perform strict control of product labeling in all steps of the manufacturing process. The conditions to be ensured during the processing and storage of blood components, organization of particular condition monitoring, limits of warning and action, procedure in case of particular condition deviation, and method of monitoring recording should be defined by a documented procedure.

Management of nonconforming blood products

An efficient system of identification, recording, labeling, storing, and reporting of nonconforming products should be established at the Department of Blood Product Manufacture. There is a number of categories of product nonconformities, the most common being lipemia, clots in RBC products, aggregates in platelet concentrates, product package damage, sterile barrier break due to poor seals, outdated blood products, and hemolytic or icteric aspect of blood product plasma. Some proportion of product nonconformities are due to nonconforming results of testing performed at laboratories for donor blood testing. Computer assistance in all or individual segments of nonconformity management greatly contributes to the overall safety. In any case, full traceability should be ensured, on the one hand to offer information on the type of product nonconformity, time of its identification, and person responsible for allocating the status of nonconformity, and on the other hand to enable traceability of the nonconforming product to its final destination.

Event/error reporting system

In line with the valid national legislative, every institution has to regulate the method of event reporting based on the national regulations and legal acts. A comprehensive and efficient system of event management, which includes the search for root causes of their occurrence, risk assessment, and consequential implementation of corrective measures, is one of the instruments in reducing risks of transfusion treatment. It is the responsibility of the blood establishment to establish and maintain such an environment where errors and other events can be reported freely and without fear. The system of error reporting should also include errors that are recognized in time and prevented (i.e., near-misses).

Errors are relatively rare in the processing of blood components and little literature data on this error category are available. These errors are a very rare cause of fatal side effects of transfusion therapy. The highest proportion ($n = 32$; 28.8%) of 111 errors (all near-miss events) recorded on the processing of blood components during a 5-year period (2003–2007) in the Croatian Institute of Transfusion Medicine in Zagreb (CITM) referred to errors on handling the automated blood component extractor, followed by errors in the method of preparation ($n = 23$; 20.7%), missed or erroneous computer records of the manufacture ($n = 16$; 14.4%), erroneous selection of the blood product unit ($n = 9$; 8.1%), incorrect handling the instruments for sterile sealing of plastic tubes ($n = 6$; 5.4%), irregular manipulation with the blood product ($n = 5$; 4.5%), and incorrectly declared blood product volume ($n = 4$; 3.6%). During the 2003–2007 period, a total of 1,003,209 blood products were manufactured at CITM, which means that the incidence of manufacture errors was 0.01% or 1/10,000 blood products.

Storage of blood products may also be the source of errors in blood product issuing or usage. Shulman and Kent[7] investigated errors in the placement of blood units in the refrigerator. The incidence of these errors was 0.12%. In one third of these errors, there was a possibility of AB0-incompatible transfusion in the case of failure of double control on unit issuing. During the 5-year period (2003–2007), 105 errors related to blood component storage, distribution, and issuing were recorded at CITM. Only seven errors were related to blood product storage, of which four errors were due to inappropriate storage conditions and three to the storage of expired units.

Blood component release

Blood components should be kept in administrative and/or physical quarantine until a decision is made on the release. An authorized person makes the definitive decision on the blood component release, based on a documented and validated procedure specifying the conditions of the release. The decision is made on the basis of quality records for each individual work segment influencing the quality of blood components. If possible, blood component release should be computer assisted.

Storage of blood products

The method and conditions of the storage of blood and blood components are of paramount importance to preserve their quality and stability. Specified conditions required in storage areas should be maintained, carefully controlled, and recorded. Timely identification of any deviation should be warranted by appropriate alert systems. There must be written instructions on the activities to be performed in the case of any deviation of storage conditions from the required ones.

The storage area should be so designed and structured to allow for safe blood component manipulation without the risk of damage. Within the storage area, blood components need to be placed so as to be easily accessible and to allow for their storage according to the "first in-first out" principle. The storage area should be regularly cleaned and maintained, with appropriate control of all these procedures. Blood components intended for release must be separated from those not intended for release. A separate part of the storage area needs to be reserved for quarantine blood components, returned blood components, nonconforming blood components, blood components intended for autologous transfusion, and so on.

Documentation of jobs: Tasks and responsibilities

All those involved in the blood transfusion chain have unique tasks and responsibilities for the achievement of optimal safety and quality of transfusion therapy; however, these goals can only be reached by their close collaboration and teamwork. In order to avoid unnecessary repetition, discussion of the tasks and responsibilities within the system of

hemovigilance in this section is based on the blood product manufacture within a blood establishment.

Personnel working in the manufacturing process are the first link in the chain of hemovigilance. Beside the manufacture and storage of blood products according to written instructions, they are responsible for conformity assessment of the input materials, intermediate products, and final products, based on macroscopic inspection, control of package and seal integrity, and control of proper blood product labeling in all phases of the manufacture process. These staff members monitor the operation of instruments and equipment, control computer and other production records, and ensure clear traceability and identification throughout the process of manufacture. In addition, they perform surveillance of environmental conditions in the manufacture and storage premises, and assess their conformity with specified requirements. They are obliged to report on any nonconformities, errors, and adverse events, in line with in-house regulations.

The head of the Department of Blood Product Manufacture is responsible for the manufacture planning, establishment and surveillance of overall processes, personnel education and evaluation of their competences, survey, maintenance, and keeping of manufacture documentation and records, reporting, and so on. This person needs to have due knowledge about quality systems in the transfusion service, including the hemovigilance system. It is this department head's responsibility to incorporate all hemovigilance components in the SOPs regulating department activities, and to regulate clearly the tasks of the personnel within this system. This person should continuously survey the correct and consistent performance of these activities and be available to staff members to solve the possible dilemmas and problems. In addition, the person should carefully consider all reports, records, and information related to his or her domain within the hemovigilance system, take appropriate measures, and forward them to the responsible people.

The person responsible for hemovigilance within a blood establishment is in charge of collaboration with the process heads, quality manager, and the entire management, for the promotion of hemovigilance as the ultimate objective. Quality education of all those involved in the process is of utmost importance to reach this objective. The hemovigilance officer is responsible for the receipt, processing, and solving reports of adverse events and adverse reactions (in collaboration with responsible persons), and then for their correct documentation, monitoring, and reporting. In addition, this officer is responsible for periodical reporting to the national board of hemovigilance or competent authority on the reports received at the institution, and for proposing system improvements based on the monitoring of results.

Successful functioning of the hemovigilance system is inconceivable without the full commitment of the institution management to the promotion of the transfusion treatment quality and safety. In addition, the management of a transfusion establishment ensures the material and financial resources needed for efficient system functioning.

Although the overall system management comes within the competence of different organizations and bodies depending on the hemovigilance system structure in different countries, the majority of experts agree that only a well-organized and efficient national system can guarantee successful service performance. Those responsible for the system management should encourage reporting of adverse reactions and adverse events, in particular near-misses, and continuously collect, timely process, and analyse data, monitor trends, compare the data collected with other systems worldwide, propose corrective and preventive measures, and perform education on all aspects of hemovigilance.

Monitoring and assessment

The manufacture process monitoring and quality assessment are crucial for the safety and efficacy of transfusion treatment. Along with the control mechanisms integrated in the work process and surveyed by those working in the manufacture department, the surveillance and assessment of the manufacturing process quality should also include an array of other tools and activities such as statistical process control, quality indicators, audits, and inspections.

Blood product quality control

Similar to the manufacturing process, the product quality control in the transfusion service differs from the product quality control in pharmaceutical and other industries. Each blood product unit is a separate batch and the stability, efficacy, amount of active substance, and sterility cannot be tested in each of them. Therefore, the release of a greater number of products of the same batch cannot be used, but a system of statistical monitoring of various parameters to maintain stability of the processes must be established instead. These parameters should be measured at a frequency that is statistically acceptable and the results obtained be used to decide on the product conformity with quality requirements. The blood product quality control procedures require close collaboration between those working in the manufacture department and quality control department.

Quality control parameters and frequency of their testing

The parameters to be assessed in each type of blood products in routine quality control and the frequency of their testing should be defined in respective documents of the blood establishment, usually in the form of blood product specifications. These requirements are included in legal provisions or professional standards. Control parameters have been chosen to be adequately informative for quality assessment of the process of manufacture and product storage stability.

Quality control planning

Quality control of blood products should be continuous to ensure appropriate statistical process monitoring. Monthly, weekly, and daily plans of quality control are designed according to the scope of manufacture and frequency of particular parameter testing required at the blood establishment. In some establishments, the statistical process control procedures are performed periodically rather than continuously for operative reasons. Such an approach to quality control is defective because the possible error in the process of manufacture may be detected with a considerable delay after its occurrence.

Quality control plans should be revised at certain intervals to adjust them to changes in the scope of manufacture. In quality control planning, care should be taken to ensure that the entire manufacturing process is covered by surveillance, including various preparation techniques and all critical equipment used thereby (e.g., blood centrifuges, devices used on blood separation into blood components, cell separators, and so on). Such an approach guarantees surveillance over the quality of blood products and also can be considered as a part of materiovigilnce.

Blood product sampling for quality control

The sample intended for quality control should be representative in its contents irrespective of the mode of sampling. The sample identification and traceability needs to be ensured throughout the process of quality control. Sampling of blood product to be used in transfusion treatment should be performed so as to prevent any impairment of the product integrity and/or quality. Sample volume should be adequate for the analysis required. The methods of sampling must be properly validated and the procedure described in work instructions. The sampled blood product should be left in quarantine until the end of testing and a decision on further procedures in case of result deviation from specified requirements.

Methods of testing

Blood product quality control includes a series of testing methods. The methods employed should be properly validated and described in detail in work instructions. Instruments and reagents must be used in line with the manufacturers' instructions. The reliability of test results should be periodically verified by active participation in a formal external quality control system. The results of blood product quality control as a calculated value should be traceable to the original measuring data and documented in respective forms/work sheets.

Statistical analysis and interpretation of blood product quality control results

For the majority of parameters tested in blood products, quality requirements are defined by legal provisions. Interpretation of the quality control results cannot be done without the use of appropriate statistical methods of data processing. Results of blood product quality control can be expressed by some simple method of descriptive statistics; however, a more sophisticated statistical processing of the results obtained and continuous statistical monitoring are preferable. Calculation of the process capability to meet the specified quality requirements is desirable for critical parameters. In particular, this applies to residual leukocytes in leukocyte-depleted blood products.

Monitoring of quality control results and corrective measures

Quality control results should be submitted to continuous evaluation. When these results deviate from the specified requirements, investigation/additional testing is to be performed to identify the reasons for aberrations. Appropriate corrective measures are then taken based on the underlying causes of nonconformities detected, followed by testing of their performance.

Quality indicators in blood product manufacture

Quality indicators are defined as measurable, objective, numerical indicators of efficiency of the key segments of a system. In addition to allowing for the evaluation of an institution against the others, quality indicators also enable the institution management to assess the quality system compatibility with the preset goals.

The following activities are crucial for the setting and efficient management of quality indicators:[8]

• *Defining the indicators:* Quality indicators are defined on the basis of scientific concepts, personal experience, literature review results, debate with professionals within and outside the institution, and so on. Such indicators should be clear, comprehensible, and unambiguous. The number of quality indicators depends on the size of the institution and the extent of the activities performed, but they should preferably cover all services performed within the institution. When setting quality indicators, the numerator and denominator need to be precisely defined first. Quality indicators are liable to both qualitative and quantitative modifications. In the case of changes in the institution structure and work organization, a particular indicator may be abandoned or a new one introduced as being more appropriate in the new situation.

• *Setting quality goals and critical action limits:* Experiences of other blood transfusion institutions and literature data can be used; however, the specificities arising from the manufacture modality, blood donor selection, and so on at a particular institution need to be taken into account. Therefore, the goals and critical limits are best based on the results of the institution's own process measurements over a period of time. At the CITM, the indicators are set after 2–3 years of data monitoring (retrospectively or prospectively, depending on whether the indicators have to be set for the already existing activities or for the activities to be implemented). The n-charts and p-charts have been used in quality indicator monitoring, the former being employed for the indicators presented as absolute values and the latter for the indicators presented as a proportion (%). The mean value calculated from monthly values of quality indicators during the period of monitoring is used as the initial goal. Later on, the quality goal is defined according to the results achieved per year. If the mean value of the results achieved in a year exceeds the preset goal, the previously set goal is replaced by this higher quality value. If not, the goal remains unchanged for the next 1-year period. The upper and lower action limits are based on the calculated 2 or 3 mean standard deviations for the monitoring period, and in the case of n-charts these are corrected for the factor of sample size. Two standard deviations are used for more critical quality indicators, and three standard deviations for less critical quality indicators.

• *Defining the method of data collection and processing:* The method of data collection must be strictly defined, primarily as applies to defining the source of data and the people responsible for data collection and processing. The statistical methods used on data processing should also be defined.

• *Monitoring, interpretation (trends) and reporting:* Quality indicators should be continuously surveyed, observing the trends and detecting deviations. The significance of any deviation is to be assessed and further activities decided. Appropriate corrective actions should always be taken when considered necessary. Quality indicators are part of the periodic reports submitted to the institution management by the people in charge of indicator collection and monitoring. Institution management usually use the quality indicators to assess system conformity with the preset requirements.

• *Corrective/preventive actions:* These are the most important ultimate goal of quality indicator monitoring. Corrective/preventive actions have to be documented, and their goal is the reduction of nonconformities and errors to an acceptable level. Upon completion of the corrective/preventive action, its effectiveness is monitored by further indicator surveillance.

There are a number of processes, sub-processes, and activities in the field of blood product manufacture that can be used to collect and process numerical data in order to monitor trends, thus enabling early detection of deviations that may have adverse effects on the blood product quality, safety, or availability. Efficient process surveillance and management requires the selection of an optimal number of quality indicators that will be useful and informative. Some indicators that may in the author's opinion prove useful in the manufacture surveillance are discussed below.

Product nonconformities

This indicator shows the rate of product nonconformities according to the total number of blood products manufactured (primary manufacture and modified products). It is one of the most important indicators because it unifies all types of nonconforming products and points to the total rate of nonconforming blood products at the respective transfusion institution.

Platelet concentrate outdating

This indicator represents the proportion of platelet products discarded due to shelf life expiry and can prove useful in the surveillance of manufacture planning, that is, appropriate management of this product stock. However, note that this indicator should not be considered separately from the indicators that point to the level of meeting the requirements placed by the orders for platelet concentrates.

RBC concentrate outdating

This indicator points to the frequency of RBC blood products discarded due to shelf life expiry. The management of this blood product supplies is considerably easier and consequentially the discarding rate lower because of the longer shelf life as compared with platelet concentrates. Therefore, unfavourable trends recorded on monitoring this indicator may point to serious problems in planning or managing the blood product stocks.

Poor seals in blood product manufacture

This quality indicator shows the frequency of poor seals relative to the number of blood products manufactured (monitoring relative to the total number of seals performed is a far more complicated and difficult task). Unfavourable trends recorded in this indicator point to the need to search for the possible causes (faults or reduced operating capacity of some devices for sterile sealing or sterile plastic tube connection, errors in device handling, and so on). This indicator indirectly points to the risk of bacterial contamination of blood products during the process of manufacture.

Errors

Monitoring of the number, types, and causes of errors provides an important quality indicator that points to process weaknesses and the need of undertaking particular corrective/preventive measures. Although errors can be monitored as a single indicator for the overall processes in a transfusion institution, thorough analyses should always include their distribution according to organizational units or work processes.

Clots in RBC blood products

Although this type of nonconformities is generally detected during manufacture and macroscopic inspection of the blood products, the cause of their occurrence points to problems associated with the process of blood collection or the materials and equipment used thereby (inappropriate blood mixing with anticoagulant solution, composition and amount of anticoagulant in the blood collection systems, and so on).

Aggregates in platelet concentrates

This quality indicator shows total frequency of platelet concentrates discarded due to the presence of aggregates. The frequency of this type of nonconformities differs according to the method of platelet concentrate manufacture from whole blood (BC or PRP method) and apheresis (according to the technique of platelet separation).

Damage to blood product packaging

This indicator points to the frequency of blood product nonconformities due to package damage. This type of nonconformities is generally recorded on the storage of blood products, however, part may also occur during the process of manufacture (on centrifugation, blood product handling, and so on). By monitoring this type of nonconformities, the possible defects in the quality of blood bags (materiovigilance), inappropriate blood product manipulation, inappropriate storage conditions, and so on can be identified in a timely fashion.

Positive findings on blood product bacteriological testing

The incidence of bacterial contamination of blood products is an indicator of the process ability to meet the requirements of microbiological safety of blood products. Depending on the method of microbiological control employed, it may refer to all blood products or to platelet concentrates alone.

Audits

Quality improvement in transfusion medicine is impossible without implementation of regular self-inspections and internal audits. Their objective is not only identification of nonconformities but also systematic, planned, and independent evaluation of the coordination and efficiency of all organization activities with respect to the preset goals, written protocols, legal provisions, and other regulations including the quality system requirements. All activities related to hemovigilance system should be included when planning and implementing internal quality audits. Auditing activities should be documented and appropriate corrective and preventive actions taken.

Periodical reports

The quality manager is responsible for quality reporting at all levels within the blood establishment. This person is responsible for submitting reports to the managing board on all quality aspects in the establishment. Periodical presentations on the quality system functioning for all employees interested may prove highly useful. If a hemovigilance officer has been appointed at the blood establishment, then that person submits periodical reports on this segment of quality management, including data and trend analysis, and proposals for improvement. Besides reporting to the institution management, according to legal provisions, these reports should also be submitted to the central hemovigilance office or another competent body authorized for data collection at the national level.

Implementation and evaluation of measures for improvement

According to its definition and objectives, the system of hemovigilance promotes improvement of the quality and safety of transfusion treatment through efficient management of data collected by process surveillance. The process of improvement begins with the identification of the problem, which is only possible if informative, accurate, and objective indicators have been used to make certain conclusions. An array of activities for quality measurement, collection and analysis of process data, and process surveillance have been mentioned in the previous section; the objective of all those activities is to ensure reliable assessment of the quality and safety of products, processes,

and services by use of objective, measurable, and numerical quality indicators. This is the first step in quality improvement. Successful implementation and maintenance of the hemovigilance system is warranted by collection of a greater amount of data; that is, such an approach that covers all (and not only serious) adverse events and reactions, and ensures surveillance of the overall chain of blood transfusion, from the donor to the recipient, while also promoting collection of data on near-miss events.

Problem identification is followed by investigation of the possible causes and optimal problem solution. There are a variety of tools available for problem solving. Appropriate knowledge of these tools and correct choice of the mode of problem solving are preconditions for efficient quality improvement.

Although the investigation of the possible causes of the problem identified and search for an optimal solution may frequently be a painstaking and demanding task, it generally relies on the knowledge, competences, and enthusiasm of the people involved in this process. And yet, implementation of the measures for improvement may be hampered or even prevented by a number of obstacles. In settings with reduced financial resources, the measures that imply financial investments frequently are not feasible. Therefore, results of cost-benefit or cost-effectiveness analyses should be presented on proposing and elaborating such measures for quality improvement. By the use of simple economic indicators, it may occasionally be clearly demonstrated that restricted financial investment will in the long run prove beneficial for patients and for the transfusion service in general.

Another quite common obstacle is the resistance shown by some individuals when the measures for quality improvement require modification of the rooted work habits and attitudes. Overcoming this type of obstacles usually requires a longer period of time, during which the work culture is gradually changed by systematic education of the personnel, while stimulating teamwork, transparency, and multidisciplinarity. Stimulating teamwork and the involvement of all employees in the implementation of the QMS implies informing them consistently on the quality status and results achieved, and on future planned activities. Meetings with heads of particular processes should be regularly organized on a weekly or monthly basis and improvements and modifications be proposed in collaboration with them.

Training and assessment

The knowledge and competences of personnel are vital to the success in any job, and are crucial when performing activities upon which human health and lives depend. The errors that occur in transfusion medicine frequently arise from inadequate knowledge and training of the personnel. Therefore, promoting education and training in transfusion medicine are of utmost importance. Unfortunately, planned and properly structured education is lacking in many settings. Such a situation is sometimes caused by objective circumstances (inadequate financial resources, inadequate number of educators, inappropriate premises for education, and so on), but a failure to pay due attention to education is not uncommon either.

A comprehensive and efficient personnel education should include both professional training and education in the field of quality management and hemovigilance. Like those in other segments of the transfusion service, those working in blood product manufacture need to have appropriate qualifications. As the professional qualification requirements vary from country to country, it should best be stated that the qualification should meet the employer's requirements and be adjusted with legal provisions in a particular country. Employees that start working in the manufacture process should receive initial education and training for the tasks they will perform. Education should be performed according to the preset and approved plan of education. During initial education, new employees should be supervised by experienced personnel until their newly acquired knowledge and skills are found to meet the regulated requirements. Upon completion of the education, new employees should receive formal permission to carry out independent work.

Although initial education is of paramount importance, the need of planned continuous education should be emphasized. Transfusion medicine is a very dynamic field where changes are quite frequent, thus entailing greater need for continuous education and training. Education should be planned and approved, the knowledge checked regularly, and records kept on all these activities. In settings faced with inadequate or inappropriate education due to the lack of educators, premises, or other reasons, problems can nowadays be compensated for by various computer-based programs or distant learning courses suitable for personnel education in an economical, uniform, and efficient way.

The goal of personnel education for work in the manufacture process is to acquire the necessary knowledge and skills for the manufacture of quality and safe blood products, in line with legal and other provisions. Those working in the manufacture process should be familiar with GMP principles and the fundamentals of microbiology and hygiene. They should be educated for work according to the valid work instructions and manufacture procedures. The transfusion service increasingly relies on computer technology, which has improved the efficiency, economy, and safety of its overall activities. Therefore, appropriate knowledge of the computer technology is obligatory for all employees in transfusion medicine. Proper education on the safe and correct use of transfusion software in all segments to which the worker has authorized admittance is of the utmost importance.

In addition to professional education, staff members should also be included in the program of initial and continuous education on the quality system implemented in the respective transfusion establishment, and on hemovigilance as an integral part of this system.

References

1 Faber JC, 2004, Worldwide overview of existing haemovigilance systems. *Transfus Apher Sci* **31**(2): 99–110.
2 Dhingra N, Hafner V, and Xueref S, 2003, Hemovigilance in countries with scarce resources—A WHO

Perspective. *Transfusion Alternatives in Transfusion Medicine* **5**: 277–84.

3 de Vries RRP, 2009, The International Haemovigilance Network (IHN). *Blood Transfus* **7**(Suppl 1): LE19, 36–7.

4 European Directorate for the Quality of Medicines and HealthCare of the Council of Europe (EDQM), 2010, Guide to the Preparation, Use and Quality Assurance of Blood Components, 15th edition, Strasbourg, France.

5 PIC/S Secretariat, 2007, GMP Guide for Blood Establishments (PE 005-3), September, Geneva, Switzerland.

6 Seifried E, and Seidl C (eds), 2010, European Standard Operating Procedure (SOP) Manual Edition 1.1. Project participants. Available as an e-book from http://www.eubis-europe.eu/blood_manual_details.php [accessed February 24, 2010].

7 Shulman IA, and Kent D, 1991, Unit placement errors: a potential risk factor for ABO and Rh incompatible blood transfusions. *Lab Med* **22**: 194–6.

8 Vuk T, 2010, Quality indicators in blood establishments: CITM experience. *Blood Transfusion.* **8**(Suppl 1): LE14, 20–24.

CHAPTER 6

Establishment of Hemovigilance for the Testing, Storage, Distribution, Transport, and Issuing of Blood and Blood Components: The Example of Greece

Constantina Politis

Hellenic Coordinating Haemovigilance Centre (SKAE), Athens University, Athens, Greece

Introduction

The testing, release, storage, distribution, transport, and issuing of blood components are essential functions of the blood establishment (BE) and the hospital blood bank (hBB) within the transfusion chain. For this reason, European Directive 2002/98/EC[1] requires Member States to take all necessary measures to establish and maintain harmonized quality and safety standards for BEs, based on principles of good practice throughout the blood transfusion chain so as to ensure a high level of health protection.[1] In addition, an efficient hemovigilance system must be set up, helping to ensure that the right blood component is transfused to the right patient and that transmission of diseases by blood is prevented.[1] One prerequisite for the implementation of a hemovigilance network is to build-up operational linkages between clinical departments, hospital blood banks, blood establishments, and national authorities.

This chapter presents the example of Greece in establishing an effective hemovigilance system for collecting and analyzing information on unexpected or undesirable events as well as nonconformance with technical requirements related to pretransfusion testing of donor blood, release, storage, distribution, transport, and issuing of blood components. Hemovigilance was developed as part of a quality system at an institutional level integrated into regional and national levels in conformity with the provisions of Directives 2002/98/EC[1] and 2005/61/EC[2] as well as the Recommendations of the Council of Europe[3] and guidance of the European (now International) Hemovigilance Network and the International Society of Blood Transfusion.

Establishment of the Coordinating Haemovigilance Centre

The Coordinating Haemovigilance Centre (abbreviated as SKAE in Greek) was founded by the Hellenic Centre for Disease Control and Prevention (KEELPNO) in November 1995 on a voluntary basis.[4] It was established in line with European efforts to promote the strictest possible standards

Hemovigilance: An Effective Tool for Improving Transfusion Safety, First Edition. Edited by René R.P. De Vries and Jean-Claude Faber.
© 2012 John Wiley & Sons, Ltd. Published 2012 by John Wiley & Sons, Ltd.

for quality in blood donation and transfusion medicine, and particularly to limit the risks that arise in this area of public health, thus helping to improve the safety of the blood transfusion chain from donor to patient.

Ministerial Resolution 261 of February 2011[5] resolved that SKAE would be responsible for the development and implementation of the hemovigilance system under the aegis of KEELPNO of the Ministry of Health and Social Solidarity. SKAE collects, records, and processes reports of adverse reactions (ARs) and adverse events (AEs) related to the transfusion of blood components and the donation of whole blood or apheresis products.

The hemovigilance system includes networks between hospital clinical departments and hospital blood banks, blood establishments, and the National Blood Centre (EKEA).

SKAE performs epidemiological surveillance of infectious and noninfectious ARs and AEs associated with blood transfusion as well as of ARs and injuries or accidents to donors during or after donation, and also carries out surveillance of transfusion transmissible infections (TTIs). Traceability studies and retrieval of potential infectious donations as well as look-back programs and other functions such as blood logistics and management of blood supply, quality management indices, crisis management, and training are also among SKAE's activities (see Figure 6.1).

National hemovigilance network

The national hemovigilance network that has been developed to accomplish these tasks, collects information through six regional networks of local hospital hemovigilance units (abbreviated as TODIA in Greek; see Figure 6.2).

Flow chart of information

Following a bottom-up approach, a report of an AR or AE reaches SKAE through the following bodies:

• *Level 1 (local)—Hospital:* Hemovigilance data are collected by a hemovigilance officer, who is usually the medical director of the blood bank or an experienced clinician, or in some cases the senior nurse of the blood service. The responsibility for hemovigilance matters lies with the hospital blood transfusion committee and the hemovigilance officer.

• *Level 2 (region)—Regional Hemovigilance Network:* The head of each regional hemovigilance section cooperates with the medical director of every local blood bank.

• *Level 3 (national)—Coordinating Haemovigilance Centre:* SKAE cooperates with the six regional sections and often also with the local hemovigilance bodies. SKAE reports to EKEA and KEELPNO.

This chapter is confined to discussing activities connected to the testing, storage, distribution, transport, and issuing of blood components.

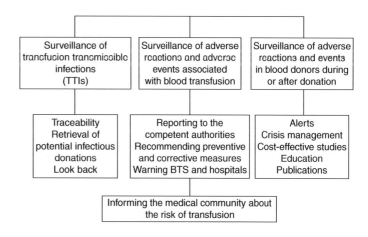

Figure 6.1 Basic functions of SKAE.

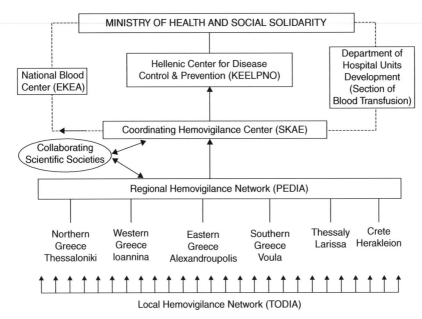

Figure 6.2 The Greek national hemovigilance network.

Quality issues and hemovigilance procedures for testing, storage, distribution, transport, and issuing

Testing for transfusion transmissible Infections (TTIs)

One of SKAE's major activities is quality management of blood donors and their donations. For this purpose, comprehensive surveillance has been implemented, covering the whole transfusion chain "vein to vein." It applies to traceability procedures, collection, and evaluation of epidemiological data of blood donors, donations, blood components, and patients, as well as notification of ARs and AEs in donors and in recipients.

Pre-transfusion screening of donor blood for infectious markers includes HBsAg, anti-HIV I/II, anti-HCV, syphilis, and anti-HTLV I/II, as well as HCV-RNA, HIV-RNA, and HBV-DNA. Anti-HBcore and additional HBV markers as well as other emerging infectious agents are tested when required. Testing is performed following a national algorithm and guidelines based on the "Guide" of the Council of Europe.[3]

SKAE has been systematically applying detailed *epidemiological surveillance* of TTIs for the last 16 years. Box 6.1 summarizes the protocol used for the collection and analysis of data on TTIs and the examined parameters for the epidemiological surveillance of whole blood and apheresis donors, quality management indices, and hemovigilance procedures in case of post-transfusion infection and look-back studies.

Box 6.1 Epidemiological protocol for the surveillance of TTIs

Collection of data on:
- infectious markers in blood donors;
- infections in tested units of whole blood and apheresis components;
- laboratory methods for blood screening;
- implementation of quality control programs
- quality parameters and Standard Operating Procedures (SOPs);
- quality management indices.

Analysis of data in relation to:
- participation of blood establishments;
- number of tested blood units;
- number of blood donors (demographic characteristics, first time, repeat);

- serological screening for infectious agents (HBsAg, anti-HIV 1/2, anti-HCV, syphilis and anti-HTLV I/II);
- molecular screening with Nucleic acid amplification technology (NAT) (HCV-RNA, HIV-RNA, HBV-DNA);
- profile of the seropositive blood donor;
- geographical mapping of infections;
- estimation of residual risk for TTIs.

Other activities:
- tracing and retrieval of potential infectious donations and a look-back program;
- conducting cost-effectiveness studies of measures for preventing TTIs.

Figure 6.3 shows the increasing participation of BEs in the epidemiological surveillance for TTIs over the period 1996–2009 and the corresponding volume of tested blood units.

Data on the profile of the seropositive donor and trends of infectious markers during the period 1996–2008 and NAT-only positive rates per 100,000 donations of HIV, HBV, and HCV in first-time donors and in repeat donors are provided in Chapter 10 of this book. It is noted that the driving force is HBsAg, the most prevalent infection.[6] The frequency of anti-HBcore antibody at national level is 4%, varying between 3–11% in different regions of the country.

With the introduction of NAT testing, one of the main issues emerging from the epidemiological surveillance of TTIs is the high prevalence of *occult HBV* (1 per 6080 blood units).[7] These alarming data demonstrate that Greece is an area of medium endemicity for HBV infection, especially of the occult type.

Transfusion-transmitted HIV infection in recipients in relation to implicated blood donors' sexual-risk behavior, and the impact on the public and subsequently on the health authorities' policies regarding the implementation of new testing strategies, has also been described.[8]

As regards *quality indicators* in recent years, improvements have been noted in laboratory screening methods and in basic preconditions for quality: written guides and protocols, records of equipment maintenance, reagents, samples, and results. However, there are still deficiencies in exterior quality control and obtaining accreditation (see Figure 6.4).

In the context of hemovigilance in testing procedures for infectious markers, BEs are required to notify SKAE of any deviations from good manufacturing practices (GMP) and applicable standards or established specifications—such as product defect, equipment failure, and human error—that may affect the quality and safety of the blood product, as well as errors in the choice of and/or use of out-of-date SOPs. SKAE regularly conducts training programs for the quality assurance of the screening process for TTIs focusing on validation of testing assays, reagents, and equipment as well as internal quality control, external quality assurance, and documentation of all these actions.

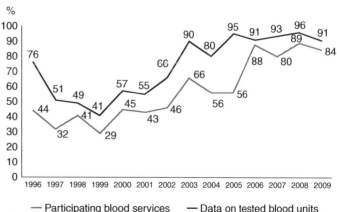

Figure 6.3 Participation in surveillance.

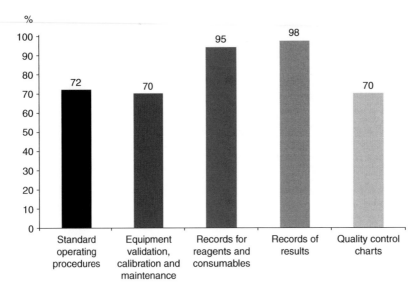

Figure 6.4 Quality indices.

Traceability studies and look-back procedures

Traceability studies and look-back procedures systematically requested by SKAE are described in Chapter 10. These hemovigilance procedures have proved to be very helpful for the BEs in performing a risk analysis to assess whether a post-transfusion infection in a recipient indicates a potential infectious blood product. For look-back studies, whenever a blood donation may have taken place within the window period of a (repeat) donor with confirmed HIV, HBV, or HCV infection, SKAE uses a standardized protocol for tracing recipients of blood components from the potentially infectious blood donation and notifying them through their treating physicians. Implicated donations include those within a time frame equal to the maximum test-specific window period of the infection, preceding a negative screening test result in the donor.[9]

According to SKAE's protocol, the BE informs the hospital in writing about the incident and advises the hospital to trace the recipients of the implicated blood product and inform them of the potentially infectious transfusion. It is the responsibility of the treating physician to inform the recipient about the potentially infectious transfusion, unless there are medical arguments not to do so.

If the recipient is tested in order to establish or exclude the infection, the hospital should notify the BE of the test results. If the recipient is not tested, this should also be notified to the BE.[9]

Blood group serology-compatibility

Guidelines for pre-transfusion testing

National guidelines updating pre-transfusion testing protocols are recommended by EKEA.[10] These protocols include ABO and Rh(D) grouping, antibody screening, group and screen, crossmatching, sample validity, selection of RBC and non-RBC products for transfusion, emergency transfusion, and quality control. Guidelines for massive transfusion, and transfusion recommendations in pregnancy, as well as selection of blood components for neonatal and infant use and autologous pre-deposit transfusion are also provided in line with the "Guide" of the Council of Europe.[3] (SKAE produced a Greek edition of the 14th English edition in 2009.) Guidance on identification of the patient at blood sampling, compatibility testing, and transfusion safety measures conforms to Council of Europe recommendations[3] and the *EU Manual of Optimal Blood Use* (Greek edition by the Hellenic Society of Blood Transfusion, 2010).[11] Standardization of patient identification, sample collection, and labeling, as well as pre-transfusion testing records, transfusion records, and laboratory records, is recommended by SKAE to ensure quality and safety in blood group serology and compatibility.

Technical procedures for pre-transfusion testing (reagents, tube techniques, microplate, and other techniques), as well as quality assurance programs (personnel, records, reagents, equipment, computer validation, storage requirements, transport, and administration of blood components), should be applied, following the recommendations of the Council of Europe and the relevant national guidelines.[3,7,10] The aim of any blood transfusion laboratory is to perform the right test on the right sample and obtain the right results.

Hemovigilance procedures

SKAE has set up hemovigilance procedures for blood group serology and compatibility in order to identify failures in correct patient identification at the time of sample collection, prescription of the wrong blood component or transfusion to the wrong patient, and generally any error that could lead to transfusion of incompatible or inappropriate blood with serious clinical implications for the recipient's health. Every BE and hBB should have a system in place to identify and record any incidents, discrepancies, and "near-misses" that had, or potentially had, an AE on the patient.[3,12] All transfusion reactions that are considered potentially hemolytic or are due to bacterial contamination are reported to the laboratory that performed the pre-transfusion testing.[12] Serious ARs are reported to SKAE and subsequently to EKEA.

Box 6.2 summarizes SKAE's protocol for the epidemiological surveillance of incorrect blood component transfused.

○ site of primary error
  – blood unit (wrong donor group label, wrong recipient identification on unit);
  – patient sample (wrong name of tube, including wrong patient collected);
  – transfusion (ABO-incompatible transfusion, wrong patient but ABO-compatible, wrong product type plasma versus platelets).

Several automated technologies such as an upgraded Column Agglutination Technology and a Solid Phase System for the immobilization of human erythrocytes have been implemented for pre-transfusion testing. These technologies apply to antibody screening, crossmatching, or antibody identification problem resolution and red cell antigen phenotyping and other immunohematological tests (i.e., indirect antiglobulin test). Standardization of test performance in pre-transfusion testing and computerization of test results are advantages offered in comparison to the classical manual methods.

Blood typing and matching with donor blood for at least the ABO, Rh, and Kell systems (small phenotype) are routinely applied and screening for the detection and identification of irregular antibodies before each transfusion is recommended. An extended matching policy for Kidd, Duffy, Lewis, Lutheran, MNS, P_1 and S systems (large phenotype) is applied when required. One BE issuing blood components to four of the largest general hospitals in Athens has implemented a computerized recycling program in order to provide matched phenotyped RBCs and HLA to multi-transfused patients with thalassemia.

Storage, release, distribution, and issuing of blood components

Presidential Decree 25/2008[13] implements Directives 2005/61/EC and 2005/62/EC in Greece. It imposes on the BE compliance with EU quality standards and other appropriate technical specifications and safety measures for the establishment of a quality system concerning the collection, testing, processing, storage, and distribution of blood

---

Box 6.2 Incorrect blood component transfused (IBCT)

Use of standard form for aggregate data:
- Analysis of data by category:
  ○ transfused with reaction
  ○ transfused without reaction
  ○ component not transfused (near-misses)[12]

and blood components. The aim is to ensure that the correct blood component is released from the BE and distributed to the hBB, and subsequently issued to a clinical department for transfusion to the correct patient.

SKAE recommends that institutions should have policies for pick-up and delivery of blood, and that an accurate mechanism to identify the intended recipient and the requested component at the time of issue should be in place in conformity with the relevant quality standards. Furthermore, procedures should lay down in detail the specifications for storage, release, issue, and transport of blood components with the aim of preventing ARs and AEs associated with transfusion.

SKAE also recommends that quality data should be routinely analyzed to identify product and quality problems that may require corrective action or to identify unfavorable trends that may require preventive action. SKAE's database for preventive and corrective measures has proved valuable in assessing the effectiveness after the implementation of such measures.

In line with the recommendations of the Council of Europe, SKAE advises that inter-institutional audits should be actively promoted and that external inspections and audits by approved and competent authorities are necessary to monitor compliance with the quality management system as well as implementation of preventive and corrective measures.

Storage requirements

Blood components must be stored for specified maximum periods, under conditions and at temperatures optimal for their function and safety.[3,13]

Storage conditions should be controlled, monitored, and checked.[3,13] Procedures must be validated to ensure the quality of blood and blood components during the entire storage period and to exclude mix-ups of blood components. Appropriate alarms should be present and checked regularly. Each area of storage should be secured against the entry of unauthorized persons. All storage actions including receipt and distribution should be defined by written procedures and technical specifications.[3,13]

Packaging must maintain the integrity and storage temperature of blood and blood components during distribution and transportation. Return of blood components into inventory for reissue shall only be accepted when all the quality requirements laid down by the BE are met, to ensure blood component integrity.[3,13]

Refrigerators and freezers for storage of blood components must have a temperature recording device, which is checked daily, and must have an alarm system. The alarm function of temperature recording devices shall be checked for the high and low temperature limits.

Release of blood components

The national presidential decree[13] requires that no blood component be released until all mandatory requirements set out in its provisions have been fulfilled, and that each BE is able to provide approval for release of a blood component by an authorized person in accordance with the appropriate validation, documentation, and laboratory testing criteria. In the event that the final product fails release due to a confirmed positive infection test result, a check shall be made to identify all other components from the same donation and components prepared from previous donations given by the donor. In these situations, there shall be an immediate update of the donor record.[14]

SKAE recommends a computerized control for product status. A computer system should be validated to ensure that all donor selection criteria and laboratory testing requirements are fulfilled (see Chapter 10).

Distribution and transport

National legislation[13] requires that, prior to distribution, blood components should be visually inspected, and that all distribution requirements comply with Directive 2003/94/EC.[15]

All means of transport should be validated to maintain the recommended storage temperature of the blood component over the proposed maximum time and extreme ambient temperature of transportation:[3,13]

• The containers used in transport should be well insulated, and easy to clean and handle. Where a refrigerated vehicle is used, the principles applying to control of refrigerators should be observed.

- Systems for road, rail, or air transport using controlled cooling elements should also fulfill quality standards and specifications.
- Containers must be labeled with information on blood components, place of origin, and destination.
- Platelet components must be agitated continuously and the platelets should not be used if agitation has not occurred for more than 24 hours. Therefore, transportation of this product cannot take longer than 24 hours from the time it leaves the BE.
- Transportation time between facilities should not exceed 24 hours.

SKAE recommends the use of a temperature indicator to monitor the in-transit temperature. On receipt, the blood component should be transferred to storage under recommended conditions, if it is not intended for immediate transfusion:

- Returned blood components should not be reissued for transfusion if the bag has been penetrated or damaged, if the blood component has not been maintained continuously within the approved temperature range, or if there is a leakage, abnormal color change, or excessive hemolysis.
- The proper identification, time of issue, and transit history should also be fully documented.
- hBBs receiving blood components from BEs should have a system to ensure that components are accompanied by a dispatch note with details of the donation number of each component, the components ABO and Rh(D) blood group, the signature and designation of the person responsible for the issue, and designation of the person receiving the consignment.

SKAE recommends that each BE must also have in place a system for documenting any adverse effects caused by the administration of any component or the identification of a component quality problem. This system should enable the recall, if appropriate, of all unused components from that donation or all donations that are a constituent of a component pool. SKAE further recommends that recalls should be thoroughly investigated with a view to preventing recurrence.

All transportation actions, including receipt and distribution, should be defined by written procedures and specifications.[16] BEs must have a system in place to maintain and control the storage of blood components during their shelf life, including any transportation that may be required. Temperature and hygienic conditions should be monitored continuously: Warning systems need to be used where applicable. Autologous blood and blood components should be stored separately.[14]

Issuing

The responsibility for accurately identifying a transfusion component rests with both the transfusion service personnel who issue the blood and the clinical representatives who receive it.

The steps that have to be completed by the hBB personnel before issuing a unit are described in Chapter 10.

References

1 European Union, 2003, Directive 2002/98/EC of the European Parliament and of the Council of 27 January 2003 setting standards of quality and safety for the collection, testing, processing, storage and distribution of human blood and blood components and amending Directive 2001/83/EC. *Official Journal of the European Union* 8.2.2003: L33/30.

2 European Union, 2005, Commission Directive 2005/61/EC of 30 September 2005 implementing Directive 2002/98/EC of the European Parliament and of the Council as regards traceability requirements and notification of serious adverse reactions and events. *Official Journal of the European Union* 1.10.2005: L256/32.

3 Council of Europe, 2008, Guide to the Preparation, Use and Quality Assurance of Blood Components, Recommendation R (95) 15. 14th edition. Council of Europe Publishing, Strasbourg.

4 Centre for Disease Control and Prevention, 2001, Ministerial Resolution Y1/5028, *Official Journal of Hellenic Government* **831**. Internal operational regulation.

5 Greek Government, 2011, Ministerial Resolution 261/17-Feb-2011, Definition of conditions and

procedures for the notification of adverse events to the National Blood Centre (EKEA) and the Centre of Disease Control and Prevention (KEELPNO) through the haemovigilance system.

6 Politis C, Richardson C, Damaskos P, *et al.*, 2010, Hellenic Coordinating Haemovigilance Centre, Summary report Epidemiological Surveillance of Transfusion Transmitted Infections (TTIs) (1996–2009); Surveillance of adverse reactions (ARs-TR) and adverse events (AEs-TR) associated with blood transfusion (1997–2009), Surveillance of adverse reactions (ARs-DN) and adverse events (AEs-DN) during or after donation (2003–2009), Athens.

7 Politis C, Kavallierou L, Asariotou M, *et al.*, 2010, Surveillance of transfusion transmitted infections in 1996–2008 in Hellas: The impact of individual NAT testing on blood safety. *Vox Sang* **99**: 279.

8 Politis C, Richardson C, Damaskos P, *et al.*, 2011, Risk behaviours with an impact on blood donor management in Hellas. *Blood Transf* **9**(Suppl 1): 29.

9 Politis C, Asariotou M, Koumarianos S, *et al.*, 2009, Look back programme for HIV seropositive blood donors in Hellas. Vox Sang **96**(1): 142.

10 National Blood Centre (EKEA), 2009, Guidelines for pre-transfusion testing and other technical requirements.

11 McClelland DBL, Pirie E, and Franklin IM, 2010, *Manual of Optimal Blood Use, Support for safe, clinically effective and efficient use of Blood in Europe.* EU Optimal Blood Use Project.

12 ISBT, 2011, Proposed standard definitions for surveillance of non-infectious adverse transfusion reactions. http://www.isbtweb.org/fileadmin/user_upload/WP_on_Haemovigilance/ISBT_definitions_final_2011_4_.pdf [accessed February 22, 2012]

13 European Union, 2005, Presidential decree 25/2008 implementing Directives 2005/61/EC of the European Parliament and of the Council as regards traceability requirements and notification of serious adverse reactions and events and 2005/62/EC of the European Parliament and of the Council as regards Community standards and specifications relating to a quality system for blood establishments. *Official Journal of the European Union* 1.10.2005: L256/1.

14 European Union, 2005, Commission Directive 2005/62/EC of 30 September 2005 implementing Directive 2002/98/EC of the European Parliament and of the Council as regards Community standards and specifications relating to a quality system for blood establishments. *Official Journal of the European Union* 1.10.2005: L256/41.

15 European Union, 2003, Commission Directive 2003/94/EC of 8 October 2003 laying down the principles and guidelines of good manufacturing practice in respect of medicinal products for human use and investigational medicinal products for human use. *Official Journal of the European Union.* 14.10.2003: L262/22–25.

16 National Law 3402/2005—Restructuring the blood transfusion system.

CHAPTER 7

Medical Decision, Ordering, Administration of Component, and Monitoring of the Patient

Mickey B.C. Koh[1,2], Ramir Alcantara[2], Mark Grumbridge[1], and Ai Leen Ang[2,3]

[1]Department of Haematology, St George's Hospital and Medical School, London, UK
[2]Blood Services Group, Health Sciences Authority, Singapore
[3]Department of Haematology, Singapore General Hospital, Singapore

Introduction

The optimal and appropriate use of blood products is widely regarded as a crucial aspect of the hemovigilance system. Although not traditionally captured in the initial design of many hemovigilance systems, inappropriate transfusion leads to wastage and, more importantly, the unnecessary exposure to blood products and its attendant risks. This will invariably require the development of transfusion guidelines/protocols, education of the hospital clinicians, and close collaboration between the hemovigilance team, transfusion medicine physicians, and clinicians.

After a decision has been made to proceed with blood transfusion, the blood products have to be ordered. This involves several important steps that are prone to errors and may in turn lead to serious complications from the transfusion of incompatible blood. Therefore, the monitoring and reporting of errors related to ordering of blood also forms an integral part of the hemovigilance system

Overarching these aspects is the establishment of a quality system that examines the organizational structure, procedures, processes, and resources needed for implementation. These policies and procedures will guide all personnel involved in the proper administration of blood and blood products and any deviation should be detected by the hemovigilance system. Since the goal of hemovigilance is to increase the safety and quality of blood transfusion, hemovigilance in the hospital needs to be linked not only to the hospital transfusion committee, but also form an integral component of quality management of the entire hospital.

Medical decision and ordering

Most hemovigilance systems were initially designed to survey the efferent arm of the transfusion chain, when a particular unit of blood has already been transfused into the patient. This continues to be important and the pivotal results of Serious Hazards of Transfusion (SHOT; see Chapter 14), for example, defined the importance of Transfusion Related Acute Lung Injury (TRALI) both to the transfusion and clinical community, leading to fundamental changes in practice.[1] The hemovigilance field, however, has subsequently matured into not only examining the entire transfusion chain, but also encompassing the afferent arm (donor hemovigilance) as well as near-misses.

Hemovigilance: An Effective Tool for Improving Transfusion Safety, First Edition. Edited by René R.P. De Vries and Jean-Claude Faber.
© 2012 John Wiley & Sons, Ltd. Published 2012 by John Wiley & Sons, Ltd.

The next point in this progression is to ask whether a unit of blood component has been appropriately transfused. An international comparative survey of differing practices for the optimal use of blood products underscores the increasingly recognition to incorporate this aspect into existing hemovigilance systems and its fundamentally crucial role for safer transfusion practice.[2]

The first step in deciding whether a transfusion event is appropriate is the establishment of clinical guidelines for transfusion.

Red cell utilization has been shown to vary between countries and regions. This is due to complex factors including population demographics, standard of medical care, and complexity of medical procedures, among other reasons. One attributable and significant factor is the inappropriateness of blood usage. The influence that clinical guidelines and policies have on this has been looked at in some hemovigilance systems.

The significant reduction in red cell utilization in England is thought to be due to the greater awareness of transfusion risks as well as hospital and national policies to encourage appropriate blood usage.[3]

Single center audits in Singapore and Malaysia have found that only 27%[4] and 47.4%[5] of fresh frozen plasma requests respectively were appropriate.

A retrospective study of cryoprecipitate usage, even allowing for a more liberal usage in massive transfusion, has demonstrated that just under half of all cryoprecipitate transfusions are not indicated. Significantly, only 37% of requests are appropriate against clinical guidelines.[6]

Products and processes

Setting standards or guidelines for transfusion is therefore necessary to tackle this issue of inappropriate use. As transfusion is a medical procedure, making decisions on transfusion will also involve assessing the clinical condition of the patient; determining whether transfusion is indicated; and the type and amount of blood products to be given.[7]

The indications for transfusing any particular blood component must therefore be defined: thresholds for when it is needed and clinical scenarios where it is clearly not helpful. Fresh frozen plasma, for example, should never be used as a volume expander and any such use must be deemed inappropriate.

Established guidelines on the appropriate transfusion and indications of various blood components are needed to serve as a benchmark against which deviation from standard practice can be determined. There is a wealth of information and published material to refer to. Several international and regional guidelines on the appropriate use of blood for various groups of patients in different circumstances are available. Some examples are guidelines from

- EU Optimal Blood Use Project;[7]
- British Committee for Standards in Haematology (BCSH);[8]
- Australia and New Zealand Society of Blood Transfusion;[9]
- World Health Organization (WHO).[10]

There are also other guidelines, such as those published by The Association of Anaesthetists of Great Britain and Ireland[11] as well as The Society of Thoracic Surgeons Blood Conservation Guideline Task Force[12], which are targeted at more specific patient groups with potentially high demand for blood. There is a close consensus among the above guidelines that aim at promoting the appropriate and safe use of blood products. This is remarkable considering that the representatives responsible for writing these guidelines come from different backgrounds, ranging from the "providers" (e.g., blood establishments) to end-users (e.g., surgeons, anesthetists).

The WHO Aide-Memoire for National Health Programmes on the Clinical Use of Blood says that there should be a national health program in developing policies for ensuring the safe and proper utilization of blood components.[13]

National guidelines should include indications for the use of blood components and alternatives to transfusion, information about available blood products and alternatives to transfusion, a standard blood request form, and guidance to hospitals on the development of a Maximum Surgical Blood Ordering Schedule (MSBOS) and standard operating procedures.[13] WHO had published its recommendations on how to develop national policies and guidelines on the clinical use of blood[14] and these include the following steps:

1 Bringing awareness to the national health authority of the need for national policies and guidelines on the clinical usage of blood. This responsibility lies with the clinicians, the country's blood transfusion society, or the National Blood Transfusion Committee.

2 Forming a Working Group comprising clinical specialists and senior personnel from the country's blood transfusion society (BTS), whose role is to oversee the planning and the implementation of the national guidelines.

3 Submitting the above draft to the national health authority for approval and endorsement.

4 Establishing a National Committee to oversee the Clinical Use of Blood. Establishing a hospital transfusion committee (comprising representatives from various clinical specialties with significant blood usage, hospital blood bank representative, nursing representative, and pharmacist) in each hospital to implement the national guidelines.

5 Disseminating the national guidelines to and developing appropriate educational and training programs for all involved in the supply and prescription of blood.

6 Monitoring key performance indicators to evaluate the success of the implementation of the national guidelines.

In essence, guidelines cannot be developed in isolation. They have to involve all stakeholders, especially the clinical end-users, and must be evidence based. These guidelines will attempt to set thresholds of safety according to the published evidence and the recommendations should be ranked or graded depending on the existing levels of evidence.

If possible, these guidelines should be peer reviewed and for successful implementation be endorsed by the existing academic bodies and organizations such as the College of Physicians or Surgeons.

It must also be accepted that these guidelines have to be subjected to regular reviews in light of new evidence and increasing knowledge. Guidelines should also not be adopted wholesale but be specific and relevant to the population at hand. For example, transfusion support for sickle cell anemia patients may be a very important issue in some countries while thalessemia is more prevalent in others. The indications for the usage of Rhesus negative blood products may be vastly different in East Asian countries where the incidence of Rhesus negativity is low and the blood resource for this scarce. There are specific guidelines for the use of Rhesus negative blood products in the national guidelines from Singapore that take into consideration the relative scarcity of the product.[15]

Individual hospitals should largely follow national guidelines if they exist, but should also take into account their infrastructure, laboratory support, rapidity of access and availability to blood products, population mix, and the nature of their clinical disciplines.

The hospital transfusion committee is usually responsible for drawing up hospital-based guidelines or adapting the national guidelines for its specific use, as well as ensuring that these guidelines are adhered to appropriately. The hospital's guidelines should, if possible, specifically address certain situations such as major hemorrhage and preoperative optimization, and special patient groups such as neonates, bone marrow transplant patients, hematology patients, and patients with bleeding disorders where relevant.[7]

The MSBOS and the massive transfusion protocol (MTP) are two examples that can help to enhance the appropriate use of blood components within hospitals. The MSBOS serves as a guide to the amount of blood components that are generally required for each particular type operation,[13] and this in turn guides the hospital blood bank in crossmatching and reserving the appropriate amount of blood components. Blood is usually ready for patients undergoing high-risk surgeries, while a group and screen for patients undergoing surgeries with low-risk of bleeding is sufficient.[16] The MSBOS is set for each hospital.

MTPs are especially useful in hospitals that often manage patients with massive hemorrhage, such as major trauma and obstetric patients. It involves rapid communication between the clinician, hematologist, and blood bank staff, thereby allowing the prompt release of prepacked blood components (red cells, fresh frozen plasma, platelets) to the patients. The protocol must clearly indicate who is responsible for initiating and stopping the protocol, how to initiate the protocol, what information needs to be communicated to the blood bank laboratory staff, the quantity and type of components to be included in the MTP pack at various phases, what laboratory parameters to monitor, and conditions for further release of blood products after the initial MTP pack had been issued. All this can then be embedded into the hospital hemovigilance system

There must be a team leader (usually the most senior doctor at the scene) who will initiate the MTP and appoint a team member to be in charge of communications with the laboratories and various departments. When the MTP is initiated, the switchboard should ensure that all the following people are informed: blood bank laboratory staff; coagulation laboratory staff; hematologist; intensive care unit senior doctor and nurse; and the surgical senior doctor and radiologist on duty.[17–23]

Other processes and documentation involved in setting up a hospital hemovigilance system are the need to document the prescription of the dose of blood components and the reasons for transfusion. Information on the lack of documentation on transfusion indications and patients' consent can be collected during regular audits. Based on the latest UK Serious Hazards of Transfusion report, the most common cause of inappropriate transfusion in 2009 was due to decisions based on spurious blood results. Other major causes include poor judgment and knowledge, resulting in errors such as excessive or under-transfusion of blood components, excessive transfusion rates, inappropriate prophylactic transfusion of platelets, and inappropriate transfusion of fresh frozen plasma when coagulation parameters were normal.[24]

Although much has been said about inappropriate transfusion linked to medical ordering, information on under-transfusion or failure to transfuse is more difficult to capture. This will often have to be reported by senior medical personnel of the clinical team and may often be picked up during daily work or mortality and morbidity meetings. Some-

times, inappropriate transfusion of blood products (either non-indicated transfusion or transfusion of the wrong component) may not be detected until mortality or morbidity occurs and these must be reported too. There should be a system in place for the clinicians to report all the above incidents to the hospital transfusion committee. Such a reporting system can most easily be incorporated into the hospital's general incidents reporting system. It can be an electronic system if technology permits and it should allow inputs from the involved clinician, senior clinicians, or other medical staff. It should be kept confidential and not entail blame on the clinician involved.

In the wards, nursing staff can help to ensure that there is proper documentation of the transfusion indication and patient's consent in the case notes before blood transfusion takes place. They can help to note down these items and provide the information to the hemovigilance officer for audits.

Jobs and responsibilities

A hospital transfusion committee led by a senior medical personnel, usually a transfusion specialist or other specialist with the relevant interest and experience, is necessary to facilitate the execution of the hospital transfusion guidelines and policies, and monitoring their adherence. The other members of the transfusion committee may include nurses and major end-users of blood products such as surgeons, obstetricians, anesthetists, and hematologists.[7] If resources permit, a hemovigilance officer or transfusion practitioner, who may be any of the experienced medical, nursing, or blood bank laboratory staff, can be appointed to further enhance transfusion safety and improve transfusion practice.

The responsibilities of the committee pertaining to optimal blood use would involve promoting appropriate clinical transfusion practices according to recognized guidelines (including setting up of the hospital's own guidelines), regularly reviewing and auditing the clinical transfusion practices within the hospital, implementing policies to improve practices based on findings of audits, and promoting education among medical and laboratory staff. There should be regular meetings among members of the hospital transfusion committee to achieve these aims.[7]

The hemovigilance or transfusion practitioner officer can play an important role in helping to take the lead in ensuring that the policies or recommendations made by the hospital transfusion committee are carried out. The person can also help in educating clinical staff, assisting in auditing clinical transfusion practices, and providing patient information.[7]

The blood bank laboratory may be best placed to assist in the monitoring of optimal blood use. A designated staff from the blood bank laboratory can help to collect information on inappropriate requests and patients with high transfusion requirements, and submit this information to the hospital transfusion committee or hemovigilance officer for review and audits.

The clinical hematologists are critical in defining guidelines for optimal use. Their help should be enlisted in a collaborative and leadership role in clinical blood usage and staff education.

Hemovigilance in the hospital can be successful only if it is endorsed by the hospital administration. One practical way is to embed it into the overall quality management of the hospital. The same tools used in the quality management of drug prescription and hospital acquired infection can then be applied into hemovigilance.

There may be involvement of the government or national authorities in the monitoring of optimal blood use and good transfusion practices although this is currently not mandatory in most countries.[1] These national authorities could be used to drive national programs and clinical initiatives. There is, for example, a proposed national protocol in development in Singapore for the support of massive transfusion across all its hospitals. Highlighting the importance of these policies will help to drive both clinical and patient awareness.

Monitoring and assessment

Information on deviation in blood usage from the hospital guidelines and policies, as well as information on massive transfusion patients, should be collected regularly (e.g., weekly or monthly) by the blood bank laboratory. Adherence to the

MTP including the logistics and rapidity of support could be assessed. The above information should be analyzed and audited by the hospital transfusion committee on a regular basis. If there is a national authority governing the optimal use of blood products, the analyzed data from each hospital could be submitted to this authority annually.

Audits on other aspects of medical decisions in transfusion practice include the proportion of transfused patients who do not have proper documentation of transfusion indications and consent. These data could be collected by the hemovigilance officer with the help of the ward nursing staff.

Blood product use is a powerful tool to assess appropriate usage. As mentioned above, however, has to be interpreted in the light of other complex factors that may influence blood component utilization. There is not only inter-country variation but also inter-hospital differences. A tertiary hospital with capabilities for organ and stem cell transplantation would have an entirely different pattern and level of usage compared to a district or community hospital. Utilization can be examined not only for red cells but also platelets and plasma containing components. How this information is to be captured and monitored will depend on the individual structure of different hospitals, but should ideally be driven in the entire hospital and led from the hospital transfusion committee. If not, individual departments could drive this aspect internally, especially if an interventional measure such as thresholds or guidelines for transfusion have recently been put in place.

Implementation, training, and evaluation of measures for improvement

Benchmarking against other comparative practices is important and can be very useful. Many hospitals have guidelines that can be readily accessed. The Royal Children's Hospital has a blood transfusion guideline available for use by its staff involved in giving blood transfusion informed consent and consumer information. The guideline provides a framework for clinicians prescribing fresh blood products for all patients and explains the elements of informed consent, frequency of informed consent, a guide in giving informed consent, as well as general risks of transfusion.[25]

Another good example of SOPs for transfusion services is The Transfusion Ontario Standard Work Instruction Manual (SWIM), which was developed with funding from the Ministry of Health and Long-Term Care (MOH-LTC) Blood Conservation Program. The SWIM is a comprehensive working tool that provides procedure templates from transfusion medicine written in accordance with the current standards and has 134 procedures divided into 10 sections with visual work aids and forms that accompany each procedure.[26]

The transfusion guidelines and policies, as well as any updates, need to be made readily available to all medical staff, by having them in each ward and department, either on the hospital intranet or as hardcopies. Every new medical staff member who joins the hospital should be briefed on these guidelines and policies, and informed on how to access them. It may be necessary to mandate all medical staff involved in making clinical decisions regarding transfusion to undergo regular online trainings and assessments, if technology permits. There should also be a means of easy communication between the clinician and the transfusion specialist or hemovigilance officer because this will help to enhance optimal blood use.

The requirement for documentation on the indications for transfusion, before blood is approved, is also a way of instilling a more formal approach to transfusion. This can take many forms and at its simplest could be some form of documentation into the patient's medical records. It could also be in the form of a checklist where blood is not automatically issued unless the relevant boxes are ticked in order to denote that it complies with guidelines or threshold values

As the success of any hemovigilance program is critically dependent on the number and quality of reports received, one way is to streamline this reporting process. Within St George's Hospital in the UK, the hospital transfusion committee, following discussions with the risk management team, created a "short" reporting version for transfusion incidents, which is a subset of the general hospital

internal incident reporting system. Simplifying this process has reduced the time spent inputting data to the system. The shortened version of the form allows the incident to be reported promptly, and thus investigated promptly (see Box 7.1).

Box 7.1 Simplified report for transfusion incidents

Only use this form to report all incidents related to the following issues:

* Problems with Blood / Blood Products / Transfusion, e.g., Delay in administration of blood products, incorrect blood product transfused etc.

* Laboratory tests documentation, e.g., Specimens unlabelled/mislabelled, test results/report misfiled etc.

* Laboratory investigations, e.g., Delay in receiving/sending specimen, Specimen lost etc.

PLEASE NOTE IF YOU NEED TO REPORT ANY OTHER TYPE OF INCIDENT THEN PLEASE COMPLETE THE MAIN TRUST ELECTRONIC INCIDENT FORM. Forms that are completed and submitted inappropriately will be required to be re-entered on the Main Electronic Incident Form which can be accessed via the Trust intranet by clicking on the Applications link then choosing the Electronic Incident Form icon.

Embedding the transfusion reporting as part of the hospital incident reporting system has the advantage of allowing access to *all* grades of staff, enabling all incidents in the transfusion chain to be reported. In addition, the risk management team is able to produce a report from the database specifically for transfusion-related incidents. The database can also produce reports for specific transfusion incident categories by clinical area such as sample labeling and the cold chain. Producing incident specific reports allows the transfusion team to concentrate on those specific areas with high numbers of transfusion incidents.

We now describe three other practical areas being implemented at St George's Hospital.

Provision of irradiated blood

Certain clinical situations exist where medical ordering could be better linked to hospital systems to prevent the occurrence of errors. One example is the provision of irradiated blood. Traditionally, this has been required mainly for patients undergoing stem cell transplants and other conditions associated with profound T-cell immunodeficiency. The advent of purine analogs means that a large proportion of nontransplant patients also require irradiated blood and may actually now form the larger group. This area is prone to errors and newer generation of purine analogs may require doctors and transfusion medicine physicians to keep continually up with the latest developments.

Traditionally, the blood transfusion laboratory at St George's Hospital was given written or verbal notification of such patients. This notification enabled lab staff to "flag" these patients on the LIMS (Laboratory Information Management System). Recently a more robust system has been developed which enables an electronic notification. This project highlights two issues: it was accomplished with the help of information technology support, a powerful tool in implementation of hemovigilance programs, and by enlisting the right experts in the right clinical scenario, in this case the pharmacist.

When patients are prescribed drugs such as purine analogs, they are dispensed from a pharmacy stock control system. This system associates the issue of the particular drug with the specific patient. The Pharmacy IT manager then produces an electronic report as soon as these drugs are dispensed. The report is then sent electronically to transfusion, which enables a rapid and accurate update of the LIMS system enabling lab staff to again "flag" the special requirements on the database.

The innovation is cost neutral, can be used in any organization, and merely requires a simple report to be produced. Since the introduction of the new reporting system, no incidents have been documented where a patient has not received irradiated products following the prescribing of purine analogue drugs.

Transfusion traceability

The Blood Safety and Quality Regulations 2005 transposes the European Blood Safety Directive into UK law. This law imposes significant new requirements on hospital transfusion. The law requires "unambiguous traceability" of all blood and blood products from donor to patient.

Implementing such legislation in a large academic teaching hospital initially proved problematic due to the sheer volume of blood and blood products issued and subsequently transfused on a daily basis. A system at St George's was devised where the traceability of blood and blood products is separated into clinical areas within a spreadsheet. This sheet acts as a "league table" for traceability. Wards and clinical areas that do not return traceability tags are documented within the table. This information is circulated to all wards, clinical areas, and clinical managers on a weekly basis along with the hospital numbers of the patients whose traceability tags are missing.

Prior to the implementation of this system the traceability percentage for all transfused blood and blood products was 75–80%; since the implementation of the new traceability "league table" system the traceability of all blood and blood products transfused has risen to and is maintained at around 99–99.5% (see Box 7.2). As per EU legislation, all blood and blood products have a traceability tag attached. Following transfusion it is the responsibility of the person completing the transfusion to complete the following data on the tag and return it to the blood bank:

- transfusion start time;
- transfusion end time;
- signature of person completing the transfusion.

A monthly summary is then circulated to all clinical areas detailing the following information:

- number of blood and blood products issued;
- number of traceability tags *not* returned;
- conversion of totals into a percentage.

Box 7.2 Traceability data for September 2010

TRACEABILITY DATA
Tracer Tag Returns
MONTH – SEPTEMBER 2010
TRACEABILITY – 99.9%
2574 COMPONENTS ISSUED
3 TAGS MISSING

Surgical blood ordering schedules

In 2009–2010, the transfusion laboratory noted an increase in the numbers of blood units issued and subsequently returned unused. St George's Hospital has a maximum blood ordering schedule for surgical teams to follow, which outlines the requirements for specific surgical procedures. The evidence gathered suggests that this protocol was not sufficiently evidence based and not routinely followed. This led to large volumes of blood being returned unused on a daily basis putting pressure on the cold chain, increasing costs of performing crossmatches, and increasing staff workload, which can all contribute to errors.

An audit undertaken over seven days in November 2010 showed the following information:

- Total = 52 elective pre-ops
- Total units requested = 144
- Total crossmatched = 124
- Total used = 25
- Ratio = approx 5:1 (issued) 6:1 (requested)

A total of seven return audits have been undertaken in the past year, as detailed in Table 7.1.

St George's is now pioneering a system on a trial basis of issuing two units per request for all procedures that requires at least two units of blood previously. The provisos are the presence of a valid sample and the absence of any significant antibodies. It is envisaged that if less lab time is spent on unnecessary samples, more focus, greater efficiency, and less errors would result from the laboratory without compromising clinical support. Clear SOPs are important when detailing this workflow as are, crucially, deviations from the defined clinical scenarios where these are bypassed.

With regards to training, this should not only involve theoretical knowledge, but also encourage the development of practical skills. Clinical scenarios depicting real-life examples or "practice" sessions for emergency situations, such as massive transfusion, may help to develop practical competency.

There should preferably be regular assessments (e.g., annually) of all medical staff and the hemovigilance officer, and this can be incorporated into the annual training and accreditation.

Physicians, nurses, and other hospital staff involved in the transfusion process must be trained to perform job-related tasks. A formal introduction program should be included in the training to provide an opportunity to explain policies and procedures, introduce hospital quality principles, and provide an overview of transfusion. The staff must be familiar with these concepts so that they understand that everyone involved has their own role in assuring compliance with regulations and improving quality. They should also have adequate technical skills and theoretical knowledge about the indications, risks, benefits, and contraindications for all blood and blood components including modifications done on the unit (e.g., leukoreduction, irradiation, washing, and so on).

The hospital must identify the training needs and provide continuous education programs and training for personnel performing critical tasks. Evaluations of competence shall be performed of assigned activities and at specified intervals as defined in the institutions' SOPs.

There are some useful online tools for e-learning and assessment, and these websites are listed in the Manual of Optimal Blood Use by the EU Optimal Blood Use Project.[7]

14–18 September 2009	233 units returned	Cost of X match = £1817.40
21–25 September 2009	170 units returned	Cost of X match = £1326.00
12–16 October 2009	346 units returned	Cost of X match = £2698.80
16–20 November 2009	285 units returned	Cost of X match = £2223.00
18–22 January 2010	271 units returned	Cost of X match = £2113.80
28 June–2 July 2010	208 units returned	Cost of X match = £1622.40
15–21 November 2010	293 units returned	Cost of X match = £2285.40

Table 7.1 Audit of returned crossmatched units and cost incurred in a single institution over seven one-week periods (total number of units returned during the seven weeks of audit was 1806).

Blood administration and monitoring

SOPs and protocols for blood administration should include preparation of the patient for blood transfusion in addition to the actual administration itself. Much effort and progress have been made in the actual administration and monitoring of the patient with hemovigilance systems in place. This includes double checking of the blood at the time of administration and monitoring for transfusion reactions.

When preparing any patient for transfusion, the relevant points to consider include:
- checking for adequate venous access;
- obtaining baseline vital signs;
- informed consent;
- prescription for the blood component ordered;
- competency on which administration sets to use, filter (if needed) for the different blood products, and gauge of needle to use.

According to the AABB Primer of Blood Administration,[27] an order to prepare a blood component does not necessarily mean that a transfusion is ordered. Orders for blood administration should mention the start time and rate of transfusion. Other important details that must be included are special requirements or modifications (e.g., leukoreduced, irradiation, and so on), quantity or volume to be transfused, and any special instructions (e.g., premedications).

The stage of greatest risk in the transfusion chain is the collection of the component from the blood bank or satellite refrigerator and its administration to the patient. Errors at these stages constituted 40% of "wrong blood" events reported to SHOT in 2003 and resulted in 12 ABO incompatible transfusions.[28]

A retrospective review of 1005 patient charts in two tertiary teaching hospitals in Canada was carried out by G. Rock and coworkers to determine whether the documentation for transfusion was adequate. Their study showed that in 75% of cases, the physician had not documented that any discussion had occurred regarding the risks and/or benefits or the availability of alternatives. Only 12% of charts included information relayed to patients on the nature and process of what blood components were given to them. The discharge summary recorded transfusion information in 32.1% of cases whereas the consultation note had this information in 26.3%. *The authors concluded that even though it is widely agreed upon within the transfusion medicine community that patients should be well informed about the risks and benefits of transfusion, in practice, these consent discussions are not properly and appropriately documented.*[29]

An important aspect of documentation is a note by the physician in the progress note or other appropriate part of the patient record stating the indications for transfusion and the expected results. Friedmann and coworkers did a retrospective review of red blood cell transfusions in adult patients in two hospital facilities during 1-week audit periods of each month from April 2001 to March 2003. Assessment forms were used to classify the level of physician documentation of transfusions into three groups: adequately, intermediately, and inadequately documented. Transfusions were deemed justified based on existing hospital transfusion guidelines. Results of the study showed that transfusion events with suboptimal (intermediate and inadequate) documentation accounted for 49% of all medical record-reviewed transfusion events and 62% could not be justified. *There was a significant correlation between inadequate documentation and suboptimal documentation with failure to justify transfusion.*[30]

Other pertinent details needed for proper documentation are the following:
- documentation of recipient consent;
- name or type of component;
- donor unit or pool identification number, date, and time of transfusion;
- pre- and post-transfusion vital signs and volume transfused;
- identification of the transfusionist;
- any adverse events possibly related to the transfusion.

Monitoring and assessment

Staff involved in administering blood and blood components should be trained and qualified to recognize signs and symptoms of suspected transfusion reactions, when to discontinue the transfusion, and how to evaluate and manage the patient. If nursing staff recognize the presence of a suspected transfusion reaction, a member of the medical staff should be contacted immediately and the patient's vitals signs checked and recorded. Further evaluation, tests, and management of the patient depends on the type and severity of the reaction.

The hospital must have policies, processes, and procedures for the training of these staff and the timely reporting to the blood bank of suspected transfusion reactions. There should be clear procedures for the initial evaluation of transfusion reactions, which includes clerical and documentation checks as well as serologic testing of post- and pre-transfusion samples to identify hemolytic transfusion reactions. There should also be a process for the evaluation of suspected non-hemolytic transfusion reactions, which includes febrile reactions, possible bacterial contamination, TRALI, and others depending on the institution's policies.

As early as 1991, Shulman and coworkers concluded that even though institutional blood administration policies were in place at their institution (Los Angeles County + University of Southern California (LAC + USC)), about 1 of every 6000 patients undergoing transfusion received an ABO-incompatible transfusion. More than half of these incompatible transfusions resulted from deviation in proper blood administration practice (e.g., the transfusionist failed to compare the information on the patient's ID band with the information on the blood component unit label prior to transfusion). In order to address this issue, a concurrent auditing system was developed in their hospital to detect variances in blood administration practice, a monitoring instrument was created (a blood administration practices audit instrument), and personnel were assigned to the review process. When an audit documented a deviation from proper blood administration practice, the transfusion service medical director informs the appropriate supervising physician or nurse, in writing, about the circumstances and significance of the procedural violation and of the need to take appropriate corrective action. As a result of this newly implemented hospital quality improvement process, the percentage of

transfusions with an associated variance from their institutional policy dropped to nearly zero.[31]

The authors recommended that even though the transfusion of blood and blood components is usually carried out by personnel who are not under the direct supervision of the transfusion service medical director, that person should be involved in the oversight and assessment of the staff involved in blood administration. Involvement by the physician responsible for the transfusion service is appropriate and consistent with the concept that the responsibility for proper transfusion does not end with the issuance of blood and components by transfusion service personnel.

According to Sazama in her report of 355 transfusion-associated deaths, the hospital that fails to manage the entire process of transfusion of blood and blood components, including proper systems of administering blood to the correct recipient, puts itself at risk of unnecessary liability.[32]

As mentioned above, a bedside blood-administering assessment program has been in place at Los Angeles County + University of Southern California (LAC + USC) Medical Center since 1991. Implementation of this blood transfusion assessment program resulted in the improvement of transfusion practice, reduced the number of near-miss events, and prevented mistransfusions.[33] To further improve blood trans-fusion safety practices, the program has been expanded to include other steps such as patient preparation, writing orders for transfusion, requesting blood for pick-up, monitoring of patients during and after the transfusion, and documenting transfusion-related details in the patient's chart.

To monitor compliance with institutional policies, a group of registered nurses was trained to observe the dispensing and administering of blood products; special emphasis was placed on the performance of the pre-transfusion clerical check, providing information brochures to the patient, and obtaining informed consent for transfusion. The results were recorded on a standardized form (see Box 7.3), which lists all the steps outlined in the nursing, medical staff, and blood bank standard operating procedures. The authors concluded that improvements made over the past several years appear to have been quite effective in preventing mistransfusions and reducing the number of near-miss events.

Box 7.3 LAC + USC Healthcare Network Blood Transfusion Assessment Tool

Blood transfusion process	Not compliant	NA

Informed consent
1 If elective transfusion, was consent to nonsurgical blood transfusion signed?
2 If elective transfusion, did the patient receive Paul Gann Blood Safety Act brochure?

Physician order
3 A written physician order exists.
4 The doctor's order includes blood product name, number of units, and administration rate.

Blood product request (Call Card)
5 Blood Call Card shows patient's name and identification number, blood product ordered, and two signatures verifying the information.

Patient preparation
6 Patient was premedicated if ordered by doctor.
7 Vital signs were checked within 30 min before transfusion.

Blood product issuance
8 Patient name and identification number on call card and Blood Product Record form match.
9 The correct blood product was issued.

Pretransfusion identification checks
10 The patient was wearing an ID band at the start of transfusion.
11 Patient ID was checked at the bedside by matching the patient's statement of his/her own name with the information on ID band.
12 Patient name and identfication number on Blood Product Record form and ID band match.
13 Patient name and identfication number on unit label and ID band match.
14 Unit numbers, blood types, etc., on the unit label match the same items on the Blood Product Record form.
15 Items 10-14 were checked at the bedside by two licensed personnel (RN, LVN, MD).
16 Two licensed personnel (in Item #15) signed the Blood Product Record form.

Blood administering
17 Vital signs were checked within 15 min after start or after 50 cc transfused.
18 Lactated Ringer's solution, 5 percent dextrose, or hypotonic sodium chloride are not added to blood or simultaneously administered via the same IV line.
19 Blood product was transfused at ordered rate.

Posttransfusion checks
20 Vital signs were checked after completion of infusion.
21 All areas were filled out on Blood Product Record form.

Reproduced from Saxena, Ramer, and Shulman[33] with permission from Wiley-Blackwell.

Conclusions

A properly functioning and established hemovigilance surveillance system should have tools to allow the implementation of preventive/corrective actions whenever necessary and demonstrate the correlation between improved reporting and the enhancement of blood transfusion safety. The system should be able to distinguish preventable from nonpreventable errors, because the way of resolving these errors are different. Preventive actions should be undertaken in the case of near-misses, whereas corrective as well as preventive actions should be carried out in the event of transfusion errors. They have to be identified and treated differently from transfusion-related complications.

Setting up a hospital-based hemovigilance program has multiple beneficial effects. These include the potential to educate clinical staff and other healthcare professionals; help ensure compliance with regulatory requirements and accreditation standards; lower costs; reduce the risks of litigation; provide information about hospital and departmental clinical practices; conserve blood; and create, document, sustain, and demonstrate a high quality of care within the institution.

A recent WHO guideline on adverse event reporting and learning systems[34] states that the effectiveness of such a system is measured not only by accurate collection and analysis of data, but also by its use to make recommendations that improve patient safety. The value or efficiency of a hospital-based hemovigilance system can be confirmed if it will result in an immediate and detailed notification of transfusion incidents allowing rapid implementation of corrective and preventive actions.

References

1 Stainsby D, Williamson L, Jones H and Cohen H, 2004, 6 years of SHOT reporting—Its influence on UK blood safety. *Transfus. Apher. Sci.* **31**: 123–31.

2 Reesink HW, Panzer S, Gonzalez CA, Lena N, Muntaabski P, *et al.*, 2010, Haemovigilance for the optimal use of blood products in the hospital. *Vox Sang* **99**(3): 278–93.

3 Murphy L, Anderson N, and Stanworth S, 2009, International comparisons of blood component usage. *NHS Blood and Transplant Blood Matters* **27**: 10–12.

4 Chng WJ, Tan MK, and Kuperan P, 2003, An audit of fresh frozen plasma usage in an acute general hospital in Singapore. *Singapore Med. J.* **44**(11): 574–8.

5 Wan Haslindawani MW, and Wan Zaidah A, 2010, Coagulation parameters as a guide for fresh frozen plasma transfusion practice: A tertiary hospital experience. *Asian J. Transf. Sci.* **4**(1): 25–7.

6 Alcantara RM, San KK, Ng HJ, and Koh M, 2011, Who Gets Cryoprecipitate. *Blood Transfus* **9**(Suppl1), February.

7 EU Optimal Blood Use Project, 2010, Manual of Optimal Blood Use [online]. Available at http://www.optimalblooduse.eu/_assets/pdf/blood_use_manual.pdf [accessed February 24, 2012].

8 British Committee for Standards in Haematology. BCSH guidelines (transfusion) [online]. http://www.bcshguidelines.com/4_HAEMATOLOGY_GUIDELINES.html?dpage=0&dtype=Transfusion&sspage=0&ipage=0 [accessed February 24, 2012].

9 Australia and New Zealand Society of Blood Transfusion. Clinical practice guidelines and other brochures. Available at http://www.anzsbt.org.au/publications/index.cfm [accessed February 24, 2012].

10 WHO Blood Transfusion Safety, 2002, Clinical Use of Blood [online]. http://www.who.int/bloodsafety/clinical_use/en/Handbook_EN.pdf [accessed February 24, 2012].

11 The Association of Anaesthetists of Great Britain and Ireland. Blood Transfusion and the Anaesthetist: Red Cell Transfusion 2 [online]. http://www.aagbi.org/publications/guidelines/docs/red_cell_08.pdf [accessed February 24, 2012].

12 The Society of Thoracic Surgeons Blood Conservation Guideline Task Force. Society of Thoracic Surgeons and The Society of Cardiovascular Anesthesiologists, 2007, Perioperative Blood Transfusion and Blood Conservation in Cardiac Surgery: The Society of Thoracic Surgeons and The Society of Cardiovascular Anesthesiologists Clinical Practice Guidelines. *Ann Thorac Surg* **83**: S27–86.

13 WHO, 2003, The Clinical Use of Blood (Aide-Memoir for National Health Programmes) [online]. Available at http://www.who.int/bloodsafety/clinical_use/en/Aide-Memoire_23.3.04.pdf [accessed February 24, 2012].

14 WHO Blood Safety Unit, 1998, Developing a National Policy and Guidelines on the Clinical Use of Blood [online]. Available at http://www.who.int/bloodsafety/clinical_use/en/WHO_BLS_98.2_EN.pdf [accessed February 24, 2012].

15 Koh BC, Chong LL, Goh LG, Iau P, Kuperan P, *et al.*, 2011, Ministry of Health Clinical Practice Guidelines Workgroup on Clinical Blood Transfusion. *Singapore Med J.* **52**(3): 209–18.

16 McClelland DBL, 2007, *Handbook of Transfusion Medicine*. Fourth edition. HMSO, UK.

17 Association of Anaesthetists of Great Britain and Ireland, 2010, Blood transfusion and the anaesthetist: Management of massive haemorrhage. *Anaesthesia* **65**: 1153–61.

18 Delouphery TG, 2010, Logistics of massive transfusions. *Hematology* 2010: 470–3.

19 Burtelow M, Riley Ed, Druzin M, Fontaine M, Viele M, and Goodnough LT, 2007, How we treat: management of life-threatening primary postpartum hemorrhage

with a standardized massive transfusion protocol. *Transfusion* **47**: 1564–72.

20 Riskin DJ, Tsai TC, Riskin L, Hernandez-Boussard T, Purtill M, Maggio PM *et al.*, 2009, Massive transfusion protocols: the role of aggressive resuscitation versus product ratio in mortality reduction. *J Am Coll Surg* **209**(2): 198–205.

21 Cotton BA, Au BK, Nunez TC, Gunter OL, Robertson AM, and Young PP, 2009, Predefined massive transfusion protocols are associated with a reduction in organ failure and postinjury complications. *J Trauma* **66**(1): 41–8; discussion 48–9.

22 Dente CJ, Shaz BH, Nicholas JM, Harris RS, Wyrzykowski AD, Patel S *et al.*, 2009, Improvements in early mortality and coagulopathy are sustained better in patients with blunt trauma after institution of a massive transfusion protocol in a civilian level I trauma center. *J Trauma* **66**(6): 1616–24.

23 O'Keeffe T, Refaai M, Tchorz K, Forestner JE, and Sarode R, 2008, A massive transfusion protocol to decrease blood component use and costs. *Arch Surg.* **143**(7): 686–90; discussion 690–1.

24 Taylor C (ed.), Cohen H, Mold D, Jones H, *et al.*, on behalf of the Serious Hazards of Transfusion (SHOT) Steering Group, 2010, The 2009 Annual SHOT Report.

25 Royal Children's Hospital Melbourne, Clinical Guidelines for Blood Transfusion Informed consent and consumer information. http://www.rch.org.au/rchcpg/?doc_id=10012 [accessed February 7, 2012].

26 Rock G, Neurath D, Laurin M, Luke B, *et al.*, 2005, Development of a total quality system for Transfusion Medicine services in Ontario hospitals. *Transfusion and Apheresis Science* **33**: 333–42.

27 AABB, 2010, Primer of Blood Administration. Available at www.aabb.org.

28 Stainsby D, Joan Russel J, Hannah Cohen H, and Lilleyman J, 2005, Reducing adverse events in blood transfusion. *British Journal of Haematology* **131**: 8–12.

29 Rock G, Berger R, Filion D, Touche D, *et al.*, 2007, Documenting a transfusion: how well is it done? *Transfusion* **47**: 568–72.

30 Friedman M, and Ebrahim A, 2006, Adequacy of physician documentation of red blood cell transfusion and correlation with assessment of transfusion appropriateness. *Arch Pathol Lab Med* **130**: 474–9.

31 Shulman IA, Lohr K, Derdiarian AK, and Picukaric JM, 1994, Monitoring transfusionist practices: a strategy for improving transfusion safety. *Transfusion* 3411–5.

32 Sazama K, 1990, Reports of 355 transfusion-associated deaths: 1976 through 1985. *Transfusion* **30**: 583–90.

33 Saxena S, Ramer L, and Shulman IA, 2004, A comprehensive assessment program to improve blood-administering practices using the FOCUS–PDCA model. *Transfusion* **44**: 1350–6.

34 WHO, 2005, Draft Guidance on adverse event reporting and learning systems. http://www.who.int/patientsafety/events/05/Reporting_Guidelines.pdf [accessed February 24, 2012].

How the System Works

CHAPTER 8

Blood Donation: An Approach to Donor Vigilance

Peter Tomasulo[1], Madhav Erraguntla[2], and Hany Kamel[1]

[1]Blood Systems, Inc., Scottsdale, AZ, USA
[2]Knowledge Based Systems, Inc., College Station, TX, USA

Introduction

In this chapter we describe and develop the concept of *donor vigilance,* a process designed to improve the safety of blood donation and the satisfaction of the blood donor.[1] Donor vigilance is required as part of the principle of continuous improvement that is in turn part of quality systems. We have chosen to describe features of an ideal system that could be used as a road map for blood systems to design new or improve existing systems. Most current systems do not collect all the data or perform all the analyses described in this chapter, and so by providing some features of an ideal system we hope to help investigators focus on future improvements.

The term hemovigilance was originally developed to describe a continuous improvement program aimed at reducing the adverse events (AEs) associated with blood transfusion. When attempting to reduce the AEs associated with blood donation, we recognize that blood itself does not produce the AE or the threat of the AE. Instead, the risk of AEs for blood donors is associated with the process of blood donation. Therefore we recommend the use of the term *donor* vigilance to emphasize that it is donor safety and not blood (hemo-) safety that is the concern of this vigilance process.

Blood can be collected by two different techniques: Whole blood is collected via gravity drainage; plasma, platelets, red cells, and combinations of these components are collected via apheresis technology. Apheresis and manual whole blood donations take place in donor centers, on buses designed for blood donation, and in buildings with rooms adapted for the purpose of accepting blood donations. The donations take place at all hours of the day and night, though most donations take place during "business" hours.

Although blood donation is currently quite safe and rewarding, the process can be made safer. More than 100,000 times each day individuals all over the world donate blood to save the lives of patients. Moderate and severe vasovagal reactions occur at the rate of ~4/1000 donations (whole blood and apheresis). About 2/1000 donations are associated with loss of consciousness. About 2% of moderate and severe reactions lead to donor injury, and about 8% of donors with moderate or severe reactions require medical care.[2] Overall, needle-related injuries are higher in 2-unit red-cell collections and platelets and/or plasma apheresis collections compared to whole blood collections (2.4, 2.4, and 0.9/1000 donations respectively).[3]

Making improvements in the donation process depends on having data that are analyzed properly to produce evidence that can support hypotheses about cause-and-effect and the design of interventions.[4] Because AEs from blood donation are extremely rare, obtaining large databases is

Hemovigilance: An Effective Tool for Improving Transfusion Safety, First Edition. Edited by René R.P. De Vries and Jean-Claude Faber.
© 2012 John Wiley & Sons, Ltd. Published 2012 by John Wiley & Sons, Ltd.

essential. Very small centers will not have enough data; however, by using common procedures, data aggregation among centers is possible.

Goals of donor vigilance

The specific benefits for donors that can result from donor vigilance need to be specified. In broad terms, the goals of donor vigilance are to reduce AEs and the frequency and severity of the sequelae (donor injury and disability) of those AEs. The five main categories of AEs associated with blood donation (see also Table 8.1) are those associated with

- hypotension;
- physical injuries associated with the venipuncture;
- infusion adverse events;
- allergic reactions;
- iron metabolism.

Table 8.1 Reaction categorization.

Reaction type	Reaction category
Hypotensive	Prefaint, no LOC (uncomplicated or minor)
	LOC, any duration (uncomplicated)
	LOC, any duration (complicated)
	Injury
Local injury related to needle	Nerve irritation
	Hematoma/bruise
	Arterial puncture
	Compartment syndrome
Infusion	Citrate
	Hemolysis
	Air embolus
	Hematoma/bruise
	Allergic
Allergic	Local
	Systemic
	Anaphylaxis
Hemoglobin loss	Anemia
	Iron deficiency

Courtesy of AABB's Donor Hemovigilance Working Group, on behalf of the US Biovigilance Network.

The purpose of a sound donor vigilance program is to put these AEs and sequelae in priority order and reduce the frequency of the most important events first. Reducing even the mildest AEs is in order because mild and severe AEs discourage future blood donation.[5,6] A donor center with a successful vigilance program should expect improved efficiency of the donor recruitment process, increased frequency of donation, faster donor throughput, fewer incomplete donations, and more efficient blood drives/donor clinics. If the frequency of adverse events decreases, for example in secondary schools, the enthusiasm for hosting blood drives might increase and parents may be more enthusiastic supporters of blood donation.

Process cycle

Donor vigilance involves the collection and analysis of information related to donors, donations, and adverse events. Donor vigilance facilitates (i) establishment of baseline adverse event rates, (ii) understanding factors affecting adverse event rates, and (iii) provision of insights about interventions that might improve adverse event rates. An ideal, comprehensive donor vigilance process should facilitate continuous process improvement and include design of interventions and analysis of the effectiveness of these interventions.

The key steps in the donor vigilance process are demonstrated in Figure 8.1 and detailed below.

Gather data

An important requisite for effective donor vigilance is collection and organization of data related to adverse event, donor, donation, and denominator into a central data repository (data warehouse). To be statistically valid and widely applicable, data analysis should be performed on a large dataset spanning a time period long enough to prevent confounding by seasonal impact. Analysis of the effectiveness of interventions involves statistical comparison of baselines or contemporaneous samples with and without interventions.

In the case of a single blood establishment, the data necessary for donor vigilance might be stored

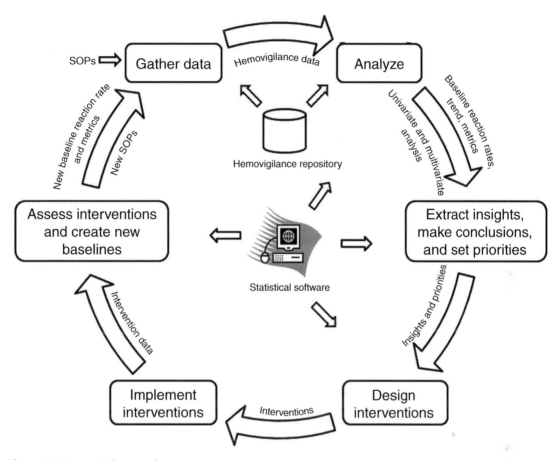

Figure 8.1 Donor vigilance cycle.

in multiple data systems. Adverse event information may be captured on a donor reaction/incident report; donor demographics and biometrics from donor screening may be captured on a donor history or donor questionnaire, and donation details such as donation type and donation technology captured on a blood donation record. In some blood establishments, adverse event information is captured in multiple systems.

A major blood establishment might be organized into a number of geographical regions with independent databases. This could be true for national systems or for very large donor collection operations such as the National Red Cross and Red Crescent Societies. The data management system could be separate for each region or centralized for the entire system. For effective donor vigilance, information from potentially different legacy database systems must be collected, integrated, and organized into a central data repository. The applicability of conclusions or hypotheses based on the analysis of donor vigilance data depends on the validity of the collected data. Thus, data validation and cleaning become integral steps in data collection in donor vigilance.

When the scope of donor vigilance covers a regional, a national, or many national blood programs, data from blood establishments in the covered areas must be similarly collected and housed in the Donor Vigilance System data repository. In cases involving data covering multiple blood establishments, it is important that the blood establishments adopt uniform definitions and classification schemes and use them consistently.

Analyze

Analysis occurs after data validation. The basic analysis involves rate calculations for different adverse event types on subsets of donors and collection procedures. This gives insights into the prevalence of different adverse event rates and serves as a baseline for comparing the adverse event rates of different entities (single or multiple blood establishments), evaluating the effectiveness of interventions, and for trend analysis. Stratified analysis involves collecting denominator data using stratified denominator classes (e.g., male/female, pre-determined age groups, different collection procedure, and so on). Odds ratio are then calculated to analyze how the different denominator dimensions (demographic, donation, anatomic, procedural, devices) affect adverse event rates.

Insights, conclusions, and priorities

Donor vigilance involves extracting insights, drawing conclusions, and setting targets and priorities for continuous process improvement. Comparing the basic adverse event rates of different adverse event types, as well as unadjusted and adjusted odds ratios from univariate and multivariate analysis, can provide insights into sources of risk and identify statistically significant associations. Comparison with literature and peers (blood establishments) can also give valuable insights into the process steps that might increase risk. Trend analysis is useful in identifying patterns over a period of time. It can provide insights into whether the interventions are effective or whether Standard Operating Procedures (SOPs) are being followed. The outputs of this step in donor vigilance should be identification of the metrics that need to be closely monitored and, potentially, improved (by designing and implementing interventions). When associations are identified, it is important to determine sources of systematic and random confounding.

Interventions

A crucial step in donor vigilance involves identification and design of interventions. Based on the priorities identified in the previous step, a set of potential interventions is identified. Brainstorming, root cause analysis (Fishbone/Ishikawa diagrams) may be used to identify the candidate interventions.[7] Consulting with experts and review of literature from different fields are invaluable at this stage. Physiologists, anatomists, neurologists, psychologists, and so on can evaluate data with the donor vigilance team and shed light on the significance of the data and possibly causes of AEs. Each candidate intervention is analyzed for feasibility, cost-benefit, and likelihood of success. Based on the feasibility, cost-benefit, and likelihood of success, a subset of interventions is selected for detailed design and implementation. Detailed design involves the application of design-of-experiment principles to identify the blood collection centers, devices, human resources, or processes that will participate in the intervention. Appropriate design of the implementation ensures that the results of intervention can be extrapolated to the other parts of the organization, region, or nation.[8] Changes to SOPs, training that needs to be performed, and measures of the effectiveness of intervention are identified and detailed in the designing intervention phase.

Implement interventions

The next step in the donor vigilance process involves implementing the identified intervention and collecting data identified for measuring effectiveness.

Assess interventions and create new baselines

In this step, data and rates collected during the post-intervention period are compared with control data. Control data could be historical rates or contemporary data from entities not implementing the intervention. Qualitative and quantitative assessments of the effectiveness of interventions and conclusions about the need for general application of the intervention are made. If an intervention was chosen to be extended, it becomes part of the new baseline for the blood establishment, and the donor vigilance continuous process improvement cycle repeats.

From a donor vigilance perspective, it is important to identify and tag datasets corresponding to different timelines with relevant metadata and identify the interventions and changes in baseline procedures. This will ensure that data from interventions and changes in baseline procedures over time are not confounding factors in the long-term monitoring and analysis of donor vigilance.

Blood donation process

We describe the blood donation process in this section in order to help set the stage for identifying a data gathering strategy. The entire whole blood process (see Figure 8.2) requires approximately 45–60 minutes, but it varies widely among donation sites. Apheresis procedures can last 35–120 minutes depending on the components being collected and the technology used.

The donor arrives at the donation site, is greeted, provided with written or video presentations of educational and informational material about blood donation, registers, answers health-screening questions, has vital signs taken, gives a capillary blood sample (a finger-stick), and signs an informed consent before donation. Principles for donor selection vary; generally, donors are required to be older than a specified age, weigh more than a specified weight, and have a normal pulse rate and blood pressure.[9,10] In some regions, donor vital signs are not taken to determine donor suitability. Donors are almost always questioned to establish whether they are healthy enough to donate blood without experiencing excessive risk and to determine whether the blood they donate is likely to be safe and effective for the recipient. The most significant risks to the donor are related to the donor's iron and blood volume, and to the presence of existing acute or chronic diseases. The risks to the patients concern the possibility of disease, drug, or noxious agent transmission.

The preparation for donation takes about 15 to 20 minutes. Donors sit at each station during this process and they stand and walk between steps. When they are ready for donation, they "sit/lie" on a "chair/bed." The donors' arms are inspected and a vein in the antecubital area is selected. The venipuncture site is cleansed with antiseptic solutions. Single use, sterile collection systems are used. The venipuncture is performed after a few minutes in the chair. Using a large bore (often 16-gauge) needle, the whole blood phlebotomy requires about 8 or 9 minutes (see Table 8.2).[11] Whole blood donation uses gravity drainage, is unidirectional, and leaves the donor relatively hypovolemic. The blood volume collected in each collection set varies from 200 mL per donation to 500 ml, and an additional 25–45 ml is usually collected for donor blood tests. Apheresis donation requires either one or two venipunctures and entails pumping blood from a donor into a separation chamber and separating the blood into the components to be processed for transfusion and those to be returned. When the transfusable component is captured, the remaining blood is returned through the donor's vein. Apheresis can be configured to restore the donor's original blood volume by infusing an electrolyte solution.

After removal of the needle, the subject is asked to apply pressure to the phlebotomy site and then requested to sit with feet hanging over the side of the donation chair/bed for a short period before getting up. Subjects may remain on the chair for 3–5 minutes before standing up. Donors are encouraged to stay seated in the refreshment area for 15 minutes after leaving the donor chair. They are often offered refreshments while seated after donation and usually told to drink fluids after donation and to call the center if they have questions or a reaction. Many donors leave the donation site by 15 minutes after the phlebotomy was terminated.

There are at least three different types of donation settings that collection centers can use. Some preliminary evidence suggests that rates of some reactions vary according to the donation setting or the chair configuration.[2,4]

Fixed donor sites are blood center locations furnished for the sole purpose of blood donation. These sites are operated by donor center staff on a regular schedule, and donors are recruited to these sites by telephone recruitment or other

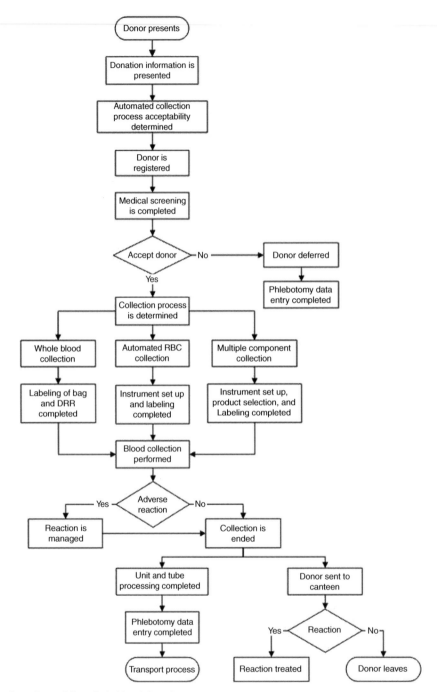

Figure 8.2 Flow chart of the whole blood donation process.

Table 8.2 Summary of donation status and whole blood collection draw time.

	Incomplete			Complete			Complete and incomplete donations		
	Male	Female	All	Male	Female	All	Male	Female	All
Donations	5564	12042	17,606	221,781	315,126	536,907	227,345	327,168	554,513
Percent of category	32%	68%	3%	41%	59%	97%	41%	59%	100%
Mean draw time in minutes (95% CI)	9.21	8.76	8.91	7.62	8.61	8.21	7.66	8.62	8.22
(records with 0–30 minute draw time)	(9.03–9.4)	(8.63–8.89)	(8.8–9.01)	(7.61–7.64)	(8.60–8.63)	(8.2–8.21)	(7.65–7.68)	(8.61–8.63)	(8.22–8.24)
25–75th percentile	3–14	2–14	3–14	6–9	6–10	6–9	6–9	6–10	6–9

mechanisms. Donors can visit these fixed donor sites on their own volition and schedule. *Mobile buses* are large motor coaches outfitted and furnished for the sole purpose of blood donation. They are self-contained vehicles with less open space, and they usually require some nearby facility to provide the donors with a site for refreshments after donation. Mobile donor buses can operate like fixed sites by appearing at the same location every day or every week. These coaches can also be used to accept donations at specially scheduled and sponsored blood drives by a local organization.

Both fixed sites and mobile buses can have substantial donor chairs designed for blood donation. The configuration of most fixed-site and mobile-bus chairs can often be altered by electric motors to raise or lower the donor's head or knees/feet.

There is also another donation site, which we can refer to as an *inside mobile set-up.*

Varying kinds of donor chairs are brought to institutions and organizations hosting blood drives (mobiles or clinics); typically, a folding lounge chair is used. In these chairs, the donors' knees may not be higher than the pelvis and their feet are at the level of or lower than the pelvis. Some blood centers use flat firm beds at inside mobile set-ups. On these beds, the donor lies in a plane and feet, pelvis, heart, and head are at the same level.

Data

Data management

The most intensive step in donor vigilance is data collection and management. Defining the data elements to be captured is critical for success and the growth of the donor vigilance program. At present, understanding of the causes of donor reactions is rudimentary. Therefore, the nature of the influence of donor characteristics, collection technology, donor position during donation, donor eating habits, and so on, on the risk of various kinds of adverse event is not clearly understood. It would be impossible and probably unnecessary to capture every data element associated with blood donation, but nevertheless, the system should be designed with attention to possible areas of future investigation.

At present, most centers do not collect enough information to do the necessary analyses, but data collection and management systems should be designed with the capacity to accept more data and more classes of data than any participant might contribute today. Then, as more is learned about the causes and risks of reactions, data collection can be altered and studies designed and implemented using the newly captured data. The key to current utility is the capacity to accept data for analysis even though the data contributed by any one center might not be "complete" according to the software specification and design.

Donor adverse event information is captured in a Donor Incident form in most organizations. In the future, hand-held devices can efficiently capture this information on-site. Information about the incident needs to be extracted from this (or an equivalent) form and captured in the Donor Vigilance System (database). Information about the donor and donation need to extracted from Donor Screening forms. Additionally, if the donor required outside medical care or suffered long-term sequelae, that information needs to be extracted from corresponding forms and entered into the Donor Vigilance System. Having two subcategories of the adverse event information, one for signs and symptoms and one for sequelae, is very helpful. Finally, the policies and procedures of the organization (amount of blood extracted, donor screening policies, donation conditions, type of devices and containers used, and so on) define the baseline conditions for evaluating the rates, metrics, and interventions. Such data must be extracted in the Donor Vigilance System.

Data processing involves consolidating data from different sources and organizing the data into schema developed for donor vigilance (see Figure 8.3). For example, information about donors from multiple forms must be collected, integrated, and maintained as a single logical entity in donor vigilance. Data validation and cleaning are necessary to ensure data completeness, consistency, and valid-

ity. This will involve using consistent date and time formats, policies for dealing with missing data, and changes to SOPs for collecting new data. Data formatting and transformation involve formatting the data into a standard format defined for the Donor Vigilance System. This step also involves capturing the denominator data, whether that refers to total number of donations or stratified denominator.

The information in the Donor Vigilance System can be logically organized into donor, donation, adverse event, and denominator tables. Each donor record can have multiple associated donation records, and each donation record can have multiple associated adverse event records. This schema allows the capturing and analyzing of longitudinal donor data. Finally, the donor vigilance database should have tables for capturing the manufacturing specifications and background conditions in the organization. When the data are collected, consolidated, validated, transformed, and organized in the donor vigilance database, they can then be exploited to create baseline rates and metrics, routine and special reports, and univariate and multivariate analyses.

In a regional or national context, the data management process is similar, but the emphasis is on different sets of issues. Figure 8.4 shows the data management flow in regional and national level donor vigilance. In the regional/national context, the users are geographically distributed, and so the donor system must be web based. Data are collected from the donor vigilance systems of individual organizations, regions, or associations. In this

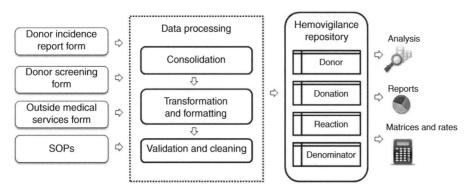

Figure 8.3 Data management flow at organization level.

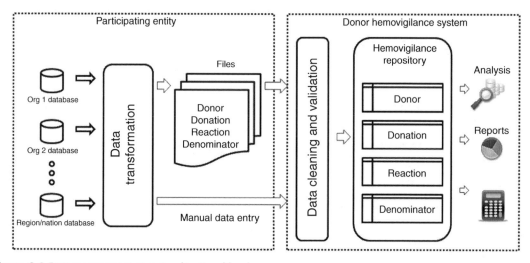

Figure 8.4 Data management at regional/national level.

context, duplicate data entry validation becomes very important: The same data might be reported by an individual organization multiple times or through different trade associations. Data can be input into the system manually or using files of a pre-defined format.

In the multi-site or multi-organization situation, it is very important that the blood establishments adopt consistent and uniform definitions and reaction classification schemes. Standards development from international organizations such as ISBT will

help move towards this goal of standardization. Sample donor complication codes developed by ISBT are shown in Table 8.3.[12]

Comparison of donor vigilance data and evaluation of the impact of interventions across system borders requires the agreement on definitions and data elements to be captured. Although most organizations realize the value of using consistent definitions and standards for rigorous analysis and comparison, consistency has not yet been achieved. The development of lists of data elements to be

Table 8.3 Sample of donor complication codes developed by ISBT.

120	Nerve injuries			
121	Injury of a nerve	Direct nerve injury by the needle	Severe, *immediate* pain when the needle was inserted, which radiates down the forearm; often associated with paresthesia	**Mild** Symptoms <2 weeks **Moderate** Symptoms >2 weeks but <1 year **Severe** Symptoms >1 year *or* required medical treatment
122	Injury of a nerve by hematoma	Neurological symptoms caused by pressure from a hematoma	Pain and paresthesia as in code 121, but symptoms develop sometime *after* the needle was inserted	**Mild** Symptoms <2 weeks **Moderate** Symptoms >2 weeks but <1 year **Severe** Symptoms >1 year *or* required medical treatment

captured and definitions of those elements has progressed in multiple locations around the globe, almost simultaneously, and significant differences in approach are present. It may be possible to adapt to these differences and produce good comparisons, but it may be necessary for some systems to make minor changes in their current plans if international collaboration is to take place.

There are genuine technical concerns and differences in relation to current donor adverse event codes. One large national program, the US Donor Hemovigilance System, developed its strategy and based the data capture process on identifying and describing the signs and symptoms (loss of consciousness, loss of bladder, bowel control, tetany, and so on) and the time of the adverse reaction in relation to the phlebotomy and duration of the reaction (loss of consciousness duration, time-to-discharge).[13] The data are captured at the fundamental element level, without being classified into arbitrary and potentially evolving classifications such as "mild, moderate, severe." Other organizations have attempted to develop specific definitions of categories in an effort to keep the system simple and manageable. This latter effort, although having the advantage of simplicity and far fewer data elements to capture, has issues that have to be resolved for international collaboration. For example, the definitions may be too narrow and thus prevent the capture of variations in duration of injury/disability. If the definitions don't recognize that the sequelae of AEs are not consistently linked to one of the classifications, then significant detail will be missed and variations in the events included in each category will result.

Consistent application of the terms "mild," "moderate," and "severe" comes into question. Adverse reactions could be quite serious even if they last only a short time. A mild reaction might be associated with a delayed cardiac event. In addition, it is possible that reactions that occur at different times during the donation process have different causes or different predictors.[14] If the vigilance system does not capture data concerning the time of the reaction during the donation process, this fact could be missed and an opportunity to improve the donor's experience also missed. By capturing the signs and symptoms of the adverse reactions as well as the details of the timing and location of the reactions, it is possible to map reactions to any simple set of classifications. In addition, as more is learned about cause-and-effect, classifications can be changed to reflect the new knowledge. Such improvements are much more difficult if one does not emphasize the data at the element level.

Mapping is necessary in the short term until the international community adopts international standards. Data interchange might be possible only from a system that captures signs and symptoms to a system with a "mild, moderate, severe" classification. If the signs and symptoms are not captured, it may not be possible to interchange information with a more detailed schema. Data mapping, transformation, and formatting are important harmonization issues that need to be addressed in multisite donor vigilance analyses.

Data validation

Ensuring the integrity and accuracy of data is a very important step in donor vigilance, especially if the data are collected from multiple collection organizations. Adequate checks need to be implemented during the data entry stage to ensure that the data being entered are complete, consistent, and accurate. Data cleaning rules should be established in advance. For example, if the data issue is serious, the entire record might need to be ignored ("Errors"); however, if the data issue is not significant and does not bias the donor vigilance data analysis ("Warnings"), the record can be captured and the issue highlighted for resolution at a later date. Table 8.4 shows sample data validations adopted by the US Donor Hemovigilance System.[15]

Denominators

In addition to capturing information about adverse events, a Donor Vigilance System needs to house information about denominators in order to calculate adverse event rates. The definition of a donation must be established. Is it the number of procedures yielding a product, venipunctures, or donor registrations? The US Donor Hemovigilance System uses the number of complete

Table 8.4 Sample data validation rules (as adopted by the US Donor Hemovigilance System[15].)

Data	Error	Warning
Required fields should be entered. Required fields are Donor ID, Donor DOB, and Sex for donor, Donation ID and Donation Date for donation, and Reaction Type and Category for a reaction	Yes	—
Dates cannot be future dates	For donor date of birth, donation date, and reaction date	Date of platelet count, protein count, and date of resolution of prolonged reaction
Reaction date >= donation date	Yes	—
If the user chooses "First Time" donor, the "number of donation in last year" should be zero	Yes	—
All numeric fields are non-negative.	Yes	—
Date of resolution of prolonged reaction >= reaction date	Yes	—
Highest pulse (pressure) >= Lowest pulse (pressure)	Yes	—
Donation Date > Date of birth	Yes	—
Donor height is in the range (48–84 inches); that is, (4–7 feet)	—	Yes
Donor weight is in the range (100–350 lbs)	—	Yes
If "Resolution of acute reaction" = "Released to outside medical care" then "Outside medical care" should have something other than "None" selected	Yes	—
In "Reaction Type" = "Infusion" the Intended Procedure Type should be "Apheresis"	Yes	—
Feasible values for pulse (20–200)?	Yes	—
Feasible range for BP (50–200)?	Yes	—
"Time needle inserted" <= "Time needle withdrawn"	Yes	—

and incomplete donations as the denominator. Basic adverse event rates can be calculated using aggregate denominator data. More comprehensive analysis can be performed using a stratified (or subset) denominator. Analysis with a stratified denominator involves collecting denominator data using pre-determined denominator classes (e.g., male and female, pre-determined age groups, and so on). Table 8.5 shows the denominator stratification used by the US Donor Hemovigilance System. Using a stratified denominator is a starting point, but in the future the system will have a complete denominator database with information on every donation event.

The advantage of the stratified denominator approach is that it allows for the analysis of factors influencing adverse events while limiting the denominator data collected and managed. However, it only allows for analyzing the effect of each factor independently. If the relative risk and the interaction effect of different factors need to be considered, multivariate analysis must be performed.

Performing multivariate analysis requires the collection of information on every donation. This is important because, although multivariate analysis can result in more accurate analysis, the approach necessarily involves the collection and management of large volumes of donor vigilance data. For example, roughly 14 million donations are collected in the USA. annually. The pressure for complete denominator data comes from the fact that adverse events are multifactorial and there is a need to consider the impact of one item on the outcome in relation to the remaining significant items. This kind of analysis is necessary in every donor vigilance analysis. If the system only has categorized denominator data, that is, the entire denominator dataset is not available, it may be

Table 8.5 US Donor Hemovigilance System denominator stratification.

Dimension name	Dimension class name	Dimension name	Dimension class name
Age (years)	1. 16–18		9. Apheresis stem cells
	2. 19–22		10. Sample only
	3. 23–29		11. Whole blood
	4. 30–39		12. Apheresis red cells
	5. 40–49	**Height (inches) (self**	1. <60
	6. 50–59	reported or	2. 60–63
	7. 60–69	measured)	3. 64–67
	8. 70–79		4. 68–72
	9. >80		5. >72
Pre-donation	1. BP <60	**Race (appropriate**	1. African American or Black
diastolic blood	2. BP 60–90	for country using	2. Asian
pressure (mm Hg)	3. BP >90	system;	3. American Indian/Alaska
Collection site	1. Mobile donor coach	international	Native
	2. Fixed site	consensus	4. Native Hawaiian/Other Pacific
	3. Mobile inside set-up	probably	Islander
Donation history	1. First	necessary)	5. White
	2. Repeat	**Sponsor group type**	1. College
Donation type	1. Allogeneic		2. High school
	2. Autologous		3. Military
	3. Directed		4. Work place
	4. Source plasma		5. Other
	5. Therapeutic		6. N/A
	6. Other	**Weight (pounds)**	1. <110
Ethnicity	1. Hispanic or Latino	**(self-reported or**	2. 110–119
	2. Not Hispanic or Latino	measured)	3. 120–129
			4. 130–139
Gender	1. Female		5. 140–149
	2. Male		6. 150–159
Procedure type	1. Apheresis double red cells		7. 160–169
	2. Apheresis leukocytes		8. 170–179
	3. Apheresis plasma		9. 180–189
	4. Apheresis platelets		10. 190–199
	5. Apheresis platelets and		11. 200–224
	plasma		12. 225–249
	6. Apheresis platelets and		13. 250–274
	red cells		14. 275–299
	7. Apheresis platelet plasma		15. >300
	red cells	**Total**	1. Total donations
	8. Apheresis plasma red cells		

Courtesy of AABB's Donor Hemovigilance Working Group, on behalf of the US Biovigilance Network

possible to perform these multivariate analyses by selecting one sample from within the population. Gathering complete denominator data on this sample will permit the necessary multivariate analyses when a specific question is being asked.

Analysis and reporting

There are two major outputs desired from donor vigilance programs. The main reason to collect and analyze donor vigilance data is to design interven-

Table 8.6 Sample high level annual report.

| | Whole blood donations | | | | | Apheresis donations | | | | |
| | Donations # | Venipuncture injuries | | Hypotensive reactions | | Donations # | Venipuncture injuries | | Hypotensive reactions | |
		#	Rate	#	Rate		#	Rate	#	Rate
Total										
Male										
Female										
First time donors										
Repeat donors										
African American or Black										
Asian										
American Indian/Alaska Native										
Native Hawaiian/Other Pacific Islander										
White										
16–19 years old										
20–23 years old										
24–65 years old										
>65 years old										
EBV <3500 mL										
EBV 3501–4000 mL										
EBV 4001–5000 mL										
EBV >5000 mL										

tions to reduce donor adverse events and continuously improve the donors' safety and satisfaction. To accomplish this objective, a robust set of analyses must be performed routinely with the goal of implementing interventions. The other reason for donor vigilance is to report the state of the operation. Just as a blood program should report the number of components collected and issued, the donor vigilance program should issue periodic high level reports (see Table 8.6). Total adverse event rates are to be reported by type periodically (annually, at minimum) to detect trends, whether positive or negative. For example, the report might include the rate/1000 donations of (i) hematomas, (ii) paresthesias, (iii) dysesthesia, (iv) compartment syndrome, (v) neurologic issues, (vi) vasovagal syncopal reaction, (vii) prefaint syndrome, (viii) tetany, (ix) incontinence, (x) donor injury requir-

ing outside medical care or with other sequelae such as disability, and so on.

In addition to these total rates, which are useful in detecting trends, analysis of the total donor database (the denominator) must also be performed on the same schedule because changes in donor demographics or biometrics can lead to changes in the adverse event rates. Research has shown that the following groups have different reaction rates: women and men; first-time donors and repeat donors; different race/ethnicity categories; and donors with different blood volumes. The annual analysis of the gender, age, race, and donation history distribution of the donation database has to be considered when assessing the total annual reaction rates. The reports should be prepared in a fashion that permits the lay public to read and understand them. These reports will inform donors, donor group sponsors, and the health system that the donor program is concerned about the safety of donation and working to make improvements on a regular basis.

A fundamental and very useful metric in donor vigilance is the adverse event rate. However, reporting global adverse event rates is meaningless in determining cause-and-effect relationships and designing interventions. To gain insights that might lead to successful interventions to reduce adverse event rates, stratified and subset analyses are essential.

Stratified analysis involves collecting denominator data using stratified denominator classes (e.g., male and female, pre-determined age groups, pre-determined estimated blood volume groups, and so on). Adverse event rates and odds ratios are then calculated to analyze how the different denominator dimensions affect adverse event rates. This approach is adopted by the US Donor Hemovigilance System.[15] Stratified analysis allows for analysis of adverse event rates based on identified layers of the denominator and keeps the denominator data collected to a subset of all denominator data. Using the selected denominator and details about the number of different adverse events (numerator), the rates of different adverse events can be calculated. These adverse event rates serve as a fundamental baseline metric in donor vigilance and measure the prevalence of different donor adverse events.

Trend analysis of this metric can also be performed by comparing the changes of adverse event rates over time. Event rates by gender, age group, estimated blood volume, donation history, arm in which venipuncture was performed, anatomic location of vein used for phlebotomy, and so on must be reported and analyzed. Manual whole blood donation has a different rate of venipuncture injury and of hypotensive reactions from apheresis donation. Two-unit red cell apheresis donations have different adverse event rates from apheresis platelet and apheresis multi-component donations.[2,3]

It is useful to report rates for each collection technology and stratify them within the technology. There may be different adverse event rates for the various apheresis devices, even when they are used to collect the same components, because these devices use different anticoagulant solutions, different separation technologies, different pump speeds, and possibly different needle manufacturers. In addition, the location of the donor collection activity may have an impact on the adverse event rates. A crowded motor coach may make it difficult to perform venipunctures in some circumstances. The bed configurations may influence the rate of hypotensive reactions through the positional impact of the bed shape on the donor's blood volume during blood donation. If donors lie completely flat on their backs, the hydrostatic pressure in the legs that is present when donors are upright disappears. The assumption of a completely flat position leads to an accumulation of intravascular fluid as the hydrostatic pressure in the legs decreases, and it may initiate diuresis. It is possible that analyzing the impact of donor position during donation on faint and prefaint rate will produce useful information. Also useful is to document whether the location of blood donation clinics (fixed sites, mobile donation buses, or inside mobile set-ups) influences reaction rates.

As donor vigilance activities grow, the list of factors to consider will undoubtedly grow as well. Does donor hemoglobin/hematocrit influence rates of needle injuries or hypotensive reactions? Does elevation above sea level, the relative humidity of the donation site, the donor dietary salt intake, or the time since the last meal influence donor-complication rates?

Although important and a fundamental requirement of a donor vigilance program, stratified adverse event rates by themselves are not enough to support the broader goal of intervention identification and design. For this multivariate analysis is required. Comprehensive *multivariate analysis* requires collecting data about every donation and developing a multivariate model to account for the interaction effects of different variables. A stepwise logistic regression model is often used to perform multivariate analysis in donor vigilance and can provide adjusted odds ratios and the relative importance of different factors.[2,4,14] Based on the goals of the donor vigilance program, data capture and analysis requirements need to be carefully identified.

An example to illustrate may be useful. In general, one starts with a process to determine which complications are most important and then designs analyses to understand when the important complications occur, to whom they occur, and, to the degree possible, why they occur. One important complication of blood donation is disability related to needle injuries. Research on mechanisms to reduce needle-induced injury has not been published sufficiently to generate interventions and continuous improvement programs. There are many factors that could influence the rates of needle injuries and data must be gathered to determine which are strongly associated. Could a multivariate model be constructed to determine the factors that affect the venipuncture-related disability rate? For apheresis donation, one would have to add such factors as whether the procedure was a 1-arm or a 2-arm procedure; the speed of withdrawal; the speed of return; whether the venipuncture was for withdrawal of blood, the return of components, or

for both; the anticoagulant solution; the manufacturer of the apheresis device; and so on. One cannot study all factors at once, and so there must be a process to establish priorities for analysis and the statistical tools used need to be appropriate for the desired results.

The fact that it is impossible to know nerve locations may lead some people to consider nerve injuries and pain at the venipuncture site unavoidable; but, without study, such a conclusion is premature. In order to implement an intervention to reduce this kind of injury, one would have to gather basic data. In which donors, during what kind of collection procedure, with what needle manufacturer is this complication common? Are these injuries common with a specific anatomic location for venipuncture? Calculating stratified rates and then creating a multivariable model with a logical set of risk factors considered in a stepwise fashion might allow one to determine the most important risk factors for this kind of complication.

The basic information to begin a focused analysis of needle injuries might be contained, for example, in a table such as the one shown in Table 8.7.

Table 8.7 Sample stratified table of needle-related injury: Collection type and the technology used for collections.

	Manufacturer	Procedures #	Hematomas Total #	Hematomas Rate/1000	Dysesthesia/ Paresthesia Total #	Dysesthesia/ Paresthesia Rate/1000	Disability cases from needle injury Total #	Disability cases from needle injury Rate/1000
Whole blood	A							
	B							
2 unit red cell	A							
	B							
Platelet	A							
	B							
	C							
Platelet + Plasma	A							
	B							
	C							
Plasma	A							
	B							
	C							
Multi-component	A							
	B							
	C							

Here the two key variables we are considering are the collection type and the technology used for collections. Knowing the number of procedures of each collection type and the technology used for those collections will provide the basic denominator information needed to calculate aggregate rates. Recording the rates of hematomas, long-term pain, paresthesia, and disability cases will give some clue about in which area an intervention might yield a positive result. Although whole blood donations may not have a high rate of complication, the fact that there are so many whole blood donations compared to apheresis donations may lead to the decision to reduce needle injuries from whole blood donation as the highest priority.

If after filling out and reviewing Table 8.7 the decision is made to further analyze whole blood donation complications, one might gather data for Table 8.8. (This is only one example; other variables could be pursued.) This table focuses on the anatomy of the arm in which the venipuncture is performed. It is assumed that the donor center involved divides the antecubital fossa into six areas, and the phlebotomy technologist indicates in which of these areas the venipuncture is performed. Filling out Table 8.8 will determine whether there is an arm or an anatomic location that has a significantly higher rate of complication than the others. This would be a clue about possible interventions for reducing donor complications.

These variables do not of course exhaust the possible risk factors for needle injuries. Could the handedness of the donor and the phlebotomy technologist be related to the risk of needle injuries and disability? Finally, there are more donor factors than the anatomic location of the venipuncture that might influence the likelihood of injury. The donor's body habitus (BMI?), age, gender, donation history (first time or repeat), may be factors. When the strength of the risk factors is understood, it becomes possible to make theories about cause-and-effect and to design interventions.

Donating red cells leads to the loss of iron. The frequency of blood donation is generally specified by voluntary standard-setting bodies, the health system, or government regulations. The permitted donation volume and frequency is not the same in every country. It has recently been observed that frequent whole blood and red cell donors have a high prevalence of iron deficiency. Ferritin levels decrease with increasing donation frequency. This decrease is more marked in men. Donation intensity, gender, weight, and age are important independent predictors of absent iron stores and iron deficient erythropoiesis.[16]

It is possible that apheresis donors experience a similar depletion of iron stores over time. Apheresis platelet and multi-component donors do not lose as much iron at one time but they donate more frequently. Because it is becoming clear that iron depletion is a complication of blood donation, donor vigilance programs must develop monitoring systems to ensure that donor iron metabolism is well-understood. Do donors with low estimated blood volume or with low body surface area have a greater risk of becoming iron deficient simply because they are smaller and have less iron? Are there ethnic factors that increase risk or provide protection? Is there a combination of diet and body habitus that protects from an impact on iron metabolism? Intervention options include dietary advice, pharmacologic intervention, changes in donation volumes, and changes in donation frequency, and so on. Data must be gathered to determine which kind of intervention is the most feasible and effective.

Publication

The detailed analyses performed by the donor center teams as part of the donor vigilance program should not only produce reports that are useful for generating theories about cause-and-effect and designing interventions, but also reports acceptable for publication in peer-reviewed literature. Pursuing the rigor that is necessary for publication in refereed journals is necessary for the analysis and will serve donor vigilance well. Publication will generate interest in donor vigilance and will create the capacity for programs to begin comparing data and practices. This will, in general, accelerate the efforts to improve the donor experience.

Table 8.8 Sample template of anatomy of arm analysis.

Donation type	Venipuncture arm	Anatomic location	Manufacturer	# Procedures	Hematoma		Dysesthesia/ Paresthesia		Disability cases from needle injury	
					Total #	Rate/1000	Total #	Rate/1000	Total #	Rate/1000
Manual whole blood	Right arm	1	A							
			B							
		2	A							
			B							
		3	A							
			B							
		4	A							
			B							
		5	A							
			B							
		6	A							
			B							
	Left arm	1	A							
			B							
		2	A							
			B							
		3	A							
			B							
		4	A							
			B							
		5	A							
			B							
		6	A							
			B							

Design interventions

Traffic lights and speeding cameras are two interventions introduced to reduce motor vehicle accidents. Although traffic lights have gained universal acceptance, controversy on the value of traffic speed cameras continues. Automobile accident rates rise and fall for many disparate reasons and data are not clear concerning a cause-and-effect relationship between cameras and accident rates. Unfortunately, with these two interventions in place, vehicular accidents including fatalities still occur every day.

Interventions to reduce AEs in blood transfusion recipients date back years and continue to be introduced: blood typing and crossmatching to component irradiation; leukocyte reduction; bacterial screening of platelet component; selective collection of plasma containing components from male donors to reduce the risk of Transfusion Related Acute Lung Injury (TRALI); and the sequential introduction of progressively more sensitive screening tests for transfusion transmitted pathogens. Few proposed interventions were universally accepted when first implemented, and some may remain controversial (e.g., pathogen reduction and screening for *T. cruzi* antibodies). Unfortunately, adverse reactions to transfusions continue to occur.

Over the years, interventions have also been introduced to protect donors including setting criteria for age, weight, percent blood volume removed per donation, hemoglobin level, pulse rate, and systolic and diastolic blood pressure. These criteria are not globally in place and the value of some is still in debate (e.g., pre-donation pulse rate and blood pressure).[9,10]

Adverse reactions to blood donations are broadly classified into five reaction types (see the earlier Table 8.1). Each reaction type encompasses additional reaction categories.

Blood collection facilities have implemented measures to minimize donor adverse reactions. For example, to protect against the development of iron deficiency, criteria for qualifying a donor are set for a minimum hemoglobin level, interdonation interval, and number of donations permitted per year. In addition, donors are informed of the importance of consuming iron-rich food, and some blood centers have implemented iron replacement programs for donors.[17] In order to reduce needle-related injury, training that covers vein selection based on visual inspection and palpation, application of a tourniquet, fist pumping, needle alignment at time of venisection, and so on have been implemented but no data are available to document a benefit from these interventions. The distribution of cutaneous veins and nerves in the cubital fossa widely varies, and no single area can be considered as suitable for all individuals. Phlebotomists should be aware of areas to avoid and areas least likely to cause nerve damage.[18,19] Citrate toxicity, a common reaction category during apheresis collections, is treated by slowing the rate of blood flow with or without calcium replacement. Intravenous administration of calcium is seldom needed in routine apheresis collections. The long-term effect of apheresis on calcium homeostasis is an area of concern and should be included in donor vigilance studies.[20]

Although syncope in blood donors has been studied since the early 1940s,[21–24] an intervention to eliminate fainting during and after blood donation remains elusive. Interventions to reduce AEs are best considered as corrective action plans. Root cause investigation and understanding of conditions potentially producing an AE should be achieved before designing an intervention. Multidisciplinary approaches, including seeking professionals in other fields, may improve the design of the intervention. Over the past seven decades, many investigators considered and identified, with some inconsistencies, a multitude of factors thought to be predictors of vasovagal reaction in blood donors (see Table 8.9).[2,4,14,21–33] Until recently a lack of consistent classification and varying study design prevented the ranking of these factors according to their importance in predicting reactions.[2,4] It is hoped that the advent of donor vigilance may speed the development of evidence-based interventions that are broadly applicable at blood programs.

Here we provide a review of the recent published literature, which reveals information about

Table 8.9 Variables studied in relation to vasovagal reactions in blood donors.

Age
Sex
Weight and body build
Blood volume
Number of donations
Race/Ethnicity
Blood pressure
Pulse
Amount of blood taken
Rate of taking blood
Nervousness/Apprehension
Anemia
Body form
Poor fluid reserve
Time from last meal
Food, rest, and sleep
Fatigue
Caffeine intake
Occupation
Time of day
Heat and humidity
History of fainting
Point of reaction
Donation site
Sponsoring group
Phlebotomist interpersonal skill

---

past and future approaches to intervention design. Strategies include one or more of the following components:

- educational/informational material to donors and others;
- limit on percent of donor blood volume donated;
- practice of applied muscle tensing during and after donation;
- restoration of plasma volume;
- post-donation observation;
- post-donation instructions.

Education/Information

Informational materials that address common donor fears and provide useful coping suggestions may result in significant improvements in attitude, anxiety, self-efficacy, and donation intention, thus improving donor satisfaction.[34]

Limit on volume of blood collected

The amount of blood collected should not exceed the limits set locally for the percent of a donor's blood volume that can be collected. The need for such a standard is based on observations made by physiologists dating back to 1941 and on more recent tilt table studies of fainting.[35] Phlebotomized or tilt-table volunteers consistently became symptomatic when cardiac filling was affected by blood loss or pooling in the lower extremities.

Muscle tensing exercises (applied muscle tensing, physical counter-pressure maneuvers)

Physical counter-pressure maneuvers are effective almost instantly and have been shown to improve dramatically the quality of life for patients with dysautonomia. The mechanism underlying the effectiveness of these maneuvers is a contraction of the skeletal muscles in the legs, buttocks, pelvic region, and abdominal wall, which squeezes the veins in these regions and pumps a bolus of blood into the thorax, producing an increase in central blood volume and an increase in cardiac filling pressures. This increases stroke volume, cardiac output, and perfusion of the brain. These maneuvers are useful in preventing most kinds of fainting whether related to blood donation, post-exercise state, orthostatic changes, and so on.

Restoration of plasma volume

Research has shown that the percentage of blood volume removed is the strongest predictor of delayed reactions that might lead to injury. It is logical that rapid restoration of blood volume, especially in physically small donors, may reduce risk of injury. It is known from clinical and physiologic studies that dietary intake of salt influences blood volume.[36] A future intervention might involve pre- and post-donation salt and fluid intake. Ideally, plasma volume restoration should start during donation.

Reducing needle-related injuries

The literature does not direct the implementation of any interventions for reducing needle injuries as yet. Only a few studies have been done to discover predictors or strong associations with needle injuries,[3] More studies need to be done before anything more specific than general training can be instituted.

One should not have to justify measures to reduce AEs, because a volunteer donor, who is donating blood freely, is entitled, at a minimum, to a pleasant experience. Donor safety is a component of donor vigilance, critical for maintaining an adequate blood supply and an ethical duty of blood collectors. The sequelae of donors' adverse events make interventions a sensible approach. AEs reduce the likelihood of future donations by the reacting donors. Delayed and off-site adverse reactions lead to potentially preventable morbidity.

Interventions may be considered for all or specific subsets of donors or donations. Alternatively, interventions may be targeted to reduce reactions associated with increased morbidity, that is, reactions with complications or delayed/off-site reactions. AEs, mild or severe, reduce the likelihood of future donations and return rates worsen with increased reaction severity.[5,6] Delayed and off-site reactions lead to increased morbidity with associated cost for outside medical care.[2] Each blood program, after thorough review of its donor population characteristics, blood and blood components collection standards, and its data on donors' adverse reactions, should tailor its own intervention priority. In making such determination, one should consider morbidity, donor loss, and cost.

Interventions should be evidence-based. When a measure has been shown to benefit non-donors and the mechanism by which the benefit is achieved is reasonably understood, one should consider the introduction of such measures to the donor population. Recently, physical counter maneuvers were successfully introduced to blood donors after demonstration of their effectiveness in preventing and aborting syncope in patients with dysautonomia and other orthostatic fainting disorders.[37–40] Similarly, a trial of prompt plasma volume restoration by providing the donor with sodium and fluid should be considered. Such protocols were shown to be effective in dysautonomic patients, athletes, and astronauts.[41]

Implement intervention

In order to implement the intervention strategy successfully, it is necessary to develop clear and detailed SOPs, task training, and educational materials.[1] The policy, its purpose, and its rationale should be shared with staff, donors, and sponsoring organizations. The goals of an intervention implementation are a reduction in adverse reactions through consistent application according to SOPs and the capacity to assess the effectiveness of the intervention. Compliance is enhanced by: (i) the commitment of the organization to the program; (ii) the supervisory staff's observing and coaching of staff and donors; and (iii) the facility's quality program as reflected in their internal audits, deviation management, and continuous improvement components.

Assessment of the effectiveness of intervention and creating new baselines are the heart of the donor vigilance program. This will be achieved by re-entering the process cycle described above: rigorous data gathering; analysis and reporting; extracting insights; and making conclusions. At this time, one should determine whether to keep, alter, discontinue, and/or design alternate interventions as well as whether to set new priorities.

Simple monitoring and measuring changes in rates of AEs before and after implementation of an intervention or a set of interventions may not be sufficient. Known and unknown factors are bound to confound the analysis. When an intervention of more than one component is introduced, determining the effectiveness of each component is rather complicated.[1] Randomized controlled trials are difficult in the highly regulated setting of blood donation: randomization and blinding are difficult to establish. To minimize known confounders, stratified and subset analyses and multivariable regression analyses are required.

Summary

Adverse events from blood donation are rare, but they can lead to morbidity and serious disability and they disrupt donor clinics. Donors deserve the benefits of an aggressive, continuous improvement program. Donor vigilance is effective when data are gathered using consistent definitions and shared so that the databases analyzed are sufficiently large to make conclusions. Because AEs are rare and because there are multiple contributing features, the study of donor AEs requires comprehensive and rigorous data analysis. By focusing on those AEs that lead to disabilities, it will be possible continuously to implement interventions and improve safety and satisfaction for blood donors.

References

1 Tomasulo P, Kamel H, Bravo M, James RC, and Custer B., 2011, Interventions to reduce the vasovagal reaction rate in young whole blood donors. *Transfusion* **51**: 1511–21.

2 Kamel H, Tomasulo P, Bravo M, Wiltbank T, Cusick *et al.*, 2010, Delayed adverse reactions to blood donation. *Transfusion* **50**: 556–65.

3 Custer B, Bravo M, James RC, Cusick RM, Tomasulo P, and Kamel H, 2009, Associations between collection procedure type and donor adverse events. *Transfusion* **49**(3S): 52A.

4 Wiltbank TB, Giordano GF, Kamel H, Tomasulo P, and Custer B, 2008, Faint and prefaint reactions in whole blood donors: an analysis of predonation measurements and their predictive value. *Transfusion* **48**: 1799–1808.

5 France CR, France JL, Roussos M, and Ditto B, 2004, Mild reactions to blood donation predict a decreased likelihood of donor return. *Transfus Apher Sci* **30**: 17–22.

6 Eder AF, Hillyer CD, Dy BA, Notary EP, and Benjamin RJ, 2008, Adverse reactions to allogeneic whole blood donation by 16- and 17-years olds. *JAMA* **299**: 2279–86.

7 Ishikawa, K (translator: J.H. Loftus), 1990, *Introduction to Quality Control*. 3A Corporation, Tokyo.

8 Ghosh S, and Rao CR (eds), 1996, *Design and Analysis of Experiments. Handbook of Statistics 13.* North-Holland.

9 Eder A, Goldman M, Rossmann S, Waxman D, and Bianco C, 2009, Selection criteria to protect the blood donor in North America and Europe: Past (dogma), present (evidence), and future (hemovigilance). *Transfus Med Rev* **23**(3): 205–20.

10 Karp JK, and, King KE, 2010, International variation in volunteer whole blood donor eligibility criteria. *Transfusion* **50**(2): 507–13.

11 Tomasulo P, Bravo M, and Kamel H, 2010, Time course of vasovagal syncope with whole blood donation. *ISBT Science Series* **5**: 52–8.

12 ISBT, 2008, Standard for Surveillance of Complications Related to Blood Donation. http://www.isbtweb .org/fileadmin/user_upload/WP_on_Haemovigilance/ ISBTt_StandardSurveillanceDOCO_2008_3_.pdf [accessed February 10, 2012]

13 AABB, 2010, Donor Hemovigilance System User Manual. http://www.aabb.org/programs/biovigilance/ us/Documents/biovigilancemanual.pdf [accessed February 10, 2012]

14 Bravo M, Kamel H, Custer B, and Tomasulo P, 2011, Factors associated with fainting – before, during and after whole blood donation: Predictors of fainting across time course of blood donation. In preparation. *Vox Sang* **101**: 303–312.

15 KBSI, 2010, Whitepaper on US Donor Hemovigilance System, Knowledge Based Systems Inc. http://www .kbsi.com/COTS/DonorHemovigilance.htm [accessed February 10, 2012]

16 Cable RG, Steele WR, Wright DJ, Glynn SA, Kiss JE, *et al.*, 2010, Predicting hemoglobin deferral in blood donors: A multicenter prospective study. *Transfusion* **50**(2S): 44A–45A.

17 Gordeuk VR, Brittenham GM, Hughes MA, and Keating LJ, 1987, Carbonyl iron for short-term supplementation in female blood donors. *Transfusion* **27**(1): 80–5.

18 Rayegani SM, and Azadi A, 2007, Lateral antebrachial cutaneous nerve injury induced by phlebotomy. *Journal of Brachial Plexus and Peripheral Nerve Injury* **2**: 6.

19 Yamada K, Yamada K, Katsuda T, and Hida T, 2008, Cubital fossa venipuncture sites based on anatomical variations and relationships of cutaneous veins and nerves. *Clin. Anat.* **21**: 307–13.

20 Bolan CD, Cecco SA, Yau YY, Wesley RA, Oblitas JM *et al.*, 2003, Randomized placebo-controlled study of oral calcium carbonate supplementation in plateletpheresis: II. Metabolic effects. *Transfusion* **43**: 1414–22.

21 Poles FC, and Boycott M, 1942, Syncope in blood donors. *Lancet* **2**: 531–5.

22 Williams GE, 1942, Syncopal reactions in blood donors. *Br Med J* **1**: 783–6.

23 Boynton MH, and Taylor ES, 1945, Complications arising in donors in a mass procurement project. *Am J Med Sci* **209**: 421–36.

24 Maloney WC, Lonnergan LR, and McClintock JK, 1946, Syncope in blood donors. *N. Engl J Med* **234**: 114–8.

25 Tomasulo P, Anderson AJ, Paluso MB, Gutschenritter MA, and Aster RH, 1980, A study of criteria for blood donor deferral. *Transfusion* **20**: 511–8.

26 Trouern-Trend JJ, Cable RG, Badon SJ, Newman BH, and Popovsky MA, 1999, A case-controlled multi-center study of vasovagal reactions in blood donors: influence of sex, age, donation status, weight, blood pressure, and pulse. *Transfusion* **39**: 316–20.

27 Newman B, 2002, Vasovagal reactions in high school students: Findings relative to race, risk factor synergism, female sex, and non-high school participants. *Transfusion* **42**: 1557–60.

28 Newman B, and Newman D, 2003, The effect of blood donation status, sex, age, and weight on blood donor return rates and the further effect of physical experience [abstract]. *Transfusion* **43**(Suppl): 141A.

29 Newman B, 2003, Vasovagal reaction rates and body weight: Findings in high- and low-risk populations. *Transfusion* **43**: 1084–8.

30 Newman B, Janowicz NM, and Siegfried B, 2006, Donor reactions in high-school donors: the effect of sex, weight, and collection volume. *Transfusion* **46**: 284–8.

31 Stewart KR, France CR, Rader AW, and Stewart JC, 2006, Phlebotomist interpersonal skill predicts a reduction in reactions among volunteer blood donors. *Transfusion* **46**: 1394–401.

32 Kasprisin DO, Glynn SH, Taylor, and Miller KA, 1992, Moderate and severe reactions in blood donors. *Transfusion* **32**: 23–6.

33 Sauer LA, and France CR, 1999, Caffeine attenuates vasovagal reactions in female first-time blood donors. *Health Psychol* **18**: 403–9.

34 France CR, Montalva R, France JL, *et al.*, 2008, Enhancing attitudes and intentions in prospective blood donors: Evaluation of a new donor recruitment brochure. *Transfusion* **48**: 526–30.

35 Ebert RV, Stead EA, and Gilbert JG, 1941, Response of normal human subjects to acute blood loss. *Arch Int Med* **68**: 578–90.

36 El-Sayed H, and Hainsworth R, 1996, Salt supplement increases plasma volume and orthostatic tolerance in patients with unexplained syncope. *Heart* **75**: 134–40.

37 Krediet CT, van Dijk N, Linzer M, van Lieshout JJ, and Wieling W, 2002, Management of vasovagal syncope – Controlling or aborting faints by leg crossing and muscle tensing. *Circulation* **106**: 1684–9.

38 Ditto B, France CR, Lavoie P, *et al.*, 2003, Reducing reaction to blood donation with applied muscle tension: a randomized controlled trial. *Transfusion* **43**: 1269–75.

39 Ditto B, and France CR, 2006, The effects of applied tension on symptoms in French-speaking blood donors: A randomized trial. *Health Psychol* **25**: 433–7.

40 Ditto B, France CR, Albert M, and Byrne N, 2007, Dismantling applied tension: mechanisms of a treatment to reduce blood donation-related symptoms. *Transfusion* **47**: 2217–22.

41 Waters WW, Platts SH, Mitchell BM, Whitson PA, and Meck J.V, 2005, Plasma volume restoration with salt tablets and water after bed rest prevents orthostatic hypotension and changes in supine hemodynamic and endocrine variables. *Am J Physiol Heart Circ Physiol* **288**: H839–H847.

CHAPTER 9

Preparation of Blood Components

Erhard Seifried, Reinhard Henschler, Juergen Luhm, Thea Mueller-Kuller,
Hans-Ulrich Pfeiffer, Walid Sireis, and Markus M. Mueller

Institute for Transfusion Medicine and Immunohematology, Clinics of the Johann Wolfgang Goethe University
Frankfurt/Main, German Red Cross Blood Transfusion Service Baden-Wuerttemberg-Hessen, Frankfurt/Main, Germany

Introduction

Transfusion of safe and sufficient blood components to patients has become a cornerstone of supportive care in contemporary medicine. The mission of blood transfusion centers is to provide such quality blood components for all patients in need, "24 hours, 365 days per year," in an economic way.

In the past, virus transmission by a blood product was a major threat. Nowadays, blood donor selection and intensive modern testing of blood donations have reduced this problem for the major three transfusion-transmitted viruses HCV, HBV, and HIV to a minimal residual risk, at least in developed countries.

Hemovigilance is still focusing on recipients of blood components, however the transmission of viral diseases is a very rare event thanks to the activities mentioned above. Other threats such as transfusion of an incorrect blood component, over- or under-transfusion, bacterial contamination of the blood component or immunological incompatibilities between donor and recipients have been identified as occurring with a relatively high frequency and therefore as being more relevant for hemovigilance, although the absolute numbers of such complications are low. In addition, over recent years donor vigilance has become another important topic in hemovigilance around the world.

Although these two topics remain the main focus of hemovigilance, transfusion medicine and hemotherapy nowadays are seen as "a process" by Dzik and others, and "not only [as] a product."[1-3] The aspect of the "vein-to-vein" transfusion chain including numerous processes and complex interfaces has broadened the scope of hemovigilance.

This chapter deals with the preparation of blood components. Departments dealing with these preparation steps, regularly called *production*, are often judged as self-contained units. However, production departments rely heavily on perfectly working interfaces. Regarding the flow of blood components, incoming whole blood or apheresis donations as well as the corresponding datasets from the donation departments require both expert blood donation handling and a bilateral information flow to and from the donation departments. After preparation, the same holds true for the issuing and distribution departments as well as hospital blood banks. While the flow of products requires traceability from the donor to the patient and back, a safe and sufficient supply without an excessive waste rate requires excellent communication and data flow between blood donation, preparation,

Corresponding author: Erhard Seifried, MD, PhD, Professor of Transfusion Medicine, Chair for Transfusion Medicine and Immunhematology at the JW Goethe University Frankfurt/Main, CEO of the German Red Cross Blood Transfusion Service Baden-Wuerttemberg—Hessen, Sandhofstrasse 1, Frankfurt/Main, Germany. Phone: +49 69 6782 201; fax: +49 69 6782 231 email: e.seifried@blutspende.de.

Hemovigilance: An Effective Tool for Improving Transfusion Safety, First Edition. Edited by René R.P. De Vries and Jean-Claude Faber.
© 2012 John Wiley & Sons, Ltd. Published 2012 by John Wiley & Sons, Ltd.

technicians, and issuing and transfusing physicians in both directions.

The results from the testing laboratories authorized by the responsible testing personnel have to be securely administered and connected with other datasets, for example, from the blood donation and finally to the blood components, before release by the production head, labeling, and final release by the qualified person. Any wastage or loss of products during the production process must be documented and assessed. Traceability from the donor to the recipient in either direction has to be safeguarded. Therefore, other departments such as information technology (IT) that provide soft- and hardware and support for data management as well as quality assurance, quality control, and quality risk management supported by the quality management department are indispensable parts of the preparation of blood components.

Compliance with manufacturing and marketing authorizations, good manufacturing practice (GMP), product specifications, standard operating procedures (SOPs), and production flow charts, as well as correct management of deviations, error trends, errors, risks, product recalls, look-backs, and complaints, require well trained and highly motivated personnel as well as highly qualified supervisors and department heads.

Premises and equipment have to be kept under close surveillance and require a tight hygiene management involving technical departments, cleaning staff, and hygiene experts as well as control laboratories and suppliers.

Quality management of a certified and accredited blood transfusion service involves all members of the department and also includes the upper management through continuous supervision, regularly reporting, and annual business reviews.

This chapter cannot cover all the steps relevant for hemovigilance in the preparation of blood components. We are well aware that national legislation, local situation regarding blood donor population, as well as requirements of hospitals and transfusing physicians, force individual blood transfusion services to adapt to their local needs as they have done in the past. This is also part of the European diversity.[4] Therefore we focus on interfaces, products including specifications, processes, standards such as GMP, monitoring, reporting, assessment, documentation, quality management, as well as training and assessment of personnel. Novel techniques such as pathogen reduction require ongoing implementation and validation of new processes as well as evaluation of these measures of improvement.

Active hemovigilance measures serve to keep track with all interfaces and processes. By applying such methods, assessment and evaluation are possible including economical benefits thereof. Although the absolute number of errors or deviations in the preparation of blood components is small compared to other parts of the transfusion chain, hemovigilance in this sector nevertheless helps to achieve the major goal: a safe and secure blood component provision to all patients in need.

Products and processes: Standards, specifications, and documentation

In the production processes of contemporary blood components, high technical and preparatory standards have been reached, which enable stable processes and an internationally harmonized pharmaceutical quality.[5] The guidelines governing medicinal products in the European Union (EU) stress the importance of conformity with GMP as stated, for example, in the directive 2003/94/EC. EU guidelines to GMP (part II, basic requirements for active substances used as starting materials, 2005) formally exclude whole blood and plasma, because directive 2002/98/EC sets up "standards of quality and safety for the collection, testing, processing, storage and distribution of human blood and blood components".[6] However, since human plasma is a main starting material for numerous medicinal products throughout the EU, directive 2003/63/EC amending directive 2001/83/EC includes this common source material by implementing the concept of a plasma master file (PMF). Most blood establishments either process source plasma or sell it

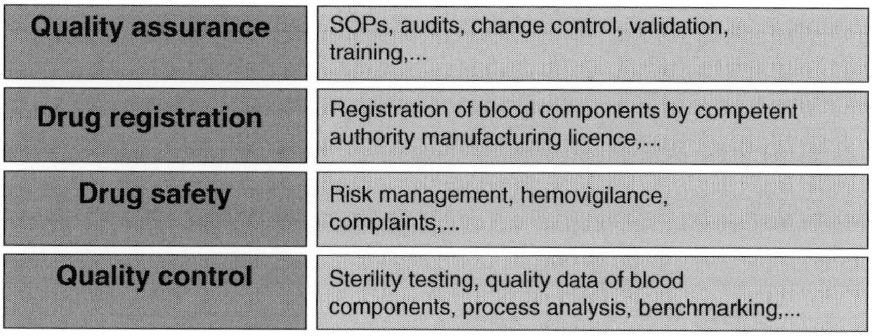

Quality assurance	SOPs, audits, change control, validation, training,...
Drug registration	Registration of blood components by competent authority manufacturing licence,...
Drug safety	Risk management, hemovigilance, complaints,...
Quality control	Sterility testing, quality data of blood components, process analysis, benchmarking,...

Figure 9.1 Structure and tasks of a contemporary quality management system.

for fractionation, and so adherence to GMP standards is mandatory for production departments as well.

In Germany, blood products are considered as medicinal drugs. That way, it is mandatory for a blood establishment to achieve manufacturing licences from the regional authorities as well as marketing authorizations by the federal authority. The preparation of blood components in Germany is regulated by the German law on pharmaceuticals (drug act) and the German ordinance for the production of pharmaceuticals and active pharmaceutical ingredients (API) called AMWHV. In addition, the German transfusion act, amended by the German guidelines for production of blood and blood components and for blood product usage (hemotherapy), defines minimal quality control parameters according to the specifications defined in the manufacturing and marketing authorizations held by the blood establishments. The Council of Europe (CoE) was one of the first institutions to set up European standards and minimal requirements for preparation of blood components.

Products and processes in preparation of blood components are tightly regulated on a regional, national, and European level. Quality management systems including quality assurance, drug registration, drug safety, and quality control (see Figure 9.1) are indispensable in this field, as are internal and external audits and inspections by authorities.

Table 9.1 shows the products and processes in the preparation of blood components.

Starting material: Whole blood donation or apheresis bags with stored information on donor clearance, donor traceability, and the donation process itself

The pharmaceutical process leading to final blood components that are ready for release for transfusion starts as early as blood donor advertising and donor selection. Directive 2002/98/EC clearly states that

voluntary and unpaid blood donations are a factor which can contribute to high safety standards for blood and blood components and therefore to the protection of human health. The efforts of the Council of Europe in this area should be supported and all necessary measures should be taken to encourage voluntary and unpaid donations through appropriate measures and initiatives and through ensuring that donors gain greater public recognition, thereby also increasing self-sufficiency. The definition of voluntary and unpaid donation of the Council of Europe should be taken into account.[6]

With this statement, the European Parliament and the Council encourage blood establishments to follow the idea of voluntary and unpaid blood donors, which is also supported by WHO and ISBT as well as many other international institutions. In times of growing demand and shrinking donor bases due to the ageing of most European populations,[7] donor management becomes an increasingly important part of contemporary blood procurement.

Table 9.1 Products and processes involved in the preparation of blood components.

Process	Product Whole blood donation	Apheresis products: PRC, PC, TP	Packed red cells (PRC)	Platelet concentrates (PC)	Therapeutic plasma (TP)	Source plasma
Incoming goods	✓	✓	–	–	–	–
Registration and documentation	✓	✓	–	–	–	–
Traceability	✓					
Data consistency	✓					
Weighing	✓	✓	–	–	–	–
Centrifugation	✓	✓	–	–	–	–
Separation	✓					
Semi-automated preparation steps	–	✓	✓	✓	✓	✓
Universal leukodepletion	–	✓	✓	✓	–	–
In-process controls	✓					
Special products (e.g., irradiation, CMV neg. etc.)	–	✓	✓	✓	✓	–
Storage	–	✓	✓	✓	✓	✓
Labeling	–	✓	✓	✓	✓	✓
Release	–	✓	✓	✓	✓	✓

Standard blood donor inclusion and exclusion criteria remain the major backbone in blood safety. While reducing the amount of blood donations for preparation of blood components, a standardized donor history using questionnaires as well an additional interview by a healthcare professional and a medical examination of each donor by far surpasses all laboratory testing in reducing risks to donor and recipient. It is therefore mandatory for production departments to get full information of the blood donor's history and examination results. This information may also guide the preparation, for example by excluding the production of platelet concentrates and therapeutic plasma in donors taking specific drugs for underlying diseases such as hypertension, which do not lead to a full deferral of the donor.

Incoming goods or starting material for the preparation of blood components have to be checked for appropriate donation information, as well as storage and transportation data coming with the blood bags as such.

Auto-sterilization of blood products occurs when the whole blood donation is kept at room tempera-ture for a certain period after donation before cooling. Single bacteria from the deep skin parts of the donor might have found their way into the donation. Most of these single bacteria will be diverted to a small pouch by pre-donation sampling, and so never reach the final blood bags; however, in rare cases, such single bacteria might end up in the donation bag. Phagocytosis by donor leukocytes will then be facilitated by room temperature. In addition, production of pooled buffy-coat derived platelet concentrates is not feasible if the whole blood donation is cooled down early to 4°C (40°F). Therefore, temperature logging is a requirement for quality control of incoming raw material to the preparation department as well.

Incoming goods comprise blood bags as well. Supplier data delivered with the batches of blood bags and release information of each specific blood bag batch have to be documented and forwarded to the production department. Blood bags have to be checked by preparation personnel for any defects, (micro-)leakage or any other untoward sign showing irregularities. Such visual checks of blood components are mandatory and are repeated throughout the whole processes starting from donation until transfusion to the patient. Results of preceding checks have to be recorded, summarized, for example by issuing a standard label, and passed on until the final check of the blood component at the patient's bedside. Micro-leakages of blood bags, for example, might only become apparent when pressure is applied to a blood bag during centrifugation or preparation steps. Donation department personnel, though they check the blood bags thoroughly as well, might not be able to detect this problem.

Apart from the donor information, blood bag, and donation data as discussed above, the weight of the whole blood donation, donation duration, and identity check data have to be processed as well. Therefore, interfaces from donation departments are multifaceted and have to be estimated accordingly by any hemovigilance approach.

After data, and raw material according to SOPs and product and production specifications, have reached the preparation department, accuracy, completeness, full traceability, and consistency have to be checked and documented. Any deviations have to be documented, reported, and decisions regarding rejections taken by competent personnel.

Preparation of blood components relies on the close adherence to specifications laid down in SOPs followed by highly motivated and well trained personnel as discussed below.

Machinery and information technology including hardware and software

For the preparation of standard blood components, machinery such as centrifuges, separators, welders, scales, freezers, etc. play a major role as do the personnel involved in these complex and labour-intensive production steps. Maintenance, validation, and in-process controls of all steps are key elements in hemovigilance in this regard. All data of these processes have to be readily available to supervisors. Any deviations must be immediately reported, assessed, and documented. In addition, such summaries have to be available for internal and external audits as well as inspections by customers and authorities. If any questions arise, details of the process in question have to be available as well.

The preparation of blood components is a complex procedure consisting of registration of incoming data and raw material, data and quality checks, centrifugation, separation, leukocyte depletion, welding, and mixing procedures as shown in Figure 9.2. It also includes several in-process control and release steps by quality laboratory and qualified personnel, labeling and (quarantine)

Figure 9.2 Error management in preparation of blood components. The scheme depicts the supervision of different production elements (left) such as employees, machinery, computer hard- and software, and the production chain of blood components (lines and dots). Important features are a formalized error report and report processing, which is simple to handle, a clear flow of information, and repetitive evaluation platforms. The latter provide instant awareness and evaluation as well as continuity through repetitive reports to, and involvement of, the upper management.

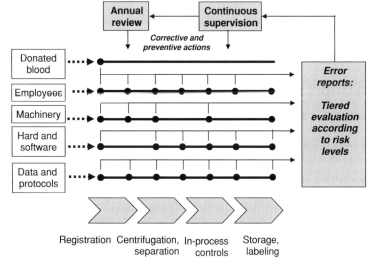

storage procedures, and finally the release for distribution to hospital blood banks by the qualified person. In most blood establishments, a distribution and issuing department is involved here. The authors' blood establishment also includes a big university hospital blood bank and the reference laboratory for immunohematology for the whole region. Therefore, labeled blood components are also directly crossmatched for specific patients.

Premises and machinery have to fulfill not only detailed hygiene requirements regularly controlled by the responsible section and department heads as well as by the quality control laboratories, but also detailed technical specifications regarding light, humidity, temperature, and so on. These technical specifications are laid down in technical SOPs and have to be controlled and documented, too. Any deviations are directly reported to the responsible technical personnel, discussed and assessed by technical and production supervisors, and countermeasures taken. It also needs to be judged whether any of these deviations might have caused damage to raw, intermediate, or final products, which have to be taken out of the preparation process in such cases immediately.

In cases of severe complications, an alarm plan must include all responsible personnel in an escalating manner up to the highest management level. Less important deviations are collated, assessed, and reported to the quality and upper management in quarterly or less frequent management reports (MR) as well as annually in product quality reports (PQR).

All the above steps have to be performed according to the specifications of each blood component, as outlined by the CoE and the national legislation and directives and specified by the individual blood establishments' manufacturing licences and marketing authorizations. Specifications of the final blood components ready for issuing include parameters and detailed specifications, the frequency and time points of parameter checks, and the expected results. These specifications also state the percentage of finally labeled blood components, which have to be within the required guard bands. These percentages range from 90% in less important details of the specification up to 100%

for the important release criteria. If the accepted percentage is below 100%, these specifications also explain the maximally acceptable deviations from the expected results.

From the complexity of the processes outlined, and as discussed in detail in the quality management section on page 104 and 105, it becomes clear that IT technology plays a crucial role in maintaining daily work in the preparation of blood components in a blood establishment. Data consistency, multiple interfaces for supplier data, incoming blood donor, donation, quality control, and donor test result information must be ascertained as well as traceability of all these data from the blood donor to the recipient and backwards, even after decades in each individual case. In addition, service and maintenance as well as in-process control data, reports from personnel, deviations, assessments by supervisors, quality, and upper management have to be collated to a full documentation. This documentation must both allow a general overview of the preparation of blood components and, in the case of deviations, an in-depth analysis of individual datasets.

Therefore, the quality management of IT including hardware as well as software has to be thorough. Validation procedures add to system security here. Any changes in hard- or software settings have to be discussed between IT and production specialists, including quality management personnel when required. Design, installation, operational, and performance qualification plans for critical steps have to be collated in a validation master plan, and then discussed, approved, and released. The validation manager in close cooperation with the IT and production department has to set up and execute the validation plans and collate a summary report. This final report has to be approved and released by production, IT, quality, and upper management.

Quality management

As depicted in the earlier Figure 9.1, quality management consists of several different facets all dealing with the main goal of blood transfusion, blood establishments, and hemotherapy. This main goal is to supply patients in need and their treating physicians with the best possible blood components regarding content and function, safety and availability. All aspects of quality management serve this goal. It is vital to provide blood components with the quality required for their intended use and that they meet the specifications laid down in manufacturing and marketing authorizations. Therefore, quality management is part of the upper management's tools in running a blood establishment.

Quality assurance comprises all activities that ensure the required quality of products and services according to specifications and intended use. All specifications, SOPs, training issues, internal and external audits, validation, and qualification, as well as change control procedures, are tools and duties covered by quality assurance.

Blood components in Germany are registered drugs according to the German drug act, and so drug registration (DR) is a second, closely related, field of quality management. Cooperation with the competent local and federal authorities is vital for a research and development (R&D) driven blood establishment. Registration of the blood establishment as such, manufacturing licences, quality and hygiene tests, internal and external audits, inspections, and marketing authorizations are the field of DR.

In addition to drug registration, blood component safety (which means drug safety (DS) in Germany) is the third facet of quality management. This covers hemovigilance with all aspects from the donor to the recipient. Furthermore, risk and deviation management (as explained on pages 105–107) is located here. Complaint and recall management as well as look-back procedures are also parts of DS duties. The competent authorities have close contact with DS. Severe and serious adverse events are reported immediately to the authorities, while working parties located at the German ministry of health and the federal authorities, such as the working party on blood (Arbeitskreis Blut), compile recommendations and guidelines, which have to be followed by the blood establishments.

Quality control (QC) is the fourth important part of quality management, dealing with quality data such as sterility testing results from the donation and preparation of blood components. Their major goal is to ensure that all specifications regarding functionality and safety of all blood components produced are met on a daily basis. Samples for quality control and sterility testing are processed here. Process and risk analysis are standard tools in QC as well as benchmarking between different institutes and organizations.

Documentation and analysis of deviations and errors in the preparation of blood components

An electronic workflow-based system is an appropriate solution for the management of production errors and deviations because all personnel involved in a single case, such as production workers, department heads, or heads of manufacturing and quality control, use the identical electronic document online. For monitoring and control of equipment and supplies, the use of an electronic system is desirable, but not mandatory.

It is important to have a cross-reference to the risk and deviation management system. All documents concerning one single risk and deviation report should be summarized in one single electronic summary file including all correspondence, e-mails, drawings, technical leaflets, and so on. Figure 9.3 depicts the absolute numbers of deviations and errors reported from eight different production departments in the authors' group during 2009.

Suppliers' self-assessments should be collated as well as a standardized assessment of all suppliers implemented by the involved departments of a blood establishment, both from the commercial and medical point of views. After a summary suppliers' assessment, the quality management department should finalize the evaluation of all important suppliers. The risk and deviation reporting system must be linked to the supplier assessment system. The most important and critical suppliers should be regularly audited, for example at 2-year intervals.

Risk management

Although the standard daily preparation of blood components is a stable and well orchestrated (albeit complex) procedure, supplier errors, production errors, near-misses, and various deviations may nevertheless occur. In order to detect such

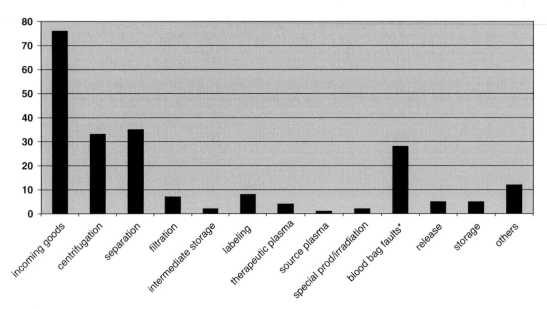

* = faults during preparation processes

Figure 9.3 Deviation and error reports from eight production departments of the authors' group of blood transfusion services in 2009.

out-of-specification procedures and products, different safety measures are implemented throughout the preparation steps of blood components. Monitoring, documentation, and assessment of near-misses and deviations are mandatory in order to identify critical steps in preparation and to alter, circumvent, or avoid them in the future.

A sophisticated deviation and risk management system covers all deviations, errors, and risks occurring from the donor to the recipient and provides a standardized documentation platform. Documented cases have then to be analyzed, evaluated, and assessed by different supervisors in the production and quality management departments. A "no punishment error culture" must be implemented within the staff, which can be achieved within a few years. Interfaces between the production and all other departments, such as IT, donor testing, blood collection and distribution/issuing, as well as hospital blood banks have to be included in the analysis. A modern management system of complaints, recalls, and returns adds to this culture. Data from quality control laboratories analyzing regular samples taken out of the

standard preparation processes must be assessable here, too.

Such systems must differentiate between the detection and the causative agent. Standardized reporting procedures up to the highest management levels in the case of severe errors should be thoroughly tested. Necessary corrective measures in preparation processes or additional training of the staff must be performed and documented as well. The quality management and production departments also assess sustainability of the measures taken.

For the preparation of blood components, an appropriate error and risk management system must involve a categorization of the various production steps such as centrifugation, separation, welding steps, labeling, and so on (see the earlier Figure 9.3). An electronic workflow-based system is useful here. All employees involved use the same online form to first report, document, and assess the deviation detected. The online form also covers incoming material or technical defects including batch and lot numbers as well and must enable cross-reference to the error reporting system of the suppliers involved, in order to allow shortest possible reaction times. It should also provide the opportunity to follow up change control procedures and process (re-)validations.

The severity of each error, deviation, or risk occurring must be rated. Assessing systems such as the failure mode/effects analysis (FMEA) system and, for example, a traffic light visualization with green for low impact, yellow for medium impact, and red for high risk problems are helpful tools. They summarize the potential impact of an error on the quality of the procedure or product and the relevance for process safety. This should also apply for minor deviations, near-misses, or errors that occur with higher frequency.

All deviation and risk reports should be statistically analyzed and results used for benchmarking processes. Analyses must be part of regular quality and management reviews with the upper management of the blood establishment.

Blood pack fault monitoring is a very good example showing the benefits of a risk management system associated with one of the most important supplies provided by external manufacturers. Blood bag systems are becoming more and more complex medicinal products, including additive solutions as well as technical parts such as in-line filters, sample diversion pouches, couplers for sampling, and so on.[8] Blood packs are critical items for the recipient's safety and a secure blood component supply, which of course are the main issues here. Economical and marketing aspects are smaller, but nevertheless more and more relevant points for consideration as well. Beckman and colleagues[8] showed that a national initiative for collection and analysis of blood bag faults and deviations, in close cooperation with the blood pack manufacturers in the UK national blood service, resulted in early identification and rectification of specific problems associated with the production and use of blood bags. Therefore, not only waste rates of the valuable donations of volunteers, but also recalls of blood components from the hospital can be reduced. Suppliers are able to start quick and efficient changes in production processes, and other blood establishments are informed early before similar errors occur at their premises.

Such monitoring of incoming goods therefore improves production safety and economy as well as collaboration with the suppliers, and adds to the stable, safe, and low-risk preparation of blood components.

Documentation of jobs: Tasks and responsibilities, training and assessment

The preparation of blood components is a complex and work-intensive production process. Requirements regarding accuracy, hygiene, and adherence to SOPs are strict and have to be followed in detail by production workers. An in-depth understanding of quality management as well as a close adherence to GMP is required, too. Therefore, such important pharmaceutical processes fully rely on highly qualified, skilled, and dedicated personnel. Production personnel of all skill levels have to be regularly trained and training success needs to be monitored and assessed.

In order to achieve such complex goals, it is mandatory to define and clearly outline the responsibilities and tasks of each person involved in writing. Functional job descriptions for each position, especially for responsible ones according to GMP, help to define tasks and responsibilities clearly and positively, as well as delimitations toward other functions. Key personnel, such as the production head, qualified person, and so on, must be full-time employed. The head of production and the head of quality control must be separate persons sharing some of the responsibilities. The qualified person is responsible for the final release of the labeled blood components.

In addition to functional job descriptions laid down in the quality management handbook of the blood establishment, it is helpful to use authorization lists for each section and department lists for every single employee with that person's detailed tasks. Whenever a new member of a single group achieves a certain level of knowledge following theoretical and practical training, the responsible head of the section or department allows this single person to perform a certain task. This is documented on the authorization list, regularly updated after each exam, or check-passed by any of the employees on this list. The responsible person signs and dates the authorization of the single task accepted for the employee who is now allowed to perform this task in daily routine.

Deviation and problems have to be reported on a daily basis. Close monitoring of all employees, as well as immediate assessment of deviations and errors by the responsible personnel, makes sense only when immediate feedback is provided as well. (Re-)training is scheduled if necessary, for single employees or whole departments.

Since technology is able to amplify greatly the consequences of human error, quality management has to assure that risk management covers the interface of machinery and human work as well as the other topics discussed above.

Monitoring and assessment

Each step in the preparation of blood components might be critical for the safety and optimal function of the blood product finally transfused. The process controls of each step (according to Table 9.1 on page 102) are being performed during night and day shifts in the production department. Figure 9.4 gives the example of the continuous monitoring of blood component separators as performed in the authors' institute. Results and deviations from specifications are documented using standard documentation forms as well as electronic documentation. Foremen and shift managers perform a first assessment of the whole documentation before the department head (or deputy) performs an assessment and prepares a release report.

The release documentation by the production manager is one of the documents relevant for the final blood product release by the responsible person. The second document required for final release of the labeled blood components is the quality control report signed by the laboratory head, stating that all donor tests were performed according to SOPs and all results were validated. The final assessment by the responsible person then leads to the release of blood components fulfilling all the specifications, tested negative for

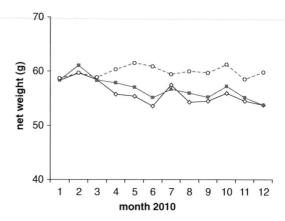

Figure 9.4 Continuous supervision of blood component separators. Semiautomated separators are monitored once a month by the weighing of ten buffy coats per machine. Plotted are the mean values (bold) of seven machines and values from two individual separators. One (quadrangles) moved along the mean values line while another (circles) developed a higher than average separation weight, providing a reason for technical adjustments.

all relevant pathogens, tested positive for blood groups, and so on.

Figure 9.5 shows results of benchmarking regarding fine-tuning of the blood component separators in two institutes of the authors' group. After implementation of several small changes identified during the benchmarking process in February and March 2008, the recovery of source plasma and the quality of the blood components improved significantly. This small example shows the impact on both the quality of the final products and the economical benefit achieved.

In addition, internal and external audits following clear-cut descriptions and rules using standard questionnaires, procedures, and final audit reports are helpful for a regular update to the upper management on potential risks in each and every department. We find it useful to perform at least yearly internal audits by department heads of collaborating blood establishments from the authors' group. Peers therefore assess the quality and performance of a department in another blood establishment and discuss their findings with the responsible department heads. A final audit report is generated by the auditor and sent to quality

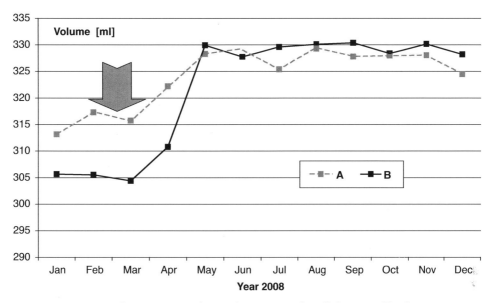

Figure 9.5 Increase in source plasma recovery after implementation of small changes in blood component separators in February and March 2008 (arrow), identified during a benchmarking process between two production departments in two different institutes (A and B).

management, which then compiles all internal audit reports and assesses the overall impact. The final summary report is then used for an upper management report.

As certified and accredited blood establishments since 2001, regular monitoring and assessments on all levels are daily routine. Standard monitoring and assessment reports are analyzed by quality management and summary reports generated. Routine staff training efficacy is controlled by staff competency assessment. Authorized bodies regularly control compliance with the certified and accredited qualifications of laboratories and donation, production, and apheresis departments.

Regular external audits and inspections by the competent authorities at regional and national level are additional checks helpful in maintaining and improving the quality of the daily work.

Implementation and evaluation of measures for improvement

New methods for improving the safety of blood components, such as pathogen inactivation, or planned alterations in standard specifications, such

as bacterial testing of platelet concentrates, must be implemented in close cooperation with all authorities involved and require novel marketing authorizations or at least change control (CC) procedures.[9–11] Such alterations must be planned and executed in accordance with annex 14 and 15 of the EU GMP guidelines with GAMP 4 or GAMP 5 concerning IT changes.

Most novel procedures require the approval of the local and federal authorities. In order to get such approvals, standard data files as requested by the different authorities must be submitted. A central component of every planned alteration is an adequate risk analysis, which should be as long as necessary and as short as possible. Before implementation, necessary re-qualifications and re-validations as well as training must be carefully planned and executed. A sophisticated CC system outlining clear-cut responsibilities, and including IT regarding hardware and software changes if applicable, is recommended.

The preparatory work including CC processes enables upper management to follow up on timelines and deliverables while keeping all involved people up to date. Planned alterations in both equipment and technical operations must follow

Project Number		☐ new ☐ change

Title			Application date
Applicant		Institute	
Project manager		Department	Planned completion

Confirmation of the existence of necessary documents and actions					Date/Signature Project manager
		Necessary	**Existing/performed**		
1	Project and measure plan		☐ yes		
2	Risk analysis (please add details on a separate additional form!)	Yes	☐ yes		
3	(Re-)validation		☐ yes	**Form**	
				Number	
4	(Re-)qualification		☐ DQ	Number	
			☐ IQ	Number	
			☐ OQ	Number	
			☐ PQ	Number	
5	IT release		☐ yes	Cross-reference ITCC-	
6	Which SOPs need an update/change?			**SOP**	**No.**	
				1		
				2		
7	Training		☐ yes, date		

Completion and release

1.	Report
2.	Change control complete:
	Date and signature of the responsible project manager _____
3.	Routine release (Date) _____ by:
	Date and signatures (according to drug law) Qualified person Responsible person

Figure 9.6 Cumulative overview form used in change control procedures.

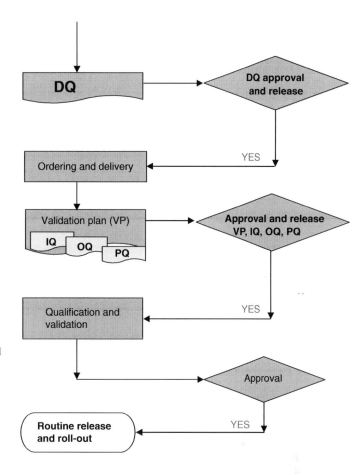

Figure 9.7 Flow chart of qualification and validation in a standard change control (CC) procedure. Elements in qualification and validation: DQ = design qualification; VP = validation plan; IQ = installation qualification; OQ = operational qualification; PQ = performance qualification.

a clearly defined path of activities. All relevant SOPs must be changed by qualified involved personnel and these changes must be supervised by department heads. Design qualification should be the focus of all owners of the project. Installation qualification, operational qualification, performance qualification, and validation must be planned accordingly. Qualification and validation processes following the validation master plan must be coordinated and conducted following a mutual agreement of all partners involved.

It is mandatory that all employees involved are fully trained including an appropriate knowledge check before introduction of the novel methodology or technique. An appropriate follow-up system for CC procedures using a logical and self-explanatory number code is helpful for keeping track.

A standardized documentation and assessment followed by the approval of relevant department heads leads to a final release of the novel process. After a final training phase and the final release of the altered SOPs involved, such alterations undergo a roll-out and implementation into routine procedures. If required, cost-effectiveness of the novel procedure can be assessed during routine use.

Figure 9.6 shows the cumulative overview form used in CC procedures and Figure 9.7 gives an overview of all the processes.

Conclusion

Modern preparation of blood components is a complex and work-intensive bundle of processes involving several interfaces to other departments.

Traceability of data and products from the blood donor to the recipient of blood components and back is mandatory. Modern hemovigilance and management procedures are used in order to fulfill the high quality and safety standards and to implement innovations.

References

1 Dzik WH, 2002, Emily Cooley Lecture: Transfusion safety in the hospital. *Transfusion* **43**(9): 1190–9.

2 Dzik WH, 2007, New technology for transfusion safety. *Br J Haematol* **136**(2): 181–90.

3 Beauplet A, 2001, [The transfusion chain: from donor to recipient.] *Rev Prat* **51**(12): 1294–8.

4 Mayr WR, 2005, Blood transfusion in Europe – The White Book 2005: The patchwork of transfusion medicine in Europe. *Transfus Clin Biol* **12**(5): 357–8.

5 Henschler R, Mueller MM, Pfeiffer HU, Seifried E, and Sireis W, 2010, Production of standard blood components. *ISBT Science Series* **5**: 190–5.

6 European Union, 2003, Directive 2002/98/EC of the European Parliament and of the Council of 27 January 2003 setting standards of quality and safety for the collection, testing, processing, storage and distribution of human blood and blood components and amending Directive 2001/83/EC. *Official Journal of the European Union* L33/30–40.

7 Seifried E, Klueter H, Weidmann C, Staudenmaier T, Schrezenmeier H, *et al.*, 2011, How much blood is needed? *Vox Sang* **100**: 10–21.

8 Beckman N, Nicholson G, Ashford M, and Hambleton R, 2004, Blood pack fault monitoring. *Vox Sang* **87**: 272–9.

9 Lee JS, and Gladwin MT, 2010, The risks of red cell storage. *Nature Med* **16**(4): 381–2.

10 Williamson LM, Stainsby D, Jones H, Love E, Chapman CE, *et al.*, 2007, The impact of universal leukodepletion of the blood supply on hemovigilance reports of posttransfusion purpura and transfusion-associated graft-versus-host disease. *Transfusion* **47**(8): 1455–67.

11 Funk MB, Gunay S, Lohmann A, Henseler O, and Keller-Stanislawski B, 2010, [Evaluation of measures aimed to reduce serious adverse transfusion reactions (hemovigilance data from 1997 to 2008).] *Bundesgesundheitsblatt Gesundheitsforschung Gesundheitsschutz* **53**(4): 347–56.

CHAPTER 10

Testing, Issuing, and Transport of Blood Components

Constantina Politis

Hellenic Coordinating Haemovigilance Centre (SKAE), University of Athens, Athens, Greece

Introduction

The blood establishment (BE) and the hospital, linked together through the hospital blood bank (hBB), play significant roles within a hemovigilance system operating at national, regional, and local level. An effective hemovigilance network collects information about errors, incidents, near-misses, and adverse reactions related to the donor, the blood product, and the transfused patient.

The Hellenic Coordinating Haemovigilance Centre (SKAE) reports that the rate of serious adverse events (SAEs) due to a deviation in whole blood collection, apheresis collection, testing of donations, processing, storage, and distribution during the period 2006–2009 was 17.5:100,000 blood components issued. The relevant rates for near-misses and uneventful transfusion errors respectively were 140:100,000 and 38.5:100,000 blood components issued for transfusion. SAEs were caused mainly by equipment failure during processing (1:6128 blood components issued) and uneventful transfusion errors were attributed mainly to human error (1:3520 blood components issued). Near-misses were associated mainly with processing (1:1086 blood components issued) and whole blood collection (1:2550 blood components issued).

Adverse events related to testing, storage, and distribution were rare <0.1:100,000, 2.2:100,000,

and 0.5:100,000 blood components issued respectively.

Better reporting methods are needed as well as further study of the factors associated with serious AEs, uneventful transfusion errors, and near-miss events.

In this chapter, quality issues and hemovigilance procedures for the testing, issuing, and transport of blood and blood components—with the ultimate goal of preventing the recurrence of adverse reactions and adverse events associated with these particular stages of the transfusion chain—is discussed.

In Europe, quality standards for all stages of donation and processes of collection, processing, testing, storage, and distribution of blood components, as well as the hemovigilance requirements allocated to the BE and to the hBB (collectively named as "reporting establishments"), are laid down by Directives 2002/98/EC,[1] 2004/33/EC,[2] 2005/61/EC,[3] and 2005/62/EC.[4]

Testing

Pre-transfusion testing of donor blood is carried out in the BE for (i) the detection of the most severe transfusion transmissible infections (HIV1/2, Hepatitis B and C), (ii) ABO and RhD grouping, and (iii) additional infectious markers and other blood types as necessary.[5] Testing is essential

Hemovigilance: An Effective Tool for Improving Transfusion Safety, First Edition. Edited by René R.P. De Vries and Jean-Claude Faber.
© 2012 John Wiley & Sons, Ltd. Published 2012 by John Wiley & Sons, Ltd.

in order to ensure the quality and safety of the blood product intended for transfusion.[1,2,4] In addition, blood group serological investigations of the intended recipient and compatibility testing with donor red cells are carried out before transfusion in the hBB, and in some cases in the BE. For these purposes, suitable strategies and technical requirements for blood screening and compatibility testing should be in place in all blood transfusion services that are involved in the pre-transfusion process.

Screening process for transfusion transmitted infections (TTIs)

Quality measures and validation of screening tests

The screening process aims to identify and remove those donors/donations that have passed the previous safety steps but present a potential risk with regard to diseases transmissible by blood.

The quality assurance of the screening of donations for infectious markers is particularly important and requires both general and specific approaches.[5] Only validated tests, reagents, and equipment that have been licensed or evaluated and considered suitable by the competent national Health Authorities can be used.[5] Screening tests for infectious markers must be performed in accordance with the instructions recommended by the manufacturer of reagents and test kits.[5]

European regulations[4,5] require that all laboratory assays and test systems used for infectious disease marker screening must be validated by the BE before their introduction, to ensure compliance with the intended use of the test. Proper validation demonstrates control, generates useful knowledge of the test, and establishes future requirements for internal quality control, external quality assurance, calibration, and maintenance of equipment, monitoring of storage conditions of test materials and reagents, and training of personnel, with documentation of all these actions.[4,5]

Current tests for the screening of donations are based on detecting the relevant antigens or antibodies and gene sequences.[1] Tests are conventionally supplied in kits that include negative and positive controls in each plate or run. The minimum performance requirement is the correct determination of these controls in accordance with the manufacturer's instructions.[6,7] It is further recommended that the tests should include an external weak positive control in order to allow for statistical process control.[6,7] Screening tests must have high sensitivity in order to be effective and sufficient specificity to avoid the unnecessary rejection of suitable donors.[7]

Initially reactive donations must be retested in duplicate by the same assay unless otherwise recommended by the manufacturer. If any of the repeat tests is reactive, then the donation is deemed repeatedly reactive and a sample should be sent to the appropriate laboratory for confirmation.[6] This donation must not be used for transfusion. In the event that the repeatedly reactive donation is confirmed positive, the donor should be counseled and a further sample be obtained in order to confirm the results and the identity of the donor.[4,6–10] Ideally, the confirmatory test should be at least as sensitive as the screening test and have higher specificity, however, some screening tests are more sensitive than the available confirmatory tests.[6]

Nucleic acid amplification technology (NAT) testing should follow the same general principle of initial screening for the presence of a pathogen in order to prevent the release of a possibly infectious donation for transfusion. A reactive screening result is followed up by testing to confirm or revoke the initial result.

The drawing-up of *national algorithms for screening* of blood for infectious markers is recommended. This enables problems associated with discordant or unconfirmed results to be resolved in a consistent fashion.[6,7]

Hemovigilance procedures relevant to testing

A set of organized surveillance procedures for the collection and analysis of information on unexpected or undesirable events, as well as for nonconformance with technical requirements related to testing for transfusion transmitted infections (TTI), should be in place in all BEs.

BEs are required to notify the competent national authorities if any of the following occur:
• Laboratory testing for infectious disease markers not carried out according to the procedures.[6]
• Deviations from good manufacturing practices (GMPs), applicable standards, or established specifications (e.g., product defect, equipment failure, human error) that may affect the quality and the safety of the blood product.[6]
• Wrong standard operating procedures (SOPs) applied (e.g., error in choice of SOP, out-of-date SOP used).[6]
• SOP designed inappropriately.
• False negative test results obtained, even though correct procedures were followed.
• Wrong interpretation of results.
• Any resultant seroconversion in a recipient that provoked and was reported as a serious adverse reaction.

Epidemiological surveillance
Epidemiological surveillance of TTIs in donors is an important hemovigilance process that informs the BE in making decisions related to safety. The BE should hold detailed records of the general donor population and its different categories (volunteers, replacement donors, paid donors, candidates to donate blood, and so on). The incidence of TTIs in blood donors and the frequency of confirmed positive screening results can be investigated in relation to factors such as donor characteristics, frequency and type of donation, and stable or mobile collection sites. This allows the monitoring of infectious markers and the analysis of trends.

Examples of follow up of quality indicators related to the systematic evaluation of annual data on donors and donations have been provided by a number of countries. The prevalence and incidence of infectious diseases vary greatly among Member States and a north-south gradient exists for hepatitis B and C virus.[11]

The example of Greece
Surveillance of TTIs by SKAE has proved to be an important tool for risk management and total quality management in the blood transfusion services.[12,13] Detailed data on positive screening tests are based on a total of 6,621,143 blood units tested from 1996 to 2008.[13] The overall incidence of any infectious marker fell quite steadily in this period, from 0.79% to 0.36% (see Figure 10.1).

This fall is largely because of the decline in incidence of HBsAg (which accounts for about three quarters of all positive tests), from 0.54%

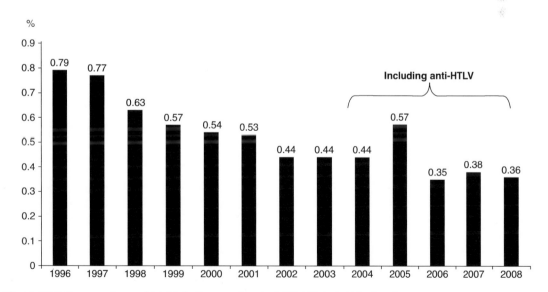

Figure 10.1 Seroprevalence of total infectious markers in 6,621,143 tested blood units.

to 0.22% (overall trend –0.025). The incidence of every infectious disease marker fell sharply in the first two years of surveillance but the other markers have not shown the same pattern as HBsAg subsequently. From 1998 onwards, the incidence of positive results for anti-HCV halved from 0.1% to 0.05% (overall trend –0.007). Positive anti-HIV tests, after an initial steep decline (1996–1999) and a stationary period up to 2003, have tended to increase slightly in frequency in the last six years to 0.009% (overall trend +0.0002). Surveillance of syphilis showed a decline in incidence to below 0.01% in the years 2001–2004, but a steady increase thereafter to 0.027% in 2008 (overall trend +0.004). Anti-HTLV testing has also been mandatory since 2003, with an overall incidence 0.002% (overall trend –0.0007).[12,13]

Prevalence of all infections is particularly high in first-time donors compared to repeat and regular donors (see Table 10.1).

These data and the unchanging profile of the seropositive donor throughout the surveillance period (male, 30–45 years of age, giving blood for the first time) showed the need for taking action in order to improve methods for blood donor recruitment and maintenance, donor deferral policy, and quality management in the laboratory.[12,13]

Furthermore, an incident occurred of transfusion-transmitted HIV infection in two recipients of red cells and plasma derived from the same blood unit of a male repeat donor with risky sexual behavior, who donated during the serologically silent window period. This had a tremendous impact on public confidence in the blood transfusion services and subsequently on

the Ministry of Health's policy regarding the implementation of NAT testing for the total blood supply.[14]

Tracing and retrieval of potentially infectious donations

In the event of confirmation of an HIV, HCV, or HBV infection in a repeat donor, the BE in cooperation with the treating physician must undertake *a look-back procedure*. The objective is to identify the recipients of any previous potentially infectious donations made by this donor, and notify them so that they can be tested and counseled.[6,7] The implicated donations are those that fall within a time frame equal to the maximum test-specific window period of the infection, preceding a negative screening test result in the donor.

Prior donations from donors who are newly identified as infected with any of the mandatorily tested infectious markers require *quarantine* of untransfused components in order to prevent possible harm to potential recipients.[6,7] Certain blood products may be re-released after proper risk analysis or additional testing. The relevant *plasma fractionation institute* must also be notified.[6,7]

The rationale for look-back is that blood donated during the window period of infection may have been infectious despite lack of reactivity on the screening assay.[8–10] In the USA, look-back was most effective after implementation of blood donor testing for HIV in the mid-1980s.[8] Retrospective HCV look-back in Canada in the late 1990s, which was intended to identify recipients of blood components that had been donated before implementation of HCV screening in 1990, yielded relatively few recipients who could be contacted and who benefited from the notification.[10] It should be stressed that without this particular hemovigilance procedure, some transfusion recipients who were unaware that they were infected, would not benefit from testing, counseling, and undergoing antiviral therapy.[7]

Traceability of blood components and look-back procedures have also proved useful in the investigation of *post-transfusion infection* in a recipient. In this situation, the blood establishment should perform a risk analysis to assess whether

Table 10.1 Rates per 100,000 donations.

Infectious markers	Serology 2005–2008		NAT only positive 2003–2008	
	1st time donors	Repeat donors	1st time donors	Repeat donors
HIV	51.9	6.8	1.65	0.2
HCV	431	17.6	3.3	0.1
HBV	2045	87.6	63.45	3.11

the incident indicates a potential infectious blood product.[7] In the Netherlands in the year 2007, there were seven reports of post-transfusion viral infection. None of these reflected a certain, probable, or possible transmission of an infection, for which the blood bank routinely tests in blood donation.[15]

The Council of Europe recommends that test results from donations of the implicated donors should be re-analysed, with additional tests (e.g., NAT) or confirmatory tests on archived samples or freshly obtained samples from the donor.[7] When an HBV, HCV, or HIV infection is confirmed, the blood establishment should defer the donor and undertake a look-back procedure on previous potentially infectious donations.

Look-back in Greece

Two multi-transfused children suffering from aplastic anemia were diagnosed anti-HCV positive and blood transfusion was incriminated for this incident. Look-back required the tracing of more than 400 donations implicated as potentially infectious for HCV involved in the transfusion of more than 600 blood components processed from these donations. Blood transfusion was eventually excluded as a root cause for the transmission of the infection.[14]

In another look-back study involving 122 repeat donors who tested seropositive for HIV in the period 2006–2008, archived samples of their previous donations were retested using an ID-NAT assay. HIV-RNA-only positive results were detected in two cases. However, possible transmission of HIV to the two recipients of the blood products derived from these infectious blood units donated in the serologically silent window period could not be investigated because both patients had died from another cause and no stored blood samples were available. The FFP unit from the first donor had been discarded due to hemolysis.[14]

Management of information and reporting hemovigilance data

Every institution that participates in a hemovigilance network should report adverse reactions and adverse events in the same way. Guidance on uniform definitions of the different types of adverse events and reactions is required. Training in the use of common report forms ensures uniform interpretation of a given type of incident.

BEs should notify to their national hemovigilance system and competent authorities all relevant information about errors, adverse reactions and adverse events, including any cases of transmission of infectious agents by blood and blood components as well as look-back positive results.

BEs should also describe the action taken with respect to other implicated blood components that have been distributed for transfusion or for use as plasma for fractionation.[3,6]

Bacterial quality control testing and hemovigilance issues

Despite all the collection and processing procedures aimed at producing safe blood components, hemovigilance reports indicate that incidents of bacterial contamination of blood components are becoming more frequent.

In 2007, TRIP reported 22 cases of post-transfusion bacteremia: 18 concerned RBC, 3 platelets, and 1 plasma.[15] There were further reports also suggesting bacterial contamination, but without a definite diagnosis because cultures had not been performed in all cases. Taking into consideration that there are not many reports with high imputability for transfusion transmitted bacterial infection, TRIP has proposed that hemovigilance reports should use two separate categories: (i) post-transfusion bacteremia and (ii) bacterial contamination of blood components.[15]

The Council of Europe recommends that bacterial quality control testing in all blood components may be appropriate. Platelets products are more likely than other blood components to be associated with sepsis due to their storage at room temperature, which permits bacterial growth. Therefore, for whole blood collection, bacterial cultures of platelets provide the best indication of the overall rate of contamination, provided that the sample for culture is obtained on a suitable sample volume and at a suitable time post-collection.[6] A variety of procedures may be used to obtain a valid platelet sample for bacterial culture. BEs wishing to establish surveillance to detect bacterial contamination rates should apply quality control testing for bacterial contamination to ensure that blood collection and processing procedures conform to current standards.[6]

Routine pre-release bacteriological testing of all platelets may also be applied by BEs as a criterion for the issue of platelets as "culture-negative to date".[6] Suitable methods of sampling and testing may significantly improve the microbiological safety of blood components.

Transfusion-transmitted bacterial infection is related to the quality and safety of the supplied blood component, and as a result should be reported to the national competent authorities. According to the UK's Serious Hazards of Transfusion (SHOT) definition for any TTI, and the recommendation of what to report, cases of bacterial transmission from blood components are reported when cultures from the patient's blood match cultures from the component bag or from the donor.[16]

Reporting confirmed positive bacterial testing where the component has been issued by the BE and transfused to a patient may fall within several specification categories (product defect, equipment failure, human errors, and others).[17]

Blood group serology: Compatibility

Quality issues

International and national bodies[6,15,18] for blood transfusion stress that the aim of any blood transfusion laboratory is to perform the right test, on the right sample, and obtain the right results. In turn this ensures that the right blood component is issued to the right patient. It is essential to obtain accurate results for tests such as ABO/RhD grouping on the donor and on the patient, antibody screening, and compatibility testing. In addition, there must be a reliable process in place for transcribing, collating, and interpreting results.

Errors at any stage of performing tests may lead to incompatible or inappropriate blood being transfused, with significant adverse effects on patients' health (see Box 10.1).

> **Box 10.1 Errors associated with blood group serology[6]**
> - Technical failure in testing.
> - Inadequate procedures:
>   - misidentification of patient or donor samples;
>   - transcription errors;
>   - misinterpretation of results.
> - Combination of factors with the original error being perpetuated or compounded by the lack of adequate checking procedures.

The implementation of a quality management system in hospital blood banks should help to reduce the number of technical and procedural errors made in the laboratory. This system includes the use of SOPs, continuous training, and evaluation of the technical competence of staff, as well as validation of techniques, reagents, equipment, monitoring reproducibility of tests results, and implementing methods to detect errors in the analytical procedure.[6,15,18–20]

The following pre-analytical, analytical, and post-analytical procedures are required:[6]

• It is necessary to ensure and document that the reagents used are in date and have been stored according to specifications.

• The donor samples must be correctly labeled and suitable for the analysis to be performed.

• Appropriate performance checks should be carried out on equipment on a daily basis.

• Analytical procedures must be performed according to the manufacturer's instructions.

An evaluation of quality must be performed on samples before purchasing batches of commercial reagents and validation of data must be provided for all lots of reagents.[6]

Quality control procedures must also be established for equipment, reagents, and techniques in blood group serology. Laboratories undertaking blood group serology testing must participate in a regular external quality assurance program.

Screening of donor blood for ABO/RhD in the BE is obligatory. Testing for clinically significant irregular red cell antibodies is also recommended for first-time donors and for donors with a history of transfusion or pregnancy since the last donation. If the ABO/RhD blood group is verified on a subsequent donation, a comparison should be made with the historically determined blood group. In the event of a discrepancy, the applicable blood components should not be released until it is resolved.[6]

Pre-transfusion testing

The blood of the intended recipient is tested to determine the person's ABO group and RhD type and to detect any clinically significant red cell antibodies. (This procedure is also called "type and screen".) If the screening test is positive, further tests may be required in order to identify the red cell antibodies so that compatible donor units can be selected.[20]

The patient's serum is tested directly in the blood bank for compatibility with the donor red cells before transfusing RBC components (crossmatch). Some countries also require a further check of the blood group immediately before the blood is transfused. The basis for compatibility is a correctly determined ABO and RhD blood type in donor and recipient. When clinically significant erythrocyte antibodies are present in the patient's circulation, only red cells that lack the corresponding antigens should be selected for transfusion.

Compatibility testing between donor red cells and the recipient's serum must be carried out in all cases with irregular erythrocyte antibodies. Although this is recommended as a routine procedure even when no antibodies have been found, it may be omitted if other measures are taken to guarantee safety.[6,9] Compatibility testing should include a sufficiently reliable and validated technique to guarantee detection of irregular erythrocyte antibodies, such as the indirect antiglobulin technique.

A type and screen procedure, when used as a replacement for compatibility testing, must include the following:[6]
• A reliable and validated—preferably by computer—checking procedure when the blood units are delivered.
• Test cells that cover all antigens, preferably homozygous, corresponding to the vast majority of clinically important antibodies.
• Sufficiently sensitive techniques for the detection of erythrocyte antibodies.

• Laboratory records of tests performed and of the disposition of all units handled (including patient identification).

Hemovigilance data and recommendations

Hemovigilance data related to testing donor blood in the BE and patient's blood and compatibility in the hBB show that the following are all common in laboratory pre-transfusion testing and in the clinical process: misidentification of the patient; wrong sampling and wrong labeling; mistakes in ABO/Rh grouping and compatibility testing because of equipment testing failures; errors in choice of SOPs; SOPs designed inappropriately; false negative results; and human errors.

In SHOT's database for Incorrect Blood Component Transfusion (IBCT), information is required for any laboratory errors concerning deviations from SOPs or testing protocols in the BE and hBB.[18] For example, blood grouping errors related to reagent/equipment failures, errors in recording results in blood grouping technique, antibody screening, antibody identification, LISS tube suspension, and so on all need to be recorded.[18] Furthermore, crossmatching errors, crossmatching techniques, and failure in checking for suitability for electronic issue of blood components should also be verified.[18]

In TRIP's Annual Report for 2007, partial administration took place in one patient of a blood component that had showed weak positive reaction in the direct antiglobulin test and upon crossmatching. Ignorance of hospital policy and failure to crossmatch blood was also noted when selecting a blood component for a child younger than one year of age.[15] In SHOT's Annual Report for 2008,[18] procedural deficiencies were predominant in a grand total of 200 laboratory-related errors, while mistakes in testing accounted for 31 errors (15.5%). Laboratory errors resulted in 39 "wrong blood" incidents, of which 20 occurred in an emergency setting while 29 occurred outside normal working hours. Of the 39 errors, 4 involved the wrong sample being tested, 5 were ABO grouping errors, and 11 were errors in D-typing; there were 14 cases of incorrect component selection and 4 cases in which units were labeled incorrectly by the laboratory.[18] One more case involved a series of procedural deficiencies for the transfusion of two patients with a similar name in two different hospitals. Fortuitously, the two patients had the same blood group and a negative antibody screen.[18]

Commenting on trends, the Annual Report stresses the significant increase in the number of "wrong blood" events, reflecting the general increase in reporting of all categories of events. The increased errors are largely in D-typing and D-typing component selection.[18] Recommendations were made by SHOT for laboratory procedures to be validated and for laboratories to be revisited following an error as part of corrective and preventive actions. It is also recommended that competency assessment in laboratories must be linked to process.[18]

SKAE reports that serious adverse reactions due to ABO incompatibility because of incorrect blood component transfused are rare.[12] Two deaths in 5,506,237 blood components transfused have been recorded, one from immunological hemolysis due to ABO incompatibility and another attributed to hyperagglutination syndrome. The frequency of transfusion of wrong blood to the wrong patient was 1:115,500 red cells units in 1997–2009. These errors arose mostly because of pre-marked sampling tubes and the failure to verify identity in the ward or operating theater. Out of 41 cases of Incorrect Blood Component Transfused (IBCT), wrong sampling and labeling and misidentification of the patient accounted for 49% and 44%, respectively. Wrong blood grouping and compatibility mistakes accounted for 4%. Mistakes in laboratory pre-transfusion testing are mostly attributable to human error. During the same period, 55 cases of incompatibility due to other alloantibodies (anti-C, anti-Cw, anti-e, anti-Kell, anti-JK^b, anti-Duffy^b, anti-Lewis^b, and unclassified allo-antibodies) were reported.

Analysis and prevention of errors in pre-transfusion testing are described in the EU Manual of Optimal Use of Blood.[20] Compliance with technical requirements and documentation of all steps in the process, understanding of what can go wrong, why it goes wrong, and an action plan for the prevention and avoidance of errors are key methods for any hemovigilance system. Audits of practice and investigation of complaints are additional methods for identifying errors, adverse events, and adverse reactions.[20]

Error management

TRIP has estimated that up to half of all serious transfusion reactions are preventable with the currently available methods.[15] Most human and system errors responsible for causing adverse reactions and adverse events associated with blood transfusion could be prevented if appropriate measures were implemented.[21,22] For example, electronic systems based on barcode-reading technologies and automated laboratory equipment with electronic interfacing reduce the risk of manual transcription and transposition errors.

A team approach and appropriate error-management tools such as "process control" to ensure that all preceding critical steps have been accomplished successfully are key factors in the risk-management process.[23,24]

The Council of Europe emphasizes the role of the Hospital Transfusion Committee (HTC) as a necessary structure for risk assessment and management.[6] The HTC should ensure that every adverse reaction associated with blood and blood products is fully investigated by a Hospital Transfusion Laboratory (HTL) and reported back to the producing BE.[6] The HTC should provide an active forum for communication between clinical and laboratory staff involved in blood transfusion, to provide solutions and education in relation to problems identified and to ensure that transfusion activities accord with best practice.[6] In this context, reporting of near-miss errors is considered to be a valuable audit tool because they often have the same root causes as actual transfusion accidents, as well as being an educational aid.[25]

SKAE estimates that most adverse reactions are preventable if appropriate measures are implemented. In its 2008 report,[12] SKAE recommends that the following safety measures should be implemented:

• The HTC is responsible for the application of safety measures in blood sampling, ordering, patient identification, and the continual

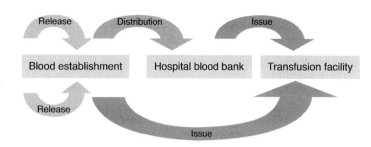

Figure 10.2 The different release/ distribution/issue scenarios. Reproduced from Reference 17 with permission from European Commission – Health and consumers directorate – General, Public Health and Risk Assessment, Unit C6 – Health Law and International.

supervision of the patient by experienced medico-nursing staff in the course of transfusion.
- Barcode-reading technologies are to be used.
- Automated laboratory equipment is to be used.
- The electronic issue of blood from the laboratory without conventional serological crossmatching is to be implemented.

Issuing and transport

The issuing and transport links in the transfusion chain are defined in EU Directives, 2002/98/EC, 2005/61/EC, and 2005/62/EC. Figure 10.2 depicts the different scenarios for release, distribution, and issue.[17]

Issuing components

General considerations

Ensuring that the correct blood component is released from the BE, distributed to the hBB,[4] and then issued to a clinical department or a transfusion facility[3] for transfusion to the correct patient is paramount in preventing adverse events, notably incidents.[5,6,19] Electronic or manual systems should be in place to check the component's unique blood number, the recipient's name and other patient identifiers, blood type, expiration data, crossmatch status or other serologic information, documentation of status of visual inspection, time and date of issue, and person to whom it is issued (or location if sending by pneumatic tube).[5,6,19]

When the component is issued to an individual, that person should conduct a second check on the correctness of the component information (label, computer, or manual log information) and manu-ally provide a signature or use an electronic badge or personnel identification number. If all checks are correct, the unit may be issued.[5,6,19]

Issuing components to more than one patient at a time is not recommended. If multiple components are required for immediate transfusion, then it is acceptable to use a validated cooler to help prevent component-recipient mix-ups before transfusion.[5,6,19]

Release of blood components

The Council of Europe recommends that each BE should be able to demonstrate that a blood component has been formally approved for release by an authorized person, preferably assisted by validated information technology systems. The specifications for release of blood components must be defined, validated, documented, and approved by quality assurance.[6]

Directive 2005/62/EC requires that there should be a system of administrative and physical quarantine for blood and blood components to ensure that they cannot be released until all mandatory requirements set out by the Directive have been fulfilled.[4]

In the absence of a validated computerized system for product status control, the following items are necessary:
- The label of a blood components should identify the product status and clearly distinguish a released from a non-released (quarantined) product.[4–6]
- Records should demonstrate that before a component is released, all current declaration forms, relevant medical records, and test results have been verified by an authorized person.[4–6]

Before the final release of blood or blood components that have been prepared from a repeat donor, a comparison with previous records should be made to ensure that current records accurately reflect that donor's history.[6]

Where release is subject to computer-derived information the following points should be checked:

• The computer system should be validated for full security against the possibility of releasing blood and blood components that do not fulfill all test or donor selection criteria.

• The manual entry of critical data, such as laboratory test results, should require independent verification by a second authorized person.

• There should be a hierarchy of permitted access to enter, amend, read, or print data. Methods of preventing unauthorized entry should be in place, such as personal identity codes or passwords that are changed on a regular basis.

• The computer system should block the release of all blood or blood components considered not acceptable for release. There should also be a means of blocking the release of any future donation from the same donor.[6]

In the event that a final product fails release due to a confirmed positive infection test result or any other potential impact on patient safety, all other implicated components should be identified and appropriate action taken.[4–6] Other components from the same donor must be identified and donor records updated immediately to ensure that the donor cannot make a further donation.[4–6]

Distribution

Directive 2005/62/EC imposes that procedures for distribution should be validated to ensure blood and blood component quality during the entire storage period and to exclude mix-ups between blood components.[4]

Blood components should be inspected visually before distribution. There should be a record identifying the person distributing and the customer receiving the components. Unused blood components should not be returned for subsequent distribution, unless the procedure for their return is regulated by a contract and it can be proved that the agreed storage conditions have been met for each component returned. Before subsequent distribution, the records should indicate that the blood component has been inspected before re-issue.[6]

Notification of adverse events

Adverse events related to the processes of release and distribution of blood and blood components should be reported to the competent national authority. They may fall under various specification categories as follows.

Product defect

As regards distribution, confirmed positive bacterial testing needs reporting, where the component has been issued by the BE and transfused to a patient.

Equipment failure

The following aspects need reporting:

• Release of a component that did not fulfill the release requirements (donor, tests, product specifications, storage).

• Release of a component from a donor deferred for reasons related to recipient safety.

• Release of a rejected component.

• Distribution of an expired blood component, a non-released component, a component showing signs of deterioration, a rejected component.

• Distribution of a blood component after detection of a safety risk or serious quality deviation (not destroyed or recalled).

• Transport under inappropriate conditions.

• Distribution of a special-requirements blood component to the wrong hospital.

• No recall after post-donation information.

Human error

The following human errors need reporting:

• Release of a component that did not fulfill the release requirements (donor, tests, product specifications, storage).

• Release of a component from a donor deferred for reasons related to recipient safety.

• Release of a rejected component.

• Distribution of an expired blood component, a non-released component, a component showing signs of deterioration, a rejected component.

- Distribution of a blood component after detection of a safety risk or serious quality deviation that should have led to destruction or recall.
- Transport under inappropriate conditions.
- Distribution of a special-requirements blood component to the wrong hospital.
- No recall after post-donation information.

Other
See Reference 17

At the time of issue[26]
Before a unit of blood is issued, hBB personnel need to complete the following steps:

1 The record that identifies the intended recipient and requested component are reviewed.

2 The name and identification number of the intended recipient, the ABO, and Rh type of the donor unit, and the interpretation of compatibility tests (if performed), are recorded on a transfusion form for each unit. This form (or a copy of it) becomes a part of the patient's medical record after the transfusion is given, but it need not necessarily be attached to the unit.

3 A tag or label with the name and identification number of the intended recipient, the component unit number, and the interpretation of compatibility tests (if performed) must be securely attached to the blood container.

4 The appearance of the unit is checked before issue and a record made of this inspection.

5 The expiration date, and time if applicable, is checked to ensure that the unit is suitable for transfusion.

6 The name of the person issuing the blood, the name of the person to whom the blood is issued, and the date and time of issue are recorded.

Transportation

Transportation of blood components
It is essential to maintain proper storage temperature during transportation. The temperature limit for refrigerated blood components is up to 10°C (50°F) during transportation, although the preferable range is 1–6°C (34–42°F).[27]

Chain of traceability
Blood components are usually transported for one of four reasons:
- to supply a hospital with blood products;
- to redistribute blood components that are nearing expiry to large hospitals for transfusion (so they do not go out of date);
- to accompany a patient en route to another facility;
- to transport components within a hospital to the patient care area.

Records that maintain the chain of traceability must be kept so that it is possible to trace all blood components from their source to final disposition.[28]

Quality requirements
Here are some quality requirements and advice to be observed:
- Validated shipping containers are critical to this process. They are necessary to ensure that blood components remain within environmental specifications at all times. The shipping container must be labeled with at least the following information:
  ○ contents;
  ○ origin;
  ○ destination;
  ○ cautions or descriptions for containers holding dry ice.
- Some hospitals and regions choose to place temperature monitoring devices in each shipment of blood and blood products in order to provide evidence that environmental specifications have been met.
- Visual inspection of each blood component to be shipped must be performed and documented. Any components that do not meet the criteria must not be shipped.
- An issue voucher or transfer record must be included with all transported blood components. This must indicate the following information:
  ○ name of the facility receiving the blood components;
  ○ unique tracking number for the shipment;
  ○ type of blood components in the shipment;
  ○ donation number of each blood component;
  ○ total number of items shipped;

○ date and time of shipping;

○ special instructions pertaining to this shipment or the units in it;

○ signature of the person responsible for packing the shipment.

• Platelet components must be agitated continuously and should not be used if agitation has not occurred for more than 24 hours. It follows that transportation of these components cannot take longer than 24 hours from the time the product leaves the blood supplier.

• SOPs must specify the training requirements for handling and transportation of components. All training must be documented and compliance with SOPs must be assessed regularly.

• Transportation between facilities should not exceed 24 hours.[28]

References

1 European Union, 2002, Directive 2002/98/EC of the European Parliament and of the Council of 27 January 2003 setting standards of quality and safety for the collection, testing, processing, storage and distribution of human blood and blood components and amending Directive 2001/83/EC. *Official Journal of the European Union* 8.2.2003: L33/30.

2 European Union, 2004, Commission Directive 2004/33/EC of 22 March 2004 implementing Directive 2002/98/EC of the European Parliament and of the Council as regards certain technical requirements for blood and blood components. *Official Journal of the European Union* 30.3.2004: L91/25.

3 European Union, 2005, Commission Directive 2005/61/EC of 30 September 2005 implementing Directive 2002/98/EC of the European Parliament and of the Council as regards traceability requirements and notification of serious adverse reactions and events. *Official Journal of the European Union* 1.10.2005: L256/32.

4 European Union, 2005, Commission Directive 2005/62/EC of 30 September 2005 implementing Directive 2002/98/EC of the European Parliament and of the Council as regards Community standards and specifications relating to a quality system for blood establishments. *Official Journal of the European Union* 1.10.2005: L256/41.

5 European Union, 1998, Directive 98/79/EC of the European Parliament and of the Council of 27 October 1998 on in vitro diagnostic medical devices (O) L 331.7.12.1998. http://eur-lex.europa.eu/LexUriServ/LexUriServ.do?uri=CELEX:31998L0079:EN:HTML [accessed February 24, 2012].

6 Council of Europe, 2008, Guide to the Preparation, Use and Quality Assurance of Blood Components, Recommendation R (95) 15. 14th edition. Council of Europe Publishing, Strasbourg.

7 Fiebig EW, and Busch M, 2008, In *Technical Manual*, Roback JD, Combs MR, Grossman BJ, Hillyereds CD, *et al.* (eds). American Association of Blood Bank 16th edition; pp. 241–78.

8 Drug Administration, 1996, Current good manufacturing practices for blood and blood components; Notification of consignees receiving blood and blood components at increased risk for transmitting HIV infection. *Fed Regist* **61**: 47413–23.

9 Food and Drug Administration, 2007, Current good manufacturing practice for blood and blood components: Notification of consignees and transfusion recipients receiving blood and blood components at increased risk for transmitting HCV infection ("lookback") final rule. *Fed Regist* 48765–801.

10 Goldman M, and Long A, 2000, Hepatitis C lookback in Canada. *Vox Sang* **2**: 249–52.

11 Van der Poel C, and Janssen MP, 2006, *Collection, Testing and Use of Blood and Blood Components in Europe.* Council of Europe Publishing, Strasbourg

12 Politis C, Richardson Cl, Damaskos P, *et al.*, 2008, Hellenic Coordinating Haemovigilance Centre, Summary report Epidemiological surveillance of transfusion transmitted infections (TTIs) (1996–2007), surveillance of adverse reactions (ARs-TR) and adverse events (AEs-TR) associated with blood transfusion (1997–2007), surveillance of adverse reactions (ARs-DN) and adverse events (AEs-DN) during or after donation (2003–2007), Athens.

13 Politis C, Kavallierou L, Asariotou M, *et al.*, 2010, Surveillance of transfusion transmitted infections in 1996–2008 in Hellas: The impact of individual NAT testing on blood safety. *Vox Sang* **99**: 279.

14 Politis C, Asariotou M, Koumarianos S, *et al.*, 2009, Look back programme for HIV seropositive blood donors in Hellas. *Vox Sang* **96**(1): 142.

15 Schipperus M, Wiersum J, Tilborgh J, *et al.*, 2007, *TRIP Annual Report.* http://www.tripnet.nl/pages/en/documents/TRIPAnnualreport2007.pdf [accessed February 24, 2012].

16 SHOT, 2009, Definition of current SHOT categories and what to report. http://www.shotuk.org/wp-content/uploads/2010/04/SHOT-Categories-2009.pdf [accessed February 24, 2012].

17 European Union, 2009, Common approach for definition of reportable serious adverse events and reactions as laid down in the blood Directive 2002/98/EC and Commission Directive 2005/61/EC version 02, **2**:11 (internal working document available only to national competent authorities).

18 Taylor C, Asher D, Davies T, *et al.*, 2009, *SHOT Annual Report 2008*. SHOT Office, Manchester Blood Centre, Manchester, UK.

19 Australian and New Zealand Society of Blood Transfusion Inc., 2002, Guidelines for pre-transfusion testing. 4th edition. http://www.anzsbt.org.au/publications/index.cfm

20 McClelland DBL, Pirie E, and Franklin IM, 2010, *Manual of Optimal Blood Use, Support for safe, clinically effective and efficient use of Blood in Europe*. EU Optimal Blood Use Project 2010.

21 Institute of Medicine, 1999, *To Err Is Human: Building a Safer Health System*. National Academy Press, Washington DC, USA.

22 McClelland DB, and Phillips P, 1994, Errors in blood transfusion in Britain: survey of hospital haematology departments. *Br. Med. J.* **308**: 1205–6.

23 AuBuchon JP, 2006, How I minimize mistransfusion risk in my hospital. *Transfusion* **46**: 1085–9.

24 AuBuchon JP, 2007, Process controls to avert mistransfusion. *ISBT Science Series* **2**: 253–6.

25 Metcalfe M, Keighley L, Jackson BR, *et al.*, 2005, Clinical audit in the speciality of transfusion medicine. NHS Trust. http://www.cmft.nhs.uk/directorates/labmedicine/clinicalgov/docs/posters/Clinical%20Audit_Transfusion%20Medicine.pdf [accessed February 24, 2012].

26 Lockwood W, Leonard J, and Liles S, 2008, *Technical Manual*. American Association of Blood Bank 16th edition, pp. 283–99.

27 The Stationary Office, National Blood Service, 2005, Guidelines for the blood transfusion services in the UK, 7th edition. http://transfusionguidelines.org.uk/Index.aspx?Publication=RB&Section=25&pageid=580 [accessed February 24, 2012].

28 Canadian blood services. Clinical guide to transfusion. http://www.transfusionmedicine.ca/resources/books/vein-vein/pretransfusion/transportation-blood-components [accessed February 24, 2012].

CHAPTER 11

Clinical Activities: Medical Decision-making, Sampling, Ordering Components, Administration, and Patient Monitoring

Clare Taylor

Former Medical Director of SHOT, Manchester Blood Centre, Manchester, UK

Introduction

The safety of blood transfusion concerns the entire process of delivering transfusion-related care to patients. Originally, hemovigilance started as a way of recording numbers of cases and data trends for recognized and defined adverse physiological reactions in patients receiving blood and blood components. In the UK the blood safety initiatives that arose during the first five years in which Serious Hazards of Transfusion (SHOT) collected data focused mainly on reduction of viral and bacterial transmissions by blood components, precautions against vCJD transmission, irradiation, and donor selection to reduce Transfusion Related Acute Lung Injury (TRALI).[1]

Over the years a great deal of resource has been invested in the safety of the blood component itself, with the involvement of regulators and the setting of standards by both external agencies and internal governance in blood establishments and hospitals. The result has been a measurable and significant reduction in the risks of transfusion transmitted infection, such that blood components are safer than they have ever been, and vastly safer than many licensed pharmaceutical agents.[2] The rate of virus transmission in the developed world is probably lower than it has ever been.[3] In addition measures in the UK, now also being put in place in other countries, have reduced the incidence of TRALI.[4] However, there is a paradox in spending vast sums on reducing the already extremely low risk of a therapy or medication when it is frequently used unnecessarily or inappropriately.[5]

More recently overall transfusion safety has been addressed, in particular the noninfectious hazards and the impact of human error. The decision to transfuse is poorly taught and documented, and there are few data from controlled trials to aid standardization of this part of the process. Several studies have documented that wrongly labeled samples are frequent, and more worryingly, "wrong blood in tube" samples continue to occur. The bedside administration of blood components is another frequent focus of errors that puts patients at high risk.

Education and training of medical staff, nurses, and other staff groups involved in the transfusion process is of paramount importance. Blood components are intrinsically extremely safe, but they must be used properly. In all hemovigilance

Hemovigilance: An Effective Tool for Improving Transfusion Safety, First Edition. Edited by René R.P. De Vries and Jean-Claude Faber.
© 2012 John Wiley & Sons, Ltd. Published 2012 by John Wiley & Sons, Ltd.

systems, human error is a major cause of adverse events.[6]

Reporting of error-based adverse incidents to hemovigilance systems

The category for "incorrect blood component transfused" (IBCT) has been used by SHOT to categorize incidents relating to blood that was transfused in error, intended for a different patient, or of the incorrect group due to laboratory error. This original core material collected by hemovigilance systems has gradually evolved and the scope has broadened. In particular the IBCT category has expanded to include errors of clinical decision-making, inappropriate or unnecessary transfusions, and knowledge-related mistakes, even though initially these were not actively requested by SHOT.[7] Also, handling and storage errors (breaches in the cold chain in clinical or laboratory areas) were gathered in this category by the UK's SHOT scheme.

In 2008 the SHOT report separated out inappropriate and unnecessary transfusion (I&U) and handling and storage errors (HSE) into completely separate categories. Incorrect transfusions due to errors in phlebotomy, laboratory testing, and issue or ward based errors remained as true IBCT events.

This widening of scope brings hemovigilance into the arena of good medical practice, medical education and training, as well as competency, and levels of knowledge and skills. Communication breakdown, between individual members of staff and different professional groups, is a recurrent theme of events in these categories. Although some errors and mistakes may be prevented by proper knowledge of and adherence to guidelines and protocols, clinical practice is complex and the exercising of informed clinical judgement of individual cases is not always readily addressed by such documents. Barcode readers and other IT systems may help to prevent some forms of human error, but are not a panacea.

This chapter highlights the different types of errors that occur in the clinical area and are reported to hemovigilance systems; cases and trends from SHOT are used in each section.

Figure 11.1 shows the incidence of error-related reports: IBCT, I&U, and HSE, and

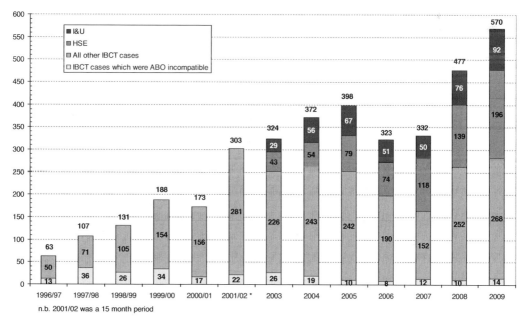

Figure 11.1 Error-related reports to SHOT from 1996 to 2009.

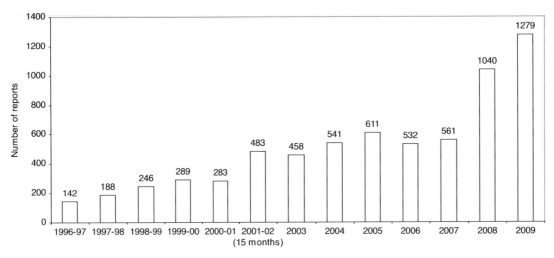

Figure 11.2 Total SHOT reports 1996 to 2009.

ABO-incompatible transfusions, in 13 years of SHOT reporting from 1996 until 2009. HAS and I&U were not collected as separate categories until 2008, but the figures for 2003 onwards were extracted retrospectively. Prior to that, the separation of data for those categories was not possible, hence the contour of the histogram. The dip in reporting in 2006 and 2007 follows the introduction of the EU Directive,[8] implemented as the Blood Safety and Quality Regulations (BSQR) 2005 in the UK.[9] Since 2007 reporting in these error-related categories has returned to join the previous curve and to increase at the predicted rate.

Overall SHOT reporting has increased very substantially because SHOT has commenced a campaign to increase awareness of transfusion errors, and striven to make reporting easy, accessible, and user-friendly, with an increase in constructive feedback to reporters (see Figure 11.2).

Categories of errors relating to clinical activities

Errors can occur in any of the stages of the clinical transfusion process as listed in Box 11.1. The three focal points for errors are the decision to transfuse, the collection of blood samples for pre-transfusion testing, and the bedside administration of components. These areas need to be recognized as critical in delivering safe transfusion care to patients, and must be embraced by the professions involved as key tasks.

Box 11.1 The clinical transfusion process

- The decision to transfuse:
  - clinical evaluation of the patient;
  - evaluation of laboratory results;
  - knowledge and experience.
- Informing the patient and documentation:
  - informing the patient about benefits and potential risk of transfusion;
  - discussion of possible alternative strategies (with colleagues and patient);
  - documentation of reason for transfusion in patient notes.
- Obtaining the patient sample for pre-transfusion testing
  - patient wristband *in situ* bearing at least three unique identifiers;
  - positive verbal identification of the patient;
  - labeling of sample tube at the bedside with three unique identifiers, plus signature;
  - use of electronic barcode reader to match wristband and print label if available.
- Ordering the component(s):
  - written (request form) or verbal request to laboratory must include at least three unique patient identifiers;
  - details of special component requirements, e.g., irradiated or CMV negative cells;

- ○ urgent or emergency requests must be telephoned to the laboratory, invoking hemorrhage protocols if required;
  - ○ details of indication for request, transfusion history, obstetric history, recent blood results, known hematological conditions.
- Collecting the component:
  - check the patient's identification details on the documentation against the patient compatibility label on the blood component;
  - documentation of removal of the component by paper or electronic system.
- Checks before commencing transfusion:
  - check that the component has been prescribed by a physician, including dose and rate of administration;
  - check for any special requirements in the notes or on the prescription;
  - check the expiry data and time of the component, and visually check the unit for discoloration etc.;
  - check the donation number on the component and the compatibility label;
  - **check the patient identification using three unique identifiers on the patient's wristband and the patient compatibility label on the component;**
  - ensure these checks are fully documented with staff names and signatures in the notes, on the prescription chart, and on the traceability tag.
- Monitoring during transfusion:
  - record baseline measurements of temperature, pulse, and blood pressure;
  - repeat the observations 15 minutes into the transfusion;
  - repeat according to patients condition and/or local guidance;
  - record time of completion and observations at finish of transfusion.

In this arena, hemovigilance extends far beyond an audit function (i.e., evaluation of compliance with an agreed set of standards) because it identifies problems, errors, and deviations during parts of the process that are not easily protocol-driven.

Decision to transfuse

In the SHOT Annual Report 2009, there were 92 cases in the category of I&U transfusion[10] (see Table 11.1). This has been a new category since 2008, because previously such cases were reported sporadically under the IBCT heading. The cases

Table 11.1 Categories of 92 cases of inappropriate or unnecessary transfusion reported to SHOT in 2009.

Category of I&U transfusion	Number of cases reported to SHOT in 2009
Transfusions based on wrong results	53
Clinical causes of falsely low Hb value	36
Laboratory causes of falsely low Hb value	6
Unknown cause of erroneous count	3
Falsely low platelet count	8
Transfusion given based on poor knowledge, incorrect decision-making, or poor prescribing	37
Excessive rate or volume transfused to a child	8
Red cell transfusion to Hb above normal range	7
Inappropriate transfusion for hematinic anemia	6
Transfusion of incorrect components due to lack of knowledge	10
Other	6
Undertransfusion	2
TOTAL	92

reported are undoubtedly only a fraction of the errors and mistakes in clinical practice that occur, but tend to be those in which there was a degree of patient harm rather than purely a breach of good medical practice. In a review in 2006 of ten years of SHOT reporting, it was stated that these cases were not encompassed by SHOT at the time, though the role of wrong clinical decision-making was acknowledged together with erroneous, misdocumented, and misinterpreted results.[11]

Most cases of inappropriate and unnecessary transfusion were the result of errors of judgment, lack of knowledge, or lack of procedural awareness among medical staff (56 cases across all categories). These errors were made predominantly by junior doctors, but included those made by more senior doctors and consultants. A further 18 cases were of "clinical" origin, although exactly which staff group was primarily involved is unclear (doctor, nurse, possibly phlebotomist). Ten of these were phlebotomy-related problems (diluted or drip arm samples), but it is not known who took the samples. There were also cases illustrating problems of confusion between types of component, and clinical requirement for components. In five cases there were communication failures between the laboratory and the clinical teams regarding the need to repeat inadequate (short, clotted, clumped) samples. There were two cases of undertransfusion owing to multifactorial clinical errors, including communication and knowledge (see below).

In ten cases there was clear responsibility for the error in a member of the nursing staff; four of these cases involved transfusion of blood to an infant or small child at a volume and/or rate which was much greater than that prescribed. There was one case of an excessive rate of transfusion of red cells to an adult. A fatal case was multifactorial, involving a mislabeled Hb sample that had been taken by a member of the nursing staff. Four further cases involved incorrect verbal relay of Hb results and misinterpretation of instructions in notes.

Hospital hematology laboratories were responsible for eight cases of inappropriate or unnecessary transfusion by issuing incorrect results to clinicians before checking for clots, platelet clumping, or short sample errors.

In many medical schools, certainly in the UK, there is very little, or even no, curriculum time available for education about clinical indications for blood transfusion, as well as little formal training about the specific use of different blood components. There appears to be a tendency for clinical evaluation of individual patients to be obscured by uncritical appraisal of laboratory results, with transfusion therapy based upon these alone. These problems are compounded by the lack of good quality clinical trials about indications for the proper use of blood components.

As stated above, the cases reported to SHOT are generally at the extreme end of a spectrum of possible scenarios for this type of error.

There were two deaths in which the transfusion of red cells possibly or probably contributed to the death. The cases often include more than one error as in Case 1 below in which there is a mislabeled full blood count sample, and a clinical failure of initial evaluation of the patient and review. There is a clear overlap between inappropriate transfusion and the occurrence of Transfusion Associated Circulatory Overload (TACO), which should be a condition that is possible to predict and avoid in many patients.

Case 1

A patient was admitted and a sample for FBC was taken by a member of nursing staff. The hospital policy for positive ID of the patient was not followed and the sample tube was labeled with a different patient's details. (The report does not state whether a transfusion sample was mislabeled at the same time, only that both patients were group O D positive.) The patient's true Hb was 10.9 g/dL and there was no indication of bleeding or hemolysis. The incorrect patient's Hb was 6.0 g/dL and based on this, a 3-unit transfusion was prescribed without querying the surprisingly low result. The patient suffered acute pulmonary complications with a drop in pO₂, and the transfusion was stopped. A CXR post-transfusion may have indicated TACO or TRALI. The patient deteriorated rapidly and died. The report stated that the death was considered to be possibly related to transfusion.

The second fatality below illustrates the consequences of communication failure, in which the person relaying the message perhaps did not have sufficient knowledge or understanding to know its importance. At the same time the doctors on the ward round did not, from a clinical perspective, assess the results to be inaccurate. No clinical assessment seems to have been made, nor basic observations. In any patient it is very rarely appropriate to transfuse 4 units of red cells back to back without review and repeat sampling—perhaps only in cases of massive active hemorrhage. It is possible that the outcome might have been different had venesection been carried out once the very high Hb was discovered.

Case 2

Following abdominal surgery a patient fell in the ward and fractured her femur. Her most recent previous Hb was 15.9 g/dL. On testing a new FBC sample, the biomedical scientist called the ward, gave an Hb of 6.1 g/dL, and requested another sample because he thought the result was incorrect. However, the result was passed to the medical team on the ward round by a nurse who did not mention the need to repeat the test. On the basis of the erroneous result, even though clinically there was not extensive bleeding, a 4 unit red cell transfusion was ordered by the consultant, and all 4 units were given without further review. The patient's Hb was 20.2 g/dL before surgery on the following day, and the anesthetist was aware of this. The patient developed cardiac failure and died. This was thought to be probably related to the excessive transfusion.

The next five cases are some typical examples in which the excessive volumes transfused posed a potential or actual risk to the patient, rather than being inappropriate purely on the basis of compliance with national guidelines or protocols.

Case 3

An elderly patient had coffee-ground hematemesis and melena, and a crossmatch request for 4 units of red cells was made. The Hb dropped but was at no time lower than 10.7 g/dL and the patient remained cardiovascularly stable throughout. All 4 units of red cells were transfused resulting in a post-transfusion Hb of 16.2 g/dL.

The junior doctor who prescribed the blood was perhaps inexperienced in assessing bleeding patients and worried by the visible blood loss. Hospitals should use the National Guidelines, for example those available from the Scottish Intercollegiate Guidelines Network[12] and local protocols and training should reflect this aspect.

Case 4

A 79-year-old female patient with CMV colitis weighing 91.5 lbs (41.5 kg) had a Hb of 6.7 g/dL. She was given a 4 unit red cell transfusion resulting in a post-transfusion Hb of 18.1 g/dL.

Case 5

A 2-year-old girl was admitted with peritonism, (possibly ruptured appendix, later found to be a ruptured tumor). Hb was 6.7 g/dL and the surgical team decided to transfuse, writing a dose of 15 ml/kg in the notes. The junior

doctor wrote up 2 units and she was given 2 adult bags over 6 hours. Hb was 18.6 g/dL post-transfusion.

Junior doctors require knowledge of the appropriate dose of red cells to correct Hb to safe levels in adults, taking account of the size of the patient, whether there is active ongoing blood loss, and comorbidities. Poor clinical assessment of the patient and the degree of blood loss continues to be a cause of overtransfusion.

Case 6

A patient was admitted for a liver biopsy and became hypotensive 2 hours after the procedure. The Hb was 7.7 g/dL (pre-procedure Hb not given) and the patient was transfused 2 units on three separate occasions over the next three days. In total 6 units of red cells were administered. No monitoring of the patient's laboratory parameters took place. A subsequent Hb was 17.1 g/dL. The patient died and no further clinical details or test results are available.

A recurrent problem is the unnecessary transfusion of patients with chronic nutritional or hematinic deficiency anemias, who should be managed without transfusion unless they are severely symptomatic.

Case 7

A GP detected an Hb of 6.6 g/dL in a young woman with chronic menorrhagia and referred the patient to the Emergency Department. The junior doctor there asked advice of the locum specialist trainee doctor who said to go ahead and transfuse, but the case was not discussed with a hematologist.

Undertransfusion

There have been very few cases of patient harm from undertransfusion reported to SHOT to date, but these cases have been actively requested only in the 2010 reporting year. It is probable that this is a more common occurrence but that it is not well documented. Data on something that does not happen can be difficult to collect. In 2010 in the UK a new Rapid Response Report (RRR) on transfusion of blood components in an emergency was produced from the NPSA[13] following reports of 11 deaths and 83 incidents between 2006 and 2010 where the patient suffered harm as a result of delays in the provision of blood. The cases were evaluated together with the SHOT team, and the causes of the problems were identified as process failures, communication failures, and logistic difficulties.

A similar problem was identified in France in a retrospective study of anesthetic-related deaths that took place in 1999.[14] Most frequent were deaths associated with intraoperative hypotension and anemia, and once again these were found to be related to deviation from standard practice and organizational failure.

It may be that there are a significant number of suboptimal outcomes in bleeding patients, whether intra-operative or emergency, because of delays in transfusion of appropriate blood components. Hemovigilance systems should develop mechanisms for collecting this important data, which may be causing more excess deaths than all other adverse incidents combined.

Sample collection

Errors at this stage, in particular collection of the sample from the incorrect patient, can result in ABO-incompatible transfusion with the potential for a fatal outcome. An estimate from the USA suggested that 15% of ABO-incompatible transfusions arose from phlebotomy errors.[15]

In 2002 the ISBT Working Party for Safer Transfusion carried out a large international audit of nearly 700,000 samples from ten countries including data from 62 hospitals.[16] It was found that 1 in every 165 samples was mislabeled and 1 in every 1986 was miscollected resulting in WBIT. The rates of error were similar in all the countries submitting data.

A study from the National Haemovigilance Office (NHO) in Ireland[17] analyzed 759 near-miss events from ten hospitals, reporting that sample collection was the most high-risk step in the transfusion process and was the first site of error in 62% of events. Of these, 13% involved samples taken from the incorrect patient, with medical staff frequently being implicated.

This finding was echoed in the "Near Miss" pilot study performed by SHOT in 2008,[18] which was carried out because previous near-miss SHOT data pointed to sampling as a focus point of errors.

In phase 1, data were analyzed on 8535 rejected samples out of 224,829 samples received in 121 hospital laboratories in the UK during April 2008. The key findings were as follows:

- The average rate of rejection of samples across the UK was 3.8% with 76% of those samples being rejected due to missing or incorrect information.
- Overall 40% of hospitals in the UK allow relabeling of incorrectly labeled samples.
- 32% of rejected samples were taken by medical staff, 25% by nurses or midwives.
- 27% of rejected samples arrived outside of core hours (generally 0800–2000 hours).
- 19% of rejected samples were received from the Emergency Department, 19% from Obstetrics & Gynaecology, and 30% from general wards.

Many hospitals have adopted the concept of "zero tolerance" toward sample errors, and insist that an erroneous sample is re-taken, but it is clear that nearly 40% of hospitals across the UK, and 50% in Wales and Scotland, still allow amendments to be made prior to testing. Of particular concern are the 271 cases (3.2% of all rejected samples) where samples have been relabeled despite not knowing who had performed the original venipuncture and labeling.

The bulk of incorrect samples where it is recorded who performed the venipuncture are taken by medical staff (31%), followed by midwives (15%) and nurses (10%). In 38% of mislabeled samples it was not documented who took the sample. Although at present there is a lack of denominator data regarding the overall breakdown of who bleeds patients for transfusion samples, it is felt that the proportion of medical staff involved in these errors is high.

In phase 2 the focus was on sample errors detected by the laboratory quality management system (QMS) after acceptance for testing. Of 214 samples included in the six-month study, 123 were samples from the correct patient but with incorrect details, while 90 were completely mislabeled "wrong blood in tube" samples with potential for ABO-incompatible transfusion and fatal outcome. The majority (74) were detected because of historical data held in the laboratory, and those remaining by various serendipitous routes. As before, the sample errors detected after acceptance for testing originated predominantly with medical staff (45%), with fewer from midwives (15%), nurses (14%), and phlebotomists (10%). The percentage of sample errors attributed to medical staff seems disproportionately high, and it would be necessary to obtain denominator data as to what proportion of all samples are taken by which groups of staff.

Wrong Blood in Tube (WBIT)

WBIT means the taking of a sample for transfusion from a different patient than the one whose details are then written on the tube label.

The causal errors and problems identified in WBIT cases reported to SHOT include:

- not checking patient ID verbally or by wristband;
- labeling the filled tube away from the bedside;
- using a computer-generated sticky ID label on a (pre-labeled) tube;
- deployment of staff not trained or familiar with standard procedures;
- reliance on bedside technology without full understanding.

Case 1

An elderly patient was bled and grouped as B D positive and transfused with 2 units of B D positive cells because of anemia (cause not given). This patient had been bled by a doctor during normal working hours. A subsequent sample grouped as A D positive, which was rechecked and proved to be the correct group. The wrong patient had been bled when the original sample was required. Fortunately the patient did not suffer any ill effects from 2 units of ABO-incompatible blood.

Case 2

A patient with anemia due to malignancy was receiving a red cell transfusion as an outpatient. After <50 ml had been transfused, he developed fever, rigors, and bronchospasm followed by a respiratory arrest 20 minutes after commencement. The transfusion was stopped and he was admitted to the ward and stabilized successfully. Upon investigation it has been discovered that the original group and screen sample had been mislabeled by a trained phlebotomist using a bedside computer-generated label, and it belonged to another patient who was group A D positive. The recipient was group O D positive. This was the patient's first transfusion and so there was no previous transfusion history.

Root causes of sampling errors include both organizational failure and human error. All WBIT errors are preventable if the person taking the sample follows national guidelines and local policy for taking transfusion samples, for instance the British Committee on Standards in Haematology (BCSH) guidelines in the UK.[19] Training must be successfully delivered to all involved staff, and systems must be in place to ensure access to training and to prevent untrained staff carrying out phlebotomy. Despite staff completing their blood transfusion training and competency assessments, work pressures can lead to staff "cutting corners" and losing sight of the reasons for completing a comprehensive ID check.

Ordering components

Once a decision to transfuse has been made, and a sample taken, blood components need to be ordered. The order may be written on a form accompanying the sample, or there may be arrangements in place for telephone or intranet ordering. The order must include as a minimum the three unique patient identifiers, the component(s) being requested, the date and time the components are required, and degree of urgency, and any special requirements. Other information as agreed by local policy will include history and indication, obstetric and transfusion history, recent blood test results, and other details.

There are several types of adverse incident arising from blood ordering errors:

- ordering for the wrong patient or with the incorrect details;

• ordering the wrong type of component due to lack of knowledge and/or communication problems;
• omitting the special requirements for the patient, from lack of knowledge or awareness;
• communication failure regarding the degree of urgency of the order, for bleeding patients.

Special requirements not met (SRNM)

In the 2009 there were 87 SRNM cases reported to SHOT due to clinical errors and omissions (and 67 cases due to laboratory causes).[10] As in previous years the majority of cases related to requests for patients who required irradiated components, but this requirement was not made clear to the laboratory by the clinical staff at the time of requesting the component.

Case 1

A baby who had been the recipient of intrauterine red cell transfusions (IUTs) was given 4 nonirradiated pedipaks of red cells on two separate occasions. The request form did state that the mother had antibodies and that there had been 3 IUTs, but the special requirements were not specified. The prescription form did not specify irradiated blood.

A smaller number of cases related to the non-communication of a requirement for CMV negative components or requiring both specifications. Generally, it appears from the information supplied to SHOT that the doctor ordering the components either did not know of the criteria for irradiated or CMV negative products or was not familiar enough with the patient to realize that this was necessary. Other clinical omissions to make a request for special requirements probably also related to a lack of transfusion medicine knowledge in non-specialized staff admitting patients through the emergency department.

Case 2

A 22-weeks-pregnant patient was admitted via the Emergency Department with status epilepticus and transferred to ITU. The Hb was 6.7g/dL and 2 units of red cells were requested. No diagnosis was given on the request form despite boxes being available to tick (i.e., pregnant yes/no/unsure). The following day it was discovered by transfusion laboratory staff that the patient was pregnant and the units were investigated. One had been, by chance, CMV negative, the other had not.

In 15 of the 87 cases linked with the clinical omission to provide special requirements, a root cause of the problem related to the fact that the patient was undergoing shared care between two hospital sites.

Case 3

A patient known to the hospital had FFP requested which was issued according to the historical blood group—O. However, the patient had received a BMT (for CLL) at another hospital and the blood group had changed from group O to group B. None of the request forms indicated that the patient had had a recent BMT.

Doctors not usually working in hematology or oncology may be required to request blood components for patients despite unfamiliarity with special requirements—this problem arises from shift working and extensive cross covering. This issue has become more significant since implementation of the EU working time directive.[20]

Doctors working in non-hematology specialties, including in the Emergency Department, must be educated sufficiently in transfusion medicine to know that certain patient groups, such as pregnant women and sickle cell patients, have important special requirements for safe transfusion.

Shared care inevitably results in a situation where communication of essential information is required, and there is a risk of communication breakdown. Again this appears frequently to be the result of lack of knowledge of the part of the referring clinicians regarding the transfusion implications arising from the diagnosis or treatment of the shared patient. Detailed information changes hands, but transfusion details may be omitted or the transfusion staff left out of the communication loop.

Administration

The bedside patient identification check is the final barrier to error in many cases of potential mistransfusion, even when the error has originated at an earlier stage in the transfusion process. Staff carrying out this task must understand that, although routine, this is an absolutely critical step. SHOT reporting has found that relatively high proportions of cases of administration error occur out of hours or in emergency situations.[10]

Case 1

An elderly patient was admitted as an emergency during the night with chest pain, ECG changes, chest infection, and iron deficiency anemia, and was deteriorating. A decision was taken to transfuse her but the incorrect unit was collected from the issue fridge of the blood-transfusion laboratory. The patients shared a first name, had a similar surname and date of birth, and were on the same ward. The recipient, who was group A D positive, had recently become unconscious at the time of transfusion and did not have a wristband. She received approximately 150 ml of group AB D positive red cells. She continued to deteriorate and died a few hours later. The report stated that it was not thought that the transfusion contributed to her death.

The single most frequent stage at which an error is introduced is when the component pack is collected from the issue fridge or transfusion laboratory. The beside check, which could prevent transfusion of this incorrect unit, then also fails and a patient receives blood intended for another patient.

Case 2

An elderly man with a lower GI hemorrhage was undergoing angiography and required emergency transfusion. A nurse took the correct documentation with her to collect the blood but did not check it formally and collected a unit for another patient with the same last name. This incorrect unit was handed to the nurse in theater who checked the unit only against the accompanying compatibility form, not against the patient's wristband. The patient, who was group B D negative, received 150 ml of group A D positive blood but did not suffer any adverse reaction. He proceeded to surgery the same day with no problems.

Although professional responsibility must be taken at every stage by the personnel involved, the final barrier to wrong blood administration is at the bedside, and this cannot be overemphasized. Patient identification is at the root of a large number of errors in hospitals—not only in transfusion practice, but also in drug administration, investigations, operative procedures, and so on. It is essential that formal bedside patient identification becomes second nature to all healthcare personnel whenever they are involved with delivery of individualized patient care.

Box 11.2 Component administration errors

- Errors in following process for collection of components:
  - poor knowledge and recognition of different component types;
  - failure to act appropriately on discovering an "unlabelled" component;
  - deployment of unqualified staff to collect components;
  - use of inappropriate documentation, or no documentation, to collect component.
- Failures of bedside checking procedure:
  - no checking done at bedside;
  - misunderstanding that ID "checking" can be performed remotely from patient's side;
  - checking against paper documents being substituted for cross check with patients ID wristband;
  - failure to check for special requirements, e.g., irradiation or CMV negative;
  - failure to observe prescribed dose and rate of transfusion;
  - failure to check expiry date and time;
  - omission of visual check of components.
- Non-recognition of a transfusion reaction:
  - lack of understanding of the imperative to monitor patients receiving blood components;
  - failure to recognize a transfusion reaction, due to insufficient knowledge or experience;
  - not responding appropriately when a patient suffers a reaction, due to lack of appreciation of the potential seriousness.

The bedside check has a role not only in correct patient identification, but also in prevention of other errors and omissions, such as ensuring that special requirements are met (see page 134), the unit is within its expiry date and time, and the visual appearance of the component is normal.

Patient monitoring

Observation and monitoring of the patient receiving the transfusion is a crucial part of the process and a key contributor to overall transfusion safety for patients. Even the most severe reactions may not be life-threatening if they are detected immediately, the transfusion stopped, and appropriate action taken. Although morbidity and mortality from transfusion in developed countries is low, this could be reduced still further by rigorous monitoring of patients at this crucial time. UK guidelines from the BCSH on blood component administration, updated in 2009,[19] state the following:

Our recommendations for *minimum* patient observations during transfusion episodes now include baseline measurement of respiratory rate. The importance of an early (15-minute) check on pulse rate, blood pressure and temperature with each component administered, repeated not more than 60 minutes after the transfusion is completed, and regular visual observation throughout the transfusion is re-emphasized. It is now recognized that adverse reactions may manifest many hours after the transfusion is completed. We recommend that patients, such as day cases, discharged within 24 hours of transfusion are issued with a *contact card* giving 24-hour access to clinical advice (as commonly used for outpatient chemotherapy).

This statement followed exactly the recommendations from SHOT in 2008[21] based on data on acute transfusion reactions (ATR). In 2008 the time between commencement of the implicated transfusion and the start of the reaction was noted in 274 cases, with an average of 66 minutes, with a range of <1 minute to 440 minutes (7 hours and 20 minutes). Crucially 199 reactions (72.6%) occurred more than 15 minutes after commencing the transfusion, which highlights the need for proper regular monitoring of the patient and

the requirement for transfusions to be carried out where there are sufficient trained staff to observe the patient. In 2009 there were 400 ATR cases reported, 366 of which gave the time of onset of the reaction. The median time was 45 minutes after commencement of the transfusion, with a median for anaphylactic reactions of 15 minutes, and 60 minutes for febrile reactions. This emphasises the need for close observation of patients throughout the period of transfusion.

National Comparative Audits of blood transfusion, UK

In the UK, the Royal College of Physicians and the blood services have joined together to perform a number of National Comparative Audits of blood transfusion practice.[22] The audit of bedside transfusion practice including blood administration and monitoring has been carried out several times over a number of years, the most recent being in 2008. This audit of 6943 transfusion episodes from 180 hospitals found that 10% (891) of patients were put at risk of an undetected transfusion reaction or a delay in detecting a reaction, because baseline observations were not recorded prior to starting the transfusion. Observations during blood transfusion were not done for 12% (1118) of patients, placing them at risk of an undetected transfusion reaction, even if they had baseline observations recorded. Over one-third of patients did not have their observations checked at the end of the transfusion. These results suggest that there is not widespread implementation of the BCSH guidelines on blood administration and raises the question of what is an optimal way to monitor a transfused patient.

In addition, in the opinion of the auditors, only 64% of patients could readily be observed. In certain hospitals patients are in side wards and cannot be observed at all times, and since the last BCSH guidelines were published the design of hospitals has changed and many more are being built with single rooms. This increases the risk to patients of suffering a transfusion reaction undetected, or detected late, and may be a particularly worrying issue at night when staff numbers are lower.

Since the series of audits commenced in 1995 the number of patients having observations within

30 minutes during transfusion has increased from 59% to 73%, but the number of patients having no observations recorded at all is unchanged at about 12%.

Under-reporting

This is a problem in any vigilance system, and reporting rates in hemovigilance are no exception. Variability in reporting rates is found between different countries and reporting systems, and within regions and institutions within a country.[3] Under-reporting may be attributed to various reasons. For an adverse event or reaction to be reported it first has to be recognized as a complication, and be related to the transfusion. Where monitoring is not rigorous, and where staffing levels are low, or education and training adequate, reactions such as fever and hypotension due to bacterial contamination can be wrongly attributed, or missed completely, or worse still a patient death can be thought to be due to underlying disease rather than transfusion.

Inevitably, even assiduous patient monitoring does not improve outcomes for patients unless the data collected is interpreted correctly and acted on appropriately—by stopping the transfusion—and treatment and investigations are carried out in accordance with the clinical picture. Education and knowledge is also therefore a prerequisite in staff carrying out the patient monitoring.

Initiatives to improve clinical transfusion activities

Two themes have emerged regularly from clinical hemovigilance data over the last decade or more. The first is the continued reports of failures of bedside-checking procedures that would have prevented the wrong blood administration; a properly carried out bedside check can prevent a large number of ABO-incompatible transfusions. The second is the prominence of knowledge gaps and lack of training and education in junior doctors; this has been instrumental in the large number of cases of inappropriate or unnecessary transfusion.

Transfusion education and training initiatives in the UK

Transfusion medicine education

In the UK there has been a multi-stranded approach to improving availability and quality of transfusion education for doctors and nurses. Much of this has been driven by the Chief Medical Officer's National Blood Transfusion Committee (NBTC),[23] a subgroup of which is working closely with the Royal Colleges and Specialist Societies to ensure that adequate transfusion medicine education and experience is a requirement across all hospital specialities. A unified curriculum is necessary for junior medical staff in training grades and completion of the module should be mandatory before a certificate of completion of specialist training (CCST) can be achieved. For junior doctors in the foundation years (first and second year after qualification) an e-Learning package has been developed and made available across the UK and is being made mandatory for accreditation and appraisal before entering specialist training grades.[24] The professional qualification and licensing bodies for nurses, midwives, and biomedical scientists need to incorporate transfusion education into the curriculum as a requirement before registration can take place.

Increasing transfusion awareness at managerial and executive level

The Department of Health has spearheaded a Better Blood Transfusion campaign in partnership with the UK blood services and the NBTC, which started in 1998, with further health service circulars directed at Hospital Chief Executive Officers and transfusion professionals in 2002 and 2007.[25]

Blood administration and component training and competency

The National Patient Safety Agency (NPSA) issued a Safer Practice Notice in 2006 (SPN 14)[26] setting out standards for training and competency assessment of all staff of all grades and professional groups that are involved in the administration of blood components. It states that all staff, medical or non-medical, qualified or unqualified, from consultants to medical laboratory assistants (MLAs), operating department assistants (ODAs), and portering staff must be trained and competency assessed before they are permitted to perform a role in the blood transfusion pathway. This includes: obtaining a venous blood sample; organizing the receipt of blood/blood products for transfusion; collecting blood/blood components for transfusion; preparing to administer a transfusion of blood components to patients; and administering a transfusion of blood components. Deadlines for achieving all staff training and competency assessments have been set, and training must be renewed every three years.

National guidelines and protocols

The UK has national guidance for the use of blood components, drawn up by the British Committee for Standards in Haematology and other professional bodies and Royal Colleges.[27] These are evidence-based documents and are used nationwide to underpin local and regional guidance.

Formal clinical handover

A significant number of cases, in several SHOT reporting categories, have occurred out of hours, at times when staffing was reduced for various reasons, or when shift working meant that junior doctors were caring for large numbers of patients with whom they were not familiar.

The European Working Time Directive (EWTD)[20] has been implemented by law across the EU but in many hospitals, certainly in the UK, there have been few practical arrangements put in place to deal with the inevitable problems for patient care that this poses. Proactive new systems are required, and need to be implemented by high-level management to ensure effective handover between shifts and teams, and continuity of patient care. This will not only enhance patient safety and satisfaction, but also reduce unnecessary prolongation of stay due to communication failures.

Despite the reduced hours, hospital doctors are increasingly stressed by being spread thinly over many patients without proper information about the clinical progress and plans for those patients. Sick leave among junior doctors has increased hugely since implementation of the EWTD, and job satisfaction has reduced.[28] A new initiative in the UK spearheaded by the Royal College of Physicians, has developed a cross-disciplinary patient handover tool that allows a rolling update of current care and problems of patients. This is then used as the basis for a formal handover session at times of changing shift or on-call team.

IT solutions

If finances are available, it may at times be worthwhile to invest in a lockable/barcode-protected issue fridge, and satellite fridges that only allow trained and accredited personnel access. This automatically releases only the correct unit of blood on presentation of the patient's details and the details of the member of staff collecting. Although reducing the risk of error, this does not reduce the burden of training and competency assessment, because involved staff must be trained in this process. Computerized refrigerator systems have been particularly effective in reducing errors in hospitals with large numbers of satellite fridges where monitoring of the audit trail, especially with regard to traceability and the cold chain, can be particularly difficult. These systems may extend to barcode readers for increased accuracy of bedside checking, together with ordering, label printing, and entry of monitoring observations.[29] These systems are expensive in terms of capital expenditure and implementation and training time. Such expenditure needs to be fully evaluated in terms of cost effectiveness for blood safety, as well as prioritized against other patient safety interventions in hospitals.

There were 61 reported incidents of IBCT errors relating to IT systems reported to SHOT in 2009, compared with 44 in 2008 and 25 in 2007. As electronic "blood tracking" systems enter more general use, SHOT is starting to receive reports of their misuse leading to IBCT.[10]

IT solutions for patient identification and for documentation of the audit trail for blood components have become more common in recent years. A variety of systems are on the market currently, with more in development. There is an enormous drive toward use of these systems from those who have implemented them successfully, from national advisory groups, and naturally from the manufacturers and retailers of the equipment.

Care must be taken to avoid the inherent problems of this approach, while maximizing the benefit to patient safety. IT-based interventions cannot eradicate error, and indeed do not directly address the problem of human error.

Undoubtedly the occurrence of certain errors can be reduced by appropriate implementation of IT-based checking systems, but new possibilities of error may also be introduced. Over-reliance on IT and believing that it circumvents human error can result in a decrease in understanding of, and engagement with, the transfusion process among the staff involved.

Box 11.3 What IT systems can and cannot do

IT can:
- Match barcodes scanned from different source material.
- Transfer data between parts of the system, parts of the same record, or between records.
- Recall data attached to specific patient ID accurately and completely.
- Print, without transcription error, labels or results on requested patient.
- Be set to produce alarms and warning messages if non-matching data is scanned.
- Display warning alarms and messages according to preset algorithms (e.g., date of birth).
- Allow specific data and high visibility warning flags to be added manually to patient records.

IT cannot:
- Ensure that the correct barcoded item is scanned.
- Ensure that data is transferred between correct records (e.g., merging incorrect patients).
- Ensure that all the patient-specific information recorded is accessed, read, and understood.
- Ensure that labels or results are requested on the correct patient.
- Ensure that alarms, warning messages, and flags are read and heeded.
- Enhance patient safety unless it is used appropriately.

IT systems have a major contribution to make in adding electronic checking at vulnerable steps in the transfusion chain, and can provide accurate and complete data at the relevant stage in the process for consideration by the users; but they cannot prevent human error. Adequate knowledge and skills are no less essential in the presence of a vein-to-vein electronic-tracking system, and education and training must be comprehensive and appropriate to the staff groups involved at each stage. All staff must be familiar with the process, able to carry it out safely (with or without an electronic aid), able to detect deviations from normal situations, and make safe, appropriate decisions as each circumstance arises. In addition, training specific to the use of electronic systems is required.

Professional responsibility

It is of concern that, by concentrating on the many issues surrounding the training and competency assessment of unqualified staff in the transfusion chain, the ultimate and overriding importance of the professional staff groups may be overlooked. Only professionally qualified staff can be held accountable and responsible for the work they carry out. It is also a professional responsibility for individual staff to ensure that they have adequate knowledge, skills, and understanding to perform the tasks that are required of them. It is through the knowledge and vigilance of professional staff that errors in transfusion can be prevented, whether at the time of the decision to transfuse and the prescription of components, in the laboratory, or at the time of blood administration at the bedside. Unqualified staff (i.e., not medical, nursing, or scientific staff) cannot be held responsible for ensuring that the correct component is transfused to a patient.

If properly conducted, the bedside check of patient identification against the intended component would prevent the vast majority of wrong blood episodes. Staff performing bedside checks must take full responsibility for correctly identifying the patient and for ensuring that the unit that they transfuse is the correct unit bearing the correct details of the patient, and that the specification of the unit and the manner of its transfusion are all in accordance with the prescription and clinical indication as documented by the medical staff.

Medical staff must possess sufficient knowledge, skills, and understanding to assess the patient fully and to make a competent decision regarding the necessity to transfuse, the correct component, and the rate of transfusion required. Only junior doctors who have sufficient knowledge to prescribe blood appropriately, effectively, and safely should be permitted to do so. Doctors must satisfy themselves that any laboratory results they use to inform the transfusion decision relate to the correct patient, and have been correctly documented.

It is also a medical responsibility to document the details of the transfusion in the notes together with the clinical indications of transfusion and intended outcome. The transfusion rate and any specific caveats relating to the patient must also be documented, together with any follow-up actions required from other staff. Effective handover is essential when going off duty.

The prescribing of the component on the prescription sheet is only the endpoint in a complex decision-making process in which a large number of variables need to have been taken into account. Who finally prescribes the blood component is therefore a much less important issue than the level of knowledge and skills of the personnel involved in the decision-making process.

Nursing staff are also professionals and fully and individually accountable for their role in transfusion safety. If nurse-prescribing of blood components is practiced, responsibility lies fully with the prescriber, who must have sufficient knowledge and skills for this task. If medical staff members are taking professional responsibility for a patient group directive, an individual prescription, or the treatment plan for a patient, the carrying out of the instruction lies with the medical or nursing staff who complete the action. Unqualified, or student nurses, or staff with no professional accountability, must not be involved in critical steps of the transfusion process.

Future hemovigilance

The inclusion of clinical practice in hemovigilance data is an important step forward in improving the safety of transfusion rather than only safety of blood components. In many developed countries components are now extremely safe, and more than half of the patient harm arising from transfusion arises from human error, in particular knowledge gaps, communication failures, and administrative mistakes.[2] Hemovigilance must continue to monitor clinical transfusion medicine, to gain an insight into areas where improvements can be made. Appropriate or optimal use of blood components is already high on the patient safety agenda, along with education and training. Alternatives to transfusion, however, are also in increasing use, such as cell salvage techniques and pharmaceutical adjuncts to reduce blood loss. Hemovigilance systems need to further expand their scope to collect adverse events data on the use of these alternative strategies.

Analysis of these data will allow standards and performance indicators to be agreed, against which blood component use can be assessed. Protocols for documentation and communication are also essential, because many adverse incidents leading to patient harm from transfusion include one or more administrative failure. Weak links in the process need to be identified and protocols should be tested in practice scenarios in hospitals to ensure that all personnel are aware of their role, of the communication pathways, and to identify any flaws in the agreed system.

Box 11.4 SHOT UK general recommendations for transfusion safety

- Mandatory participation in hemovigilance reporting schemes by all blood establishments and all hospitals where blood is transfused.
- A culture of adverse-event reporting with no fear of disciplinary action, for the improved safety of patients and the education of transfusion professionals.
- Adequate education and training of all staff involved in blood transfusion, linked to career progression where appropriate.
- Continuous review of the whole transfusion process in the light of hemovigilance data to identify areas for improvement of systems or practice.
- Broadening of the scope of hemovigilance to include patient harm from under- or overtransfusion, and to gather data on the use of some alternative strategies, e.g., cell salvage.
- To gather and learn from data from other hemovigilance systems worldwide, through the activities of the International Haemovigilance Network, the EU Commission, and the WHO.

Conclusions

Data from SHOT and from other hemovigilance schemes has demonstrated that human error is responsible for approximately 50% of transfusion-related adverse incidents reports. Although individual error may contribute to this figure, a majority of cases are related to multiple errors due to systems failure and organizational failure. The number of reports that are received by hemovigilance systems is probably still very low compared with the true number of such incidents taking place in clinical areas. It may be that some staff are still wary of reporting adverse incidents of this nature because they feel it may have implications, because of their professional accountability. It is important that a culture of incident reporting is nurtured in clinical areas. The characteristics of the ideal medical event reporting system were defined in a seminal paper by Leape in 2002:[30] nonpunitive, confidential, independent, expertly analyzed, with timely reports and a system oriented approach.

A culture shift in the clinical arena is required so that when a doctor feels unable to handle a clinical scenario, requesting and obtaining appropriate help is easy and negative judgement avoided. Doctors, nurses, midwives, biomedical scientists, and other staff should be encouraged to ask for help and clarification when they recognize that their own knowledge and skills are inadequate for a situation in which they find themselves. Failure to do so could be deemed negligent if an incident occurred. A culture of supportive, friendly surveillance and teamwork needs to be encouraged and nurtured in all clinical and laboratory areas, and any lessons learnt must be shared with the relevant Governance and Risk Management groups and users.

In fact, blood transfusion is one of the safest interventions that a patient may undergo in hospital and the actual rate of severe outcomes, that is, major morbidity or mortality, is very low. A higher incidence of adverse events is reported with pharmaceutical therapies and surgical interventions. In the SHOT report in 2009 there were 73 cases of major morbidity and 12 deaths in which the transfusion may have contributed out of a total of 1279 reports, hence in total 6.7% of patients with serious outcomes. The overall rate of adverse events reported to SHOT is 4.4 per 10,000 components transfused, or 0.04% of components that are implicated in an adverse event or reaction. A report published 2007 from the Netherlands found that 5.7% of patients out of the 1.3 million hospital admissions in 2004 suffered unintentional harm or an adverse event.[31] Worldwide this percentage ranges from 2.9% to 16.6%, according to the US Institute of Medicine's 1999 report "To Err is Human."[32] The rate of ABO-incompatible transfusion in the UK as reported to SHOT has fallen in the years since 1996 when reporting began. This may represent the impact of the collaboration between SHOT, the NPSA, and the National Blood Transfusion Committee, aimed at raising awareness and implementing a raft of strategies to improve bedside transfusion safety.

Hemovigilance systems have been proven to be an excellent tool for identifying areas for improvement of practice in transfusion medicine. Many of the problems identified that relate to human error are in no way specific to the practice of transfusion medicine but are generic problems. The most obvious of these is the perennial problem of patient identification, which is common to all areas of healthcare delivery including investigations, invasive procedures, surgery, and perhaps most importantly the prescribing of pharmaceutical agents.

Hemovigilance has set standards of data collection for patient safety purposes, and other specialties and subspecialties within medicine and surgery would do well to follow suit by developing similar systems.

References

1 Williamson LM, 2002, Using haemovigilance data to set blood safety priorities. *Vox Sang* **83**(Suppl 1): 65–9.

2 De Vries RRP, 2009, Haemovigilance: recent achievements and developments in the near future. *ISBT Science Series* **4**: 60–2.

3 Williamson LM, 2002, Transfusion hazard reporting: powerful data, but do we know how to use it? *Transfusion* **42**: 1249–52.

4 Chapman CE, Stainsby D, Jones H, Love E, Massey E, *et al.*, 2009, Ten years of hemovigilance reports of transfusion-related acute lung injury in the United Kingdom and the impact of preferential use of male donor plasma. *Transfusion* **49**(3): 440–52.

5 McClelland B, and Contreras M, 2005, Appropriateness and safety of blood transfusion. *BMJ* **330**(7483): 104–5.

6 Todd A, 2002, Haemovigilance—closing the loop. *Vox Sang* **83**(Suppl 1): 13–6.

7 Stainsby D, Williamson L, Jones H, and Cohen H, 2004, 6 years of shot reporting—its influence on UK blood safety. *Transfus Apher Sci* **31**(2): 123–31.

8 Directive 2002/98/EC of the European Parliament and of the Council, 8/2/2003. L33/30. http://eur-lex.europa.eu/LexUriServ/LexUriServ.do?uri=OJ:L:2003:033:0030:0040:EN:PDF [accessed February 14, 2012].

9 The Blood Safety and Quality Regulations 2005, http://www.opsi.gov.uk/si/si2005/20050050.htm [accessed February 14, 2012].

10 Taylor C (ed.), Cohen H, Mold D, Jones H, *et al.*, on behalf of the Serious Hazards of Transfusion (SHOT) Steering Group, 2010, The 2009 Annual SHOT Report. http://www.shotuk.org/wp-content/uploads/2010/07/SHOT2009.pdf [accessed February 29, 2012].

11 Stainsby D, Jones H, Asher D, Atterbury C, Boncinelli A, *et al.*, 2006, Serious hazards of transfusion: A decade of hemovigilance in the UK. *Transfus Med Rev* **20**(4): 273–82.

12 Scottish Intercollegiate Guidelines Network (SIGN), 2008, Management of acute upper and lower gastrointestinal bleeding: A national clinical guideline. http://www.sign.ac.uk/pdf/sign105.pdf [accessed February 29, 2012].

13 NPSA Rapid Response Report: The transfusion of blood and blood components in an emergency, http://www.nrls.npsa.nhs.uk/resources/type/alerts/?entryid45=83659 [accessed February 14, 2012].

14 Lienhart A, Auroy Y, Pequignot F, Benhamou D, *et al.*, 2006, Survey of anaesthesia related mortality in France. *Anaesthesiology* **105**: 1087–97.

15 Linden JV, Wagner K, Voytovich AE, and Sheehan J, 2000, Transfusion errors in New York State: An analysis of 10 years experience. *Transfusion* **40**: 1207–13.

16 Dzik WH, and Murphy MF, 2002, An international study of their performance of patient sample collection (abstract), *Transfusion* **42**(Suppl): 26S.

17 Lundy D, Laspina S, Kaplan H, Rabin FB, and Lawlor E, 2007, Seven hundred and fifty-nine (759) chances to learn: A 3-year pilot project to analyse transfusion-related near-miss events in the Republic of Ireland. *Vox Sang* **92**(3): 233–41.

18 Davies T, Taylor C, Jones H, and Cohen H, 2009, Serious Hazards of Transfusion (SHOT) Near Miss reporting, *BJH* **145**(Suppl S1), 45–50.

19 British Committee for Standards in Haematology, 2010, Guidelines on the administration of blood components. http://www.bcshguidelines.com/documents/Admin_blood_components_bcsh_05012010.pdf [accessed February 14, 2012].

20 Council of the European Union, 1993, European Working Time Directive (93/104/EC). http://www.eu-working-directive.co.uk/directives/1993-working-time-directive.htm [accessed February 14, 2012].

21 Taylor C (ed.), on behalf of the Serious Hazards of Transfusion (SHOT) Steering Group, 2009, The 2008 Annual SHOT Report. http://www.shotuk.org/wp-content/uploads/2010/03/SHOT-Report-2008.pdf [accessed February 29, 2012].

22 National comparative audits of blood transfusion. http://hospital.blood.co.uk/safe_use/clinical_audit/national_comparative/NationalComparativeAuditReports/index.asp [accessed February 14, 2012].

23 National Blood Transfusion Committee, UK. http://www.dh.gov.uk/ab/NBTC/DH_103433 [accessed February 14, 2012].

24 http://www.learnbloodtransfusion.org.uk [accessed February 14, 2012].

25 Health Service Circular, 2007, Better Blood Transfusion—Safe and Appropriate Use of Blood. HSC 2007/001. http://www.dh.gov.uk/en/Publicationsandstatistics/Lettersandcirculars/Healthservicecirculars/DH_080613 [accessed February 14, 2012].

26 NPSA, 2006, NPSA Safer Practice Notice 14; Right Blood Right Patient. http://www.nrls.npsa.nhs.uk/resources/?entryid45=59805 [accessed February 14, 2012].

27 NPSA, 2012, http://www.bcshguidelines.com/index.html [accessed February 14, 2012].

28 RCP, 2010, http://www.rcplondon.ac.uk/news-media/press-releases/eu-rules-working-weeks-leading-higher-rates-junior-doctor-sick-leave [accessed February 14, 2012].

29 Pagliaro P, and Rebulla P, 2006, Transfusion recipient identification. *Vox Sang* **91**: 97–101.

30 Leape L, 2002, Reporting of adverse events. *N Eng J Med* **347**: 1633–8.

31 Sheldon T, 2007, Dutch study shows that 40% of adverse incidents in hospital are avoidable. *BMJ* **334**: 925.

32 Institute of Medicine, 2009, To err is human: Building a safer health system. http://www.iom.edu/~/media/Files/Report%20Files/1999/To-Err-is-Human/To%20Err%20is%20Human%201999%20%20report%20brief.pdf [accessed February 29, 2012].

PART 3
National or Regional Hemovigilance Systems

CHAPTER 12

The French Hemovigilance Network: From the Blood Scandal to Epidemiologic Surveillance of the Transfusion Chain

Philippe Renaudier

French Society of Vigilance and Transfusion Therapeutics (SFVTT), Regional Coordination of Hemovigilance, Agence Régionale de Santé Lorraine, 4, rue Piroux, CO 80071, 54036 NANCY cedex, France

Introduction

Hemovigilance is the epidemiologic surveillance system of the transfusion chain that links a blood donor and a blood recipient. Both the word and the concept were created in France in 1992 as the medical response to the so-called "blood scandal." In this chapter, we discuss hemovigilance's epidemiologic basis, the general concept of epidemiologic surveillance, the organization of the French Hemovigilance Network, and its main results.

The blood scandal

The blood scandal (i.e., *l'affaire du sang*) began in April 1991 when doctor and journalist Anne-Marie Casteret published an article in a weekly magazine called *L'événement du jeudi* (now *Marianne*) revealing that knowingly HIV-contaminated blood products had been transfused to hemophiliacs from 1984 to 1985. Subsequently, in 1992, Dr Casteret published a book entitled *Blood Scandal (L'affaire du Sang)*, which refuted the argument that nobody was aware in 1985 that the heating of blood made the virus inactive (see Figure 12.1). The book included evidence that as early as 1983 researchers had put forth this suggestion.[1]

Scientific, commercial and political controversies surrounded French approval of the HIV-enzyme-linked immunosorbent assay (ELISA) and the use of heat-treated blood-clotting factors. From an epidemiologic point of view, France started the implementation of HIV-ELISA on blood donations around the same time as many other countries (see Table 12.1),[2,3] and hemophiliac contamination rates were very similar to other European Union (EU) States (see Table 12.2).[4] However, at the point date of March 31, 1995, 1498 cases out of 2666 HIV contaminations of blood recipients recorded within the EU (i.e., 56.23%) occurred in France.[5] An important reason for this high figure was that, because of a desire to use only domestically obtained blood products, prisoners became a major source of blood from 1983 to 1985.

Such a discrepancy points out the importance of donor selection with regards to infectious risk factors. Although Blood Banks (BBs) were requested to ask donors for their risk factors, they failed to do so because they were opposed with a huge press reaction. In addition, the social context of

Hemovigilance: An Effective Tool for Improving Transfusion Safety, First Edition. Edited by René R.P. De Vries and Jean-Claude Faber.
© 2012 John Wiley & Sons, Ltd. Published 2012 by John Wiley & Sons, Ltd.

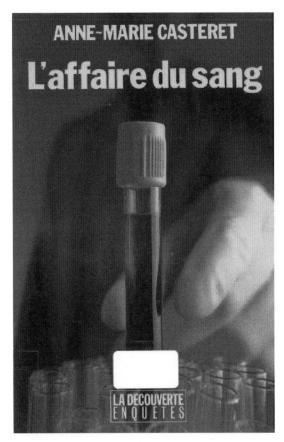

Figure 12.1 Cover of Dr Casteret's book.[1] On December 1987, she published an article "La tragédie des hémophiles" in *L'Express*, a weekly newspaper. In 1990, she wrote several articles in *L'événement du jeudi* and then this book in 1992.

Table 12.1 Date of implementation of HIV-ELISA on blood donations (adapted from[2,3]).

Date	Country
Nov 1984	New Zealand
Jan to Mar 1985	United States of America
Mar 1985	Austria
May 1985	Netherlands and Norway
Jul 1985	Italy (start)
Aug 1985	*France*
Oct 1985	United Kingdom
Nov 1985	Canada
Jan 1986	Denmark

ture, and a judiciary, and argued that these three functions of government should be assigned to different bodies, so that attempts by one branch of government to infringe on political liberty might be restrained by the other branches. The concept of separation of powers can be considered both as a model for the governance of a democratic state and a guide for public-health decisions. Powers for *l'affaire du sang* were decision (politicians), finance (paymasters), and medicine (physicians), and the

Table 12.2 Contamination rates of HIV among European countries during the 1980s.

Country	Hemophiliac patients	Transfused patients
Belgium	0.70	0.90
Denmark	6.66	0.49
France	*7.76*	*2.64*
Germany (FRG)	7.15	0.34
Greece	6.96	0.44
Ireland	8.28	0.00
Italy	4.07	0.52
Luxembourg	7.69	0.76
Netherlands	3.80	0.24
Portugal	3.94	0.74
Spain	13.75	0.65
United Kingdom	8.03	0.16
Mean	**7.20**	**0.81**

Source: European Centre for the Epidemiological Monitoring of AIDS. HIV/AIDS Surveillance in Europe: Report 31 March 1995.

the 1980s was one that was not prepared to face a viral disease being the main public health problem (see Figure 12.2). Interestingly, attention was paid to hemophiliacs rather than transfused patients, irrespective of the contamination rates.

The origin of *l'affaire du sang* can be considered to be a failure of a separation of powers within the public health arena. The concept of power separation is ascribed to the French enlightenment political philosopher Baron de Montesquieu, and appeared in a treatise on political theory entitled "the Spirit of the Laws" (*de l'esprit des lois*) published in 1748.[6] Montesquieu described the division of political powers among an executive, a legisla-

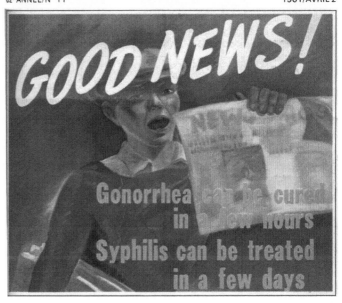

Figure 12.2 Cover of *La Vie Médicale* (*The Medical Life*) from April 1981. *La Vie Médicale* was a magazine popular with medical students who were preparing for the *Internat*, the French exam equivalent of the United States Medical Licensing Examination. The title was written in English—the international scientific tongue for physicians—probably in order to emphasize the scientific aspect of the message. I was a medical student in 1981, and remember myself receiving this issue. It appeared only two months before the Mortality and Morbidity Weekly Report of the CDCs that described the first five cases of AIDS. This discrepancy can be viewed as a reflection of the state of mind in the early 1980s, where infectious diseases were no longer considered to be a public-health problem in developed countries.

collusion of medical and financial powers during the decision process in the 1980s generated a conflict of interest (see Figure 12.3). This situation should always be kept in mind by medical experts.

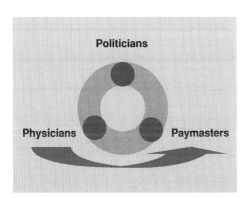

Figure 12.3 The decision process in the blood scandal depicted as the problem of powers separation. To prevent one branch from becoming supreme, systems that employ a separation of powers need a way to balance each of the branches. The National Blood Transfusion Center's physicians argued in favour of the paymasters because of its intrinsic organization, a conflict of interest.

When looking back to *l'affaire du sang*, we can see that it was as a complex event with many different components: that is, medicine, psychology, sociology, law, journalism, and politics. In addition to donor selection, the medical side includes the controversy surrounding the discovery of the Human Immunodeficiency Virus.[7] The psychology and sociology aspects included a desecration and distrust of both medicine and public health in France, a situation described in a book of Doctor and professor of health economics in the University of Paris 1 Panthéon-Sorbonne entitled "the public health failure" (*la défaite de la santé publique*). The legal and political responses were a set of laws and regulations, especially the law reforming the French transfusion system, known as the 1st Kouchner Law.

Epidemiologic surveillance

The noun *surveillance* comes from the French (*sur* = over, *veiller* = to watch) and means watchfulness or monitoring. Epidemiologic surveillance is

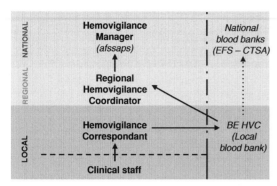

Figure 12.4 The French Hemovigilance Network (HVO = hemovigilance Officer, afssaps = *Agence française de sécurité sanitaire des produits de santé*, EFS = *Etablissement Français du Sang*, CTSA = Centre de Transfusion Sanguine des Armées).

a component of epidemiology aimed at continuously gathering, analyzing, and interpreting data about the current health status of a community or population, and disseminating conclusions of the analyses to relevant organizations. This definition is adapted from the seminal lecture by Dr Langmuir:[8]

> *surveillance, when applied to a disease, means the continued watchfulness over the distribution and trends of incidence through the systematic collection, consolidation and evaluation of morbidity and mortality reports and other relevant data.*

In order to benefit from the epidemiologic background of this concept, it is important not to forget that hemovigilance is in essence a surveillance system.

Surveillance is based on both passive and active data collection processes. In addition, sentinel surveillance systems are reporting systems based on selected institutions or individuals that provide regular, complete reports on one or more diseases occurring ideally in a defined attachment.[9] Vigilance systems such as hemovigilance are generally spontaneous reporting systems, a situation referred to as *passive surveillance* systems. When a clinician or nurse encounters a patient indicating the presence of an adverse effect of a transfusion, there is a legal obligation to report the case to the hemovigilance

officer. The result is a passive monitoring of the levels of the disease in the community and does not provide an exact numerator for incidence rates. *Active surveillance*, on the other hand, is commonly referred to as *case finding*, and occurs when the data necessary to monitor levels of a medical condition are sought out actively. This is accomplished through a variety of means. ABO accidents or red cells allo-immunizations in France can be viewed as active surveillance systems, as can the algorithm used by the University of California San Francisco Medical Center for the detection of Transfusion Related Lung Injuries (TRALI).[10,11]

The French hemovigilance system

The French Hemovigilance Network is managed by the afssaps (*Agence Française de Sécurité Sanitaire des Produits de Santé*, or French health products safety agency) and includes three levels (see Figure 12.4). At the local level, the hospital hemovigilance officer has to notify transfusion adverse effects via a website called "e-fit" and a standardized report form. Then, the information goes upwards to the Regional Hemovigilance Coordinator (RHC) for quality control, and finally to the hemovigilance manager at the national level.

Blood bank hemovigilance officers are physicians or pharmacists in charge of the transfusion safety from the blood donation to the issued Labile Blood Product (LBP) or blood component. Since 2007, they also have to notify to the afssaps incidents that occur during blood donations.

RHCs (*coordonateurs régionaux d'hémovigilance*) are physicians appointed by the regional health authority where they also participate in the general organization of health safety. They ensure that each Transfusion Incident Report (TIR) is completed according to the national guidelines, collect transfusion data in their region, and organize regional meetings for hemovigilance officers.

The Transfusion Incident Report form
The TIR form was created by a working party in 1994 and includes information on the patient as well as the symptoms, biologic investigations, and

the LBP suspected to be involved. In addition, a completion guide ensures the homogeneity of responses from hemovigilance officers. Working parties at the afssaps regularly review both the TIR and the completion guide. No major changes have been necessary since 1994, except for a new definition of Febrile Non-Hemolytic Transfusion Reactions (FNHTR) in 2002 and the addition of the item "TRALI" in October 2001.

Severity grade and imputability levels

Severity or grade has four categories adapted from the World Health Organization (WHO) classification:

- 1 for absence of immediate vital threat or long-term morbidity;
- 2 for long-term morbidity;
- 3 for immediate vital threat;
- 4 for death.

It was subsequently decided that errors resulting in the transfusion of a non-intended LBP without any harm results would also be of interest. The grade scale was recently adapted to correspond with the international definitions and so grade definitions are now as follows:

- 1 for benign;
- 2 for severe;
- 3 for life-threatening;
- 4 for fatal.

Since 2007, the notification of severe events occurring during the transfusion chain, and regardless of whether a LBP has been transfused or not, has begun.

Imputability—a term adapted from pharmacovigilance—is used as a tool to assess the causal relationship between a transfusion and an adverse reaction and includes five categories:

- 4 for certain;
- 3 for probable;
- 2 for possible;
- 1 for doubtful;
- 0 for excluded.

This classification is derived from the WHO causality assessment criteria with the addition of the category "excluded," but with less stringent criteria especially for the dechallenge/rechallenge criteria.

Traceability

Traceability is based on three legal arrangements: (i) each hospital is required to have a unique BB that provides it with the LBP; (ii) each unit of LBP must have a unique identifier; and (iii) each unit of LBP must be attributed to a definite patient. In order to fulfill this last requirement, an issuing form is given every time a LBP is issued. This form includes the identification of: (i) the LBP as defined previously; (ii) the hospital including the ward where the transfusion is planned; and (iii) the recipient (maiden name, last name, first name, date of birth, and sex).

The hospital is required to return a copy of the issuing form to the BB that includes: (i) confirmation that the LBP was effectively transfused to the scheduled patient or its final destination if not transfused (destruction or return to the BB); and (ii) the date and time of the transfusion (or destruction). The hospital also has to record the physician who prescribed the transfusion and the nurse who transfused the patient. Both the BB and the hospital are required to retain the traceability data for 30 years.

Communication of results

The afssaps publishes national data on hemovigilance online in French, and also in English at http://www.afssaps.fr/var/afssaps_site/storage/original/application/bb2a6b52bdb935954bd985d638e0e734.pdf. In addition, a specific topic is studied in the *Bulletin of Hemovigilance* edited by the afssaps twice a year, available online in French and soon in English (http://www.afssaps.fr/Afssaps-media/Publications/Bulletins). The *Etablissement Français du Sang* (EFS, the French blood establishment) also publishes some data on hemovigilance in its annual report (www.dondusang.net).

Every two years the French Society of Vigilance and Transfusion Therapeutics (*Société Française des Vigilances et de Thérapeutique Transfusionnelle* or SFVTT) holds a three-day congress dedicated to hemovigilance, alternately with a one-day meeting on a specific topic (*Journée de Montsouris*) (www.sfvtt.org).

Three times a year, a hospital transfusion safety and hemovigilance committee called CSTH *(Comité*

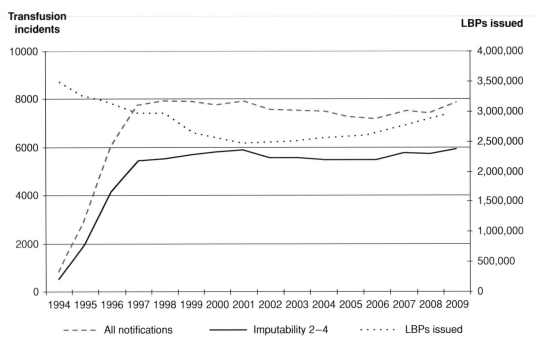

Figure 12.5 Evolution of LBPs issued and transfusion incidents notified.

de Sécurite Transfusionnelle et d'Hémovigilance) joins together the hemovigilance officers of the hospital and of the EFS, the representatives of the administrative staff of the hospital and the EFS, clinicians, nurses, and the RHC.

Selected results from 1994 to 2009

Data collection began on July 1, 1994. The TIR/1000 LBPs issued rate increased from 1994 to 1997 then reached a plateau (see Figure 12.5). The data presented below are based on TIRs with an imputability level of 2 or more (i.e., possibly, probably, and definitely associated with transfusion).

Traceability rates dramatically increased from 1995 to 2005, and reached 99.4% in 2006 (see Figure 12.6). The number of LBPs issued decreased until 2001 and then steadily increased (see Table 12.3 and Figure 12.7).

Transfusion-associated deaths are important to consider because they were the first outcome to be registered for public-health purposes. Because level

2 generally refers to complex clinical presentations where the role of the transfusion is difficult to assess, we present the distribution of diagnostics for imputability levels 3 and 4 (see Figure 12.8). Incidence rates are also presented for imputability greater or equal to level 3 (in Table 12.4). These rates are to be considered as the average for each diagnostic during the study period.

Details of Transfusion Transmitted Non-Bacterial Incidents (TTNBIs) notified in e-fit with the year of transfusion are also presented for imputability levels 3 and 4 (see Table 12.5). In France, HIV-1 and HCV NATs have been implemented on all blood donations since July 2001.

ABO-incompatibilities usually result from the failure to comply with Standard Operating Procedures (SOPs). Since 1965 in France, SOPs include the following requirements: (i) a double-independent ABO-RH typing; and (ii) for Packed Red Cells (PRCs) a "bedside blood compatibility test" i.e., a Beth-Vincent test where the pictures of agglutinations have to be identical between the PRC and the recipient. Nurses are required to

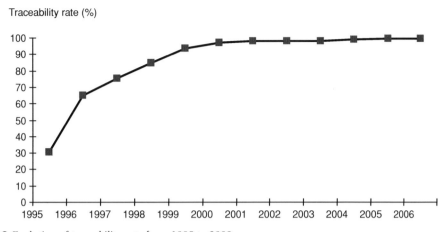

Traceability rate (%)

Figure 12.6 Evolution of traceability rate from 1995 to 2009.

ask for the referent physician in cases of discrepancy to discriminate ABO-compatible from ABO-incompatible transfusion.

Regular training for those who perform transfusions was subsequently implemented in the late 1990s after the first French Hemovigilance Congress.[12] Two successive assessments are available. From 1955 through 1978, 150 immunohemolytic accidents of variable severity have been documented in Lyon, France. An abrupt decrease

in the incidence of ABO accidents has been observed since 1966 (see Figure 12.9).[13] Subsequently, the French hemovigilance data have displayed a steady decrease since the beginning of the 2000s (see Figure 12.10).[14] (Also see http://www.afssaps.fr/var/afssaps_site/storage/original/application/7f856b43ad1bce15d2b5f5665ed3eb9d.pdf.) The sudden decrease observed in 1966 is time-related to the implementation of the two previously mentioned requirements in 1965 and it is not

Table 12.3 Number of LBPs issued in France. PRC: Packed Red Cells; APC: Apheresis Platelets Concentrates; BCPC: Buffy-Coat Platelets Concentrates; FFP: Fresh Frozen Plasma.

	PRC	APC	BCPC	FFP	Total
1994	2,507,803	120,144	80,570	246,666	3,461,349
1995	2,333,538	129,152	71,741	229,388	3,238,504
1996	2,279,979	134,132	44,105	235,813	3,125,706
1997	2,190,301	135,425	57,942	243,421	2,985,583
1998	2,180,777	147,423	46,615	242,612	2,956,653
1999	2,106,006	158,447	42,369	250,110	2,656,517
2000	2,078,342	165,578	32,746	258,782	2,535,565
2001	2,026,726	174,216	25,581	257,763	2,484,454
2002	2,031,737	173,161	24,258	261,521	2,490,781
2003	2,034,123	176,475	24,842	266,459	2,501,921
2004	2,063,613	184,848	26,041	272,118	2,546,636
2005	2,067,191	188,868	34,523	289,306	2,579,888
2006	2,108,807	190,773	43,076	293,402	2,636,058
2007	2,192,810	191,265	55,836	313,459	2,759,121
2008	2,287,350	192,784	62,139	328,562	2,870,835
2009	2,343,804	186,752	76,649	371,658	2,979,117

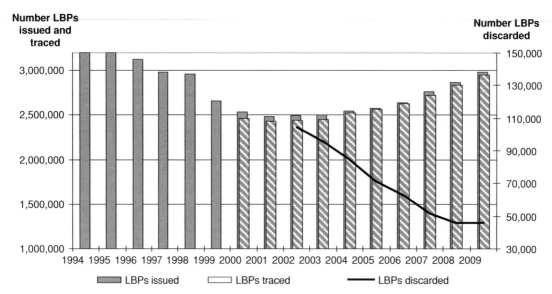

Figure 12.7 Evolution of LBPs issued and discarded.

possible to know the respective contribution of each one, whereas the slow and progressive decrease that persists since 2000 can be viewed as the effect of nurses' continuous training.

Immediate noninfectious pulmonary side effects of transfusion include Transfusion Associated Circulatory Overload (TACO) and TRALI. Because of the recognition that the pathophysiology of TRALI is likely to be due to several different mechanisms, a Canadian Consensus Conference proposed a case definition of TRALI based solely on clin-

ical and radiological parameters.[15,16] The French Hemovigilance data are to be considered according to two periods. From 1994 to 2001, TRALI cases were retrospectively retrieved by using key words on TIRs such as "TRALI," "noncardiogenic pulmonary edema," or "white lung syndrome." Since September 1, 2001, the item TRALI is explicitly present in TIRs and is used as the case definition. In order to avoid immunologic TRALIs, the donors selection criteria have been modified for obtaining LBPs: male gender, or women either without

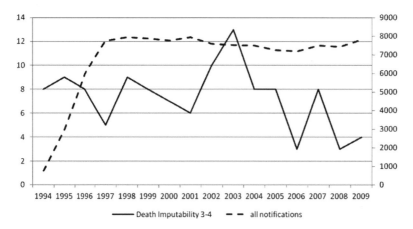

Figure 12.8 Evolution of transfusion-associated deaths.

Table 12.4 Incidence rates of transfusion-associated deaths according to the main diagnostics (the FNHTR case was misclassified by the hemovigilance officer who never modified the TIR).

	1994–1999		2000–2009		1994–2009	
	N	incidence rate 1 for x LBP	N	incidence rate 1 for x LBP	N	incidence rate 1 for x LBP
TACO	13	1,417,255	16	1,649,024	29	1,545,127
TRALI	2	9,212,156	16	1,649,024	18	2,489,372
TTBI	14	1,316,022	10	2,638,438	24	1,867,029
ABO-incompat.	7	2,632,045	7	3,769,197	14	3,200,621
Immuno others	8	2,303,039	8	3,298,047	16	2,800,543
Allergy	0		4	6,596,094	4	11,202,172
FNHTR	0		1	26,384,376	1	44,808,688
Others	3	6,141,437	6	4,397,396	9	4,978,743
Iron overload	0		1	26,384,376	1	44,808,688
Unknown	0		1	26,384,376	1	44,808,688
Sub-total	47	392,007	70	376,920	117	382,980

Table 12.5 Transfusion-transmitted non-bacterial infections.

	1994	1995	1996	1997	1998	1999	2000	2001	2002	2003	2004	2005	2006	2007	2008	2009
HCV	1	4	1	1	2		1	2	1							
HBV						1		1		1			1	1		
HIV		2			1			1	1							
CMV			1	1		2				1		1				1
HAV									1			1				
parvovirus B19		1										1				1
HEV													1			
others		2														
malaria									1				1			
Total	1	7	4	2	3	3	1	4	4	2	0	3	3	1	0	2

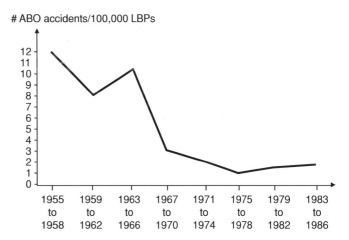

ABO accidents/100,000 LBPs

Figure 12.9 Evolution of ABO-incompatibilities in Lyon, France, from 1955 to 1986 (Adapted from Renaudier *et al.* [12] with permission from CFC).

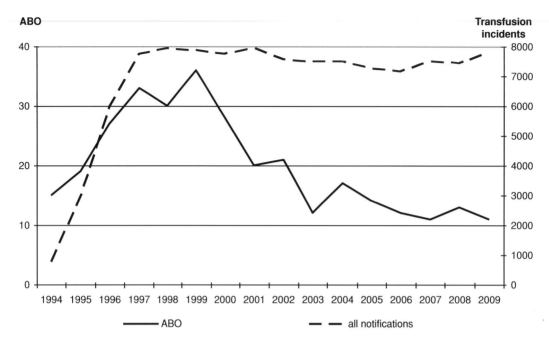

Figure 12.10 Evolution of ABO-incompatibilities since 1994 in France.

children or with children but without anti-HLA. Those not eligible are proposed for a plasmapheresis program for fractionation.

Nevertheless TRALI cases still increase (see Figure 12.11). However, the simultaneous increase of notified TRALI and TACO cases is likely to reflect the clinical staff and hemovigilance officers' better awareness rather than a true increase. Indeed, hemovigilance is a passive surveillance system and data cannot be used as a tool for incidence rates estimation, an indicator properly computed by active surveillance systems such as the one developed by the University of California-San Francisco/TRALI Study Group.[10,11,17] The main results are a special patient's profile, that is, a high disease burden and the absence of notified cases with pooled fresh-frozen plasma inactivated by solvent-detergent.[18-20]

Conclusion

Hemovigilance in France is both an epidemiologic surveillance system and a component of transfusion safety. Hemovigilance has also been a situation

for benchmarking in other fields and indirectly contributed to the reinforcement of the quality of care.

Acknowledgements

This chapter is dedicated to my colleagues, hemovigilance officers, and regional coordinators of hemovigilance for their continuous involvement in tracking information and improving transfusion safety.

I thank Maï-Phuong Vo Maï, PhD, who analyzed the national database and the staff of the afssaps hemovigilance unit: Nadra Ounnoughene, MD, Imad Sandid MD, Karim Boudjeriz MD, and Monique Carlier MD. Sylvie Schlanger, MD, reviewed the manuscript. I am also indebted to my colleagues at the SFVTT, especially Bernard Lassale, MD (Marseille), Mr Nicolas Artéro, SFVTT Webmaster (Marseille), Laurence Augey, MD (Lyon), Martine Besse-Moreau, MD (Limoges), Cyril Caldani, MD (Nice), Anne Damais-Cepitelli, MD (Le Havre), Gérald Daurat, MD (Montpellier),

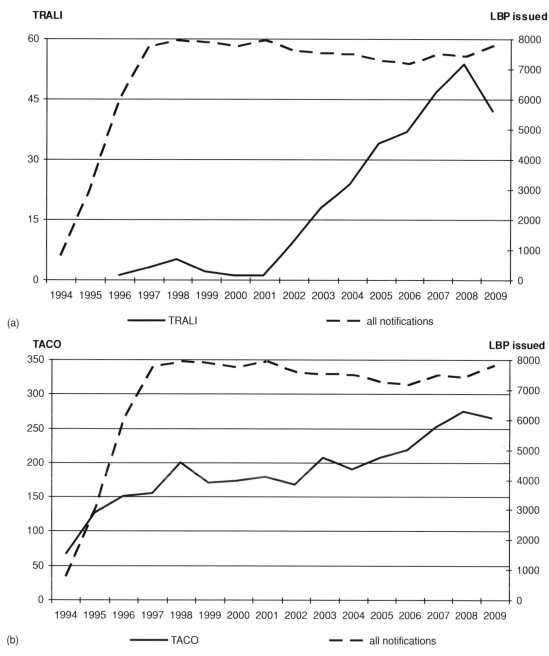

Figure 12.11 (a) Evolution of lung complications of transfusion: Transfusion Related Acute Lung Injury (TRALI); (b) Transfusion Associated Circulatory Overload (TACO).

Igor Galpérine, MD (Frontenac), Hervé Gouezec, MD (Rennes), Mrs Brigitte Le Corvaisier, chief-nurse (Clermont-Ferrand), Silvana LEO-KODELI, MD (Orléans), Mr Patrice Teterel, chief-nurse (Le Havre), Xavier Tinard, MD (Vandoeuvre-lès-Nancy), Françoise Viry-Babel, MD (Nancy), to Jean-Patrice Aullen, MD who initiated the French Hemovigilance Network, to Annie J Sasco, MD, PhD, my mentor at the International Agency for Research on Cancer, and to Mrs Béatrice Borel, my secretary.

A special thanks to Mr Jean-François Bénévise, General Director of the Agence Régionale de Santé-Lorraine, for his comments and suggestions.

References

1 Casteret AM, 1992, *L'affaire du Sang [The Blood Scandal]*. Editions La Découverte, Paris [in French].

2 Manuel C, Auquier P, and San Marco JL, 2000, [The drama of blood contamination in France. An approach to public health]. *Presse Med.* **18**: 547–52 [in French].

3 Manuel C, and Auquier P, 1996, [Look Back on the Blood Scandal]. *La Recherche* **288**: 22–31 [in French].

4 Weinberg PD, Hounshell J, Sherman LA, Godwin J, Ali Ba S, *et al.*, 2002, Legal, financial and public health consequences of HIV contamination of blood and blood products in the 1980s and 1990s. *Ann Intern Med* **136**: 312–9.

5 Morelle A, 1996, [*The Public Health Failure*]. Flammarion, Paris [in French].

6 de Secondat, Charles-Louis, Baron de La Brède et de Montesquieu, 1989, *De l'esprit des lois [Spirit of the Laws]*. Cohler AM, Miller BC, and Stone HS (eds). Cambridge Texts in the History of Political Thought. Cambridge, Cambridge, UK.

7 Barre-Sinoussi F, Chermann JC, Rey F, Nugeyre MT, Chamaret S *et al.*, 1983, Isolation of a T-lymphotropic retrovirus from a patient at risk for acquired immune deficiency syndrome (AIDS). *Science* **220**: 868–71.

8 Langmuir AD, 1963, The surveillance of communicable diseases of national importance. *N Engl J Med* **268**: 182–92.

9 Lee LM, Teutsch SM, Thacker SB, and St Louis ME, 2010, *Principles and Practice of Public Health Surveillance*, 3rd edition. Oxford University Press, New York.

10 Finlay HE, Cassorla L, Feiner J, and Toy P, 2005, Designing and testing a computer-based screening system for transfusion-related acute lung injury. *Am J Clin Pathol.* **124**: 601–9.

11 Finlay-Morreale HE, Louie C, and Toy P, 2008, Computer-generated automatic alerts of respiratory distress after blood transfusion. *J Am Med Inform Assoc.* **15**: 383–5.

12 Renaudier P, Vial J, Augey L, Garin L, and Moskovtchenko JF, 1997, [The role of the Hospital Hemovigilance Officer]. *Techniques Hospitalières* **618**: 52–6 [in French].

13 Juron-Dupraz F, Betuel H, and Jouvenceaux A, 1982, [Immunohemolytic complications observed during transfusion of more than 2 million units of blood]. *Rev Fr Transfus Immunohematol.* **25**: 101–4 [in French].

14 Renaudier P, Vo Mai MP, Schlanger S, *et al.*, 2007, The declining risk of ABO incompatibilities: Twelve years of haemovigilance in France. *Blood* **118**(Suppl 1): 851A.

15 Goldman M, Webert KE, Arnold DM, Freedman J, Hannon J, Blajchman MA, and TRALI Consensus Panel, 2005, Proceedings of a consensus conference: Towards an understanding of TRALI. *Transfus Med Rev.* **19**: 2–31.

16 Kleinman S, Caulfield T, Chan P, Davenport R, McFarland J, *et al.*, 2004, Toward an understanding of transfusion-related acute lung injury: Statement of a consensus panel. *Transfusion* **44**: 1774–89.

17 Toy P, Gajic O, Bacchetti P, Looney MR, Gropper MA, *et al.*, for the TRALI Study Group, 2012, Transfusion-related acute lung injury: Incidence and risk factors. *Blood* **119**: 1757–67.

18 Ozier Y, Muller JY, Mertes PM, Renaudier P, Aguilon P, *et al.*, 2011, Transfusion-related acute lung injury: Reports to the French Haemovigilance Network 2007 through 2008. *Transfusion* **51**: 2102–10.

19 Renaudier P, Rebibo D, Waller C, Schlanger S, Vo Mai MP, *et al.*, 2009, [Pulmonary complications of transfusion (TACO-TRALI)]. *Transfus Clin Biol* **16**: 218–32.

20 Renaudier P, Schlanger S, Vo Mai MP, Ounnoughene N, Breton P, *et al.*, on behalf of the French Haemovigilance Network, 2008, Epidemiology of Transfusion Related Acute Lung Injury in France: Preliminary Results. *Transfus Med Hemother* **35**: 89–91.

CHAPTER 13

The Japanese Hemovigilance System

Hitoshi Okazaki, Naoko Goto, Shun-ya Momose, Satoru Hino, and Kenji Tadokoro
Department of Research and Development, Central Blood Institute, Blood Service Headquarters, The Japanese Red Cross, Tokyo, Japan

History of the Japanese Hemovigilance System

Since launching the blood bank in the Japanese Red Cross (JRC) Central Hospital in Tokyo in 1952, the Japanese Red Cross Society (JRCS) has been the sole provider of the blood service until now. Because hemovigilance is a relatively new concept, there was no such term when considering the safety of donors and patients who received transfusion at that time. However, the Tokyo blood bank attached the "Transfusion Reporting Document" to each blood product for transfusion to collect data on transfusion reactions from the very beginning. In the 1960s, when paid donation was common, almost half of the blood recipients developed serum hepatitis. Yellow blood, so-called because the blood appeared yellow with low hemoglobin concentration and was associated with jaundice, became a serious social issue, particularly when the American ambassador to Japan, Edwin O. Reischauer, was hurt by an attacker and required transfusion of a massive amount of blood, and later developed hepatitis. The Japanese Cabinet decided to change from paid donation to 100% nonremunerated donation, and this was achieved in only five years. Hepatitis B virus (HBV) and hepatitis C virus (HCV) were subsequently discovered; however, the implementation of laboratory testing for these viruses markedly decreased the number of transfusion-transmitted hepatitis cases (see Figure 13.1).

In 1984, the first case of Transfusion Associated Graft-Versus-Host Disease (TA-GVHD) was reported in Japan and the subsequent vigorous investigation elucidated that TA-GVHD occurs even in non-immune compromised patients. This fatal complication caused by labile blood products reinforced the need for an effective system for gathering information about adverse events. Universal X-ray/gamma-ray irradiation of blood products has effectively eliminated this fatal reaction. This achievement further underlined the importance of establishing a national vigilance system for transfusion reactions. In 1992, the JRCS started to produce factor VIII products. This also prompted us to establish a nationwide medical representative (MR) system to identify undetected complications. MRs are usually pharmacists or laboratory technicians who visit hospitals to exchange information and data between hospitals and JRC blood centers.

The reporting system for donor complications was established in 1982. The growing awareness of the safety of blood donation prompted nurses to report complications in donors to the headquarters.

Thus, Japanese hemovigilance spontaneously developed in the JRCS as a result of the growing social awareness of the safety of donors and patients in the Society. In the meantime, the JRCS launched the voluntary reporting system for transfusion complications in 1993, leading the world in the hemovigilance field. Although the government had already set guidelines for the manufacturing of blood products and transfusion practice through

Hemovigilance: An Effective Tool for Improving Transfusion Safety, First Edition. Edited by René R.P. De Vries and Jean-Claude Faber.
© 2012 John Wiley & Sons, Ltd. Published 2012 by John Wiley & Sons, Ltd.

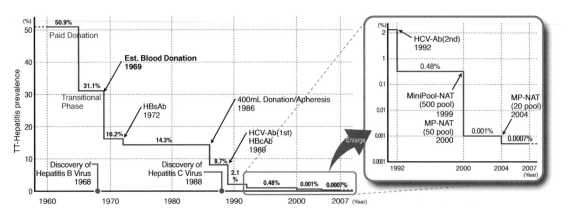

Figure 13.1 Prevalence of transfusion-transmitted hepatitis.

the existing Pharmaceutical Affairs Law (1960), the Product Liability Law was implemented in 1995, which also covers blood products.

Legal basis

The JRCS independently established the hemovigilance system in 1993, and the Japanese government notified in the same year that Good Post-Marketing Surveillance Practice should be implemented. Complying with the revised version of the Pharmaceutical Affairs Law, the organization of the JRCS was reformed and the Blood Service Headquarters (BSHQ) was established to replace the Blood Service Division in October 2004. The BSHQ in the JRCS has been realigned to meet the new licensing requirements for "marketing approval holders" following the April 2005 enactment of amendments of the Pharmaceutical Affairs Law. A Marketing Supervisor General position was established in the BSHQ and a Safety Management Supervisor in the "Safety Supervision Unit" and a Quality Assurance Supervisor in the "Quality Assurance Unit" appointed under the supervision of the Marketing Supervisor General. The "Ministerial Ordinance on Standards for Post-marketing Safety Supervision for Drugs, Quasi-drugs, Cosmetics and Medical Devices; Good Vigilance Practice (GVP)" was enforced simultaneously with the amendment of the Pharmaceutical Affairs Law.

Compliance to GVP is the licensing requirement for marketing approval holders, and we have been performing appropriate operations in accordance with GVP since April 2005.

Setting up the hemovigilance system

Because the JRCS is the only manufacturer of labile blood products in Japan, the government (Ministry of Health, Labour and Welfare; MHLW) and the JRCS should coordinate with each other and share information. Regarding the safety of blood products, this relationship between the government and the JRCS works. In 2003, the revised Pharmaceutical Affairs Law was enforced and the so-called Blood Law was enacted. This law more clearly defines the responsibility of the government, local governments, the manufacturer, and users of blood products.

The hemovigilance system was set up from its inception as a voluntary reporting system for adverse reactions and infections following transfusion. Reports on errors and near-misses, related to not only transfusion but also all other medical procedures, are collected through voluntarily participating hospitals to other independent administration agencies under the governance of the MHLW; this system is operated separately from the JRC system because we do not intend to enlarge our hemovigilance system to the surveillance of transfusion errors and near-misses.

Adverse events following transfusion are reported by hospitals through over 150 MRs nationwide assigned in JRC blood centers. The adverse event notification form and reporting form are submitted by hospital doctors, and MRs collect these forms from the hospitals and then send them to the headquarters. These forms are used for transfusion-transmitted infections and other adverse reactions/events. Because blood products in Japan are regulated by the Pharmaceutical Affairs Law, the JRCS BSHQ is also classified as a pharmaceutical company and has a responsibility to act in accordance with the law. In this sense, hemovigilance is part of pharmacovigilance. We do not actually define the types of adverse event, because some newly recognized adverse events may occur at any time. Because we must keep up to date with advances in the field of transfusion medicine, adverse reactions were classified by JRCS specialists including medical doctors.

We have been gathering data on donor adverse events from each blood center at the headquarters since 1982. Initially, the reporting system was paper-based, but it has been computer-based since mid-2004. In Japan, donor interview is performed by a medical doctor. Thus, at least one medical doctor is on standby in case of emergency at each blood donation site, such as a mobile bus or a donation clinic. However, not all reactions, particularly late reactions, are preventable; hence, the government established a no-fault relief system for donor adverse events.

Governance of the hemovigilance system

The Safety Supervision Unit of the JRCS BSHQ is responsible for data validation and analysis. Regarding the validation of data, the imputability of an adverse reaction needs to be validated. In the JRCS hemovigilance system, this validating procedure should be evaluated on the basis of objective data if possible. In order to make this possible, rigorous effort has been made to collect samples from

recipients and donors. Regarding donor samples, repository samples have been collected from all the donations and stored for 11 years since 1996.[1] Regarding patient samples, we first ask hospitals to provide us with samples in exchange for a free test to investigate the causes of adverse events or infections. This is the key step in assessing the imputability of a complication particularly in cases of transfusion-transmitted infections. However, in most cases of non-infectious complication, we rarely obtain confirmatory results concerning their causal relationship with transfusion.

Voluntary reports from hospitals were received by the manufacturer and severe cases or previously unknown cases were selected to be reported to MHLW by the manufacturer. It was not until 2003 that hospitals had responsibility to report cases that medical staff deem important for preventing the recurrence and propagation of such cases in relation to public health, such as death, sequelae, and treatment-related extension of hospitalization, congenital abnormality in the children of patients, and infections. Reporting such cases is mandatory in accordance with the revised Pharmaceutical Affairs Law.

Adverse events to be reported/ reporting system

Any type of adverse event can be reported by doctors, and the JRCS does not provide any guidelines on what to report because severe adverse events should be reported by regulation; however, mild reactions are very frequent and not likely to be reported. The JRCS has been gathering not only information on adverse events, but also the samples of affected patients and the remaining blood products (if any). The JRCS has sought to clarify the possible mechanisms underlying the adverse reactions in each case by examining in detail the samples. Hospital doctors are also eager to know the cause of adverse reactions and they make use of such information to prevent further adverse events in specific patients.

Once an adverse reaction to transfusion is suspected, hospital doctors or staff in the transfusion medicine department report the case to the MR of the local blood center. The information should be submitted in the standardized form that is provided by the Safety Supervision Unit of the JRCS BSHQ. Alternatively, hospital doctors can report the adverse reaction directly to the MHLW. Indeed, the JRCS has the responsibility of reporting some of the serious adverse reactions to the government in accordance with the Pharmaceutical Affairs Law and the government guidelines as a marketing authorization holder (drug manufacturer).

Adverse reactions are first classified by hospital doctors; however, the staff of the Safety Supervision Unit reclassify these adverse reactions into the JRCS standard categories. This reporting system has not been changed over time, but the number of MRs has been increased from 80 to 150. In the first year of our hemovigilance system, we received only 228 reports from hospitals nationwide, but the number of reports has been increasing yearly. Recently, we received approximately 1700 reports per year from hospitals nationwide; however, the rate of reporting is different from hospital to hospital. This difference is probably due to the level of awareness of the importance of hemovigilance; hence, we must continue to promote the importance of hemovigilance.

In our hemovigilance system, severe adverse events tend to be reported rather than mild adverse events. This is partly because of the current cumbersome paper-based reporting system and/or the strong desire of the doctors to know the cause of severe adverse events. A recent pilot study of the online reporting system of the trend analysis of transfusion complications in Japan showed that the rate of adverse events is 1.5% regardless of severity and imputability, which is approximately 50 times higher than that obtained by the JRCS. These systems will be integrated into a more accurate hemovigilance system in the future.

Concept and methodology of Japanese hemovigilance

The JRCS has conducted the collection and analysis of safety management information necessary for the appropriate use of drugs—including the quality, efficacy, and safety of products—and has taken necessary measures based on the results of this analysis, that is, safety measures, pursuant to GVP. The safety management information to be collected is as follows:

- information from medical and pharmaceutical professionals;
- information from look-back studies;
- information from blood donors after blood donation (post-donation information);
- information from presentations at academic meetings, published articles, and other study reports;
- information from the Ministry of Health, Labour and Welfare and other governmental agencies, local governments, the Pharmaceuticals and Medical Devices Agency, and so on;
- information from foreign governments and organizations;
- information from other marketing approval holders;
- information from the Quality Assurance Manager, other divisions, and so on.

The safety management tasks include the reporting of transfusion-related adverse reactions and infections of patients who received transfusion from medical institutions. The Pharmaceutical Affairs Law requires severe or unknown cases to be reported to the Minister of Health, Labour and Welfare through the Pharmaceuticals and Medical Devices Agency. Transfusion-related adverse reactions include hemolytic and non-hemolytic adverse reactions (fever, urticaria, anaphylaxis, and Transfusion Related Acute Lung Injury (TRALI)) and transfusion-transmitted infections including suspected HBV, HCV, HIV, and bacterial infections.

Where a blood donor becomes positive for an infection, the blood component for the transfusion obtained from the previous donation may have already been distributed to medical institutions. If such a blood component has not been transfused yet, it shall be withdrawn. If it has already been transfused, the medical institution is requested to test the patient for related viral markers to help early detection and treatment of transfusion-related infections. This process is called a *look-back study.*

To conduct look-back studies and investigations on post-transfusion infections and to verify the safety of blood for transfusion, it is important to keep frozen donor repository samples. The JRCS has been storing all donation samples since 1996 for a period of 11 years. When a donor sample turns out to be positive for a certain virus, we evaluate the causal relationship between blood donation and transfusion by comparing the viral nucleotide sequence homology between the donor sample and the recipient sample.

Information obtained after blood donation (safety information such as donors' health conditions and disqualifying information from the subsequent donor interview), including the foregoing, is handled in accordance with the "Guidelines for Lookback Studies on Blood Products," which were established by the Blood and Blood Products Division, Pharmaceutical and Food Safety Bureau, and the Ministry of Health, Labour and Welfare in April 2005.

We collect information on practices concerning blood and blood products in other countries and the latest domestic and foreign research papers on infections due to products and source materials as part of our obligation as marketing approval holders of biological products.

Data analysis and feedback

The analyzed data of each year is distributed to hospitals nationwide through MRs and also through the website of the JRCS as a brochure *Transfusion Information.* The results of individual analysis of the samples from the implicated products and patient samples are sent back to the hospital doctors in a timely manner. This information will sometimes be useful for the next transfusion to specific patients, to whom we can provide washed products or the doctors can be prepared for predictable side effects.

We have also published annual reports since 2001, but the English version is available only for 2001, 2007, and 2008.[2-4] We also give presen-

tations at the annual meetings of the Japanese Society of Transfusion Medicine and Cell Therapy, the International Society of Blood Transfusion, and the International Hemovigilance Seminar about the analyzed data of adverse events in the previous year.

Evaluation of hemovigilance system

The JRCS Blood Service is regarded as the marketing authorization holder of blood products and as such must comply with Good Vigilance Practice and Good Quality Practice (GQP). As the licenses for marketing authorization are filed or renewed every five years, we are subject to GQP and GVP inspections by the local authority, which focus on safety vigilance and quality assurance and the associated procedures and documentation.

Look-back studies

Traceability requirement is a key element for hemovigilance. Our unique and useful system for donor repository samples plays a pivotal role in our hemovigilance. As already stated, we store donor repository samples for 11 years. We also keep the records of the questionnaire for donors, testing, manufacturing, and delivery to hospitals. These records are kept until the sample storage for expiry date plus 30 years, in other words, 41 years for frozen red cell products. Hospitals are required to keep for 20 years the identifiable information of the patients who receive blood products.

This enables us to conduct look-back studies extremely easily for infectious diseases or antibody testing for TRALI without requiring the implicated donor to visit again.

Errors and near-misses

Errors and near-misses from donation to delivery at blood centers are monitored, but errors and near-misses in hospitals are currently not included in our hemovigilance system; however, a governmental organization, Japan Council for Quality Health Care, deals with errors and near-misses in all medical procedures, in which the cases related to transfusion are also included. The collection of cases of medical adverse events/near-misses is mandatory for 272 hospitals, and although the participation in this project is open to all hospitals nationwide, at present 824 are participating in this project, which is only about 13% of the total number of hospitals in Japan.

Thus, errors and near-misses are handled by separate systems.

Adverse reactions

Adverse reactions in donors

Reports on adverse reactions have been collected for 30 years in a computer-based manner. The overall rate of donor complication has been approximately 1% recently.

Adverse reactions in recipients

In accordance with the Pharmaceutical Affairs Law, doctors and pharmacists must inform the Marketing Authorization Holders of drug (including blood for transfusion)-induced severe adverse reactions and/or infection cases, or report directly to the MHLW via the Pharmaceuticals and Medical Devices Agency (PMDA). Hospital doctors are responsible for reporting adverse reactions; however, there is no penalty for not reporting. In this situation, the reporting is voluntary rather than mandatory, and which complications should be reported depends on the decision of the hospital doctors.

Data and trends

The data from donation sites are sent from all blood centers nationwide through an online system. The data are analyzed by the Quality Assurance Unit.

The trends in donor adverse events have not changed in recent years. Numbers and proportions of donor adverse events are shown in Figure 13.2,

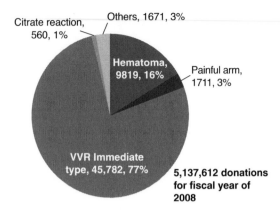

Figure 13.2 Numbers and proportions of donor adverse reaction cases in the fiscal year of 2008.

and the trends of the numbers of adverse events in donors over the last three years are shown in Table 13.1.

The data from the hospitals are categorized in the Safety Supervision Unit of the JRC. The data are

Table 13.1 Trend of numbers of donor adverse reaction cases in fiscal years 2006–2008 (donation numbers are 2006: 4,983,009; 2007: 4,955,954; 2008: 5,137,612; "–" = no data available; * = VVR Immediate/delayed types are grouped into the same category).

Adverse reaction	2006	2007	2008
Hematoma	10,141	8,912	9,438
Arterial puncture	–	–	–
Delayed bleeding	–	–	–
Nerve irritation	–	175	191
Nerve injury	441	279	248
Tendon injury	–	–	–
Painful arm	–	1,111	1,249
Localized infection	–	–	–
Thrombophlebitis	–	–	–
VVR Immediate type*	38,070	41,334	44,864
VVR Immediate,* accident	114	135	154
VVR Delayed type*	–	–	–
VVR Delayed,* accident	–	–	–
Citrate reaction	491	437	426
Hemolysis	–	–	–
Generalized allergic reaction	–	–	–
Air embolism	–	–	–
Others	2,690	1,286	1,403
Total	51,947	53,669	57,973

analyzed by a specialist in the Safety Supervision Unit and in-house medical doctors.

Transfusion records do not have to be sent back to the JRCS, and for this reason the Society does not have a complete traceability of all blood products.

In 2008, the JRCS issued 4,903,649 blood products: namely, 733 whole blood; 3,243,936 RBC (including washed red blood cells, frozen-thawed red blood cells, and blood for exchange transfusion); 727,972 platelet; and 931,008 plasma products. All these products were leukoreduced.

In 2008, two transfusion error causing adverse events were reported to the JRCS, which were ABO-incompatible transfusion. The error rate is unavailable because the JRCS does not have error reporting from hospitals, and the ministry reporting system is not mandatory.

The numbers of adverse reaction cases in 2008 are as follows: 11, AHTR; 11, DHTR; 956, Allergic reactions; 186, FNHTR; 39, TACO; 32, TRALI; 152, TAD; 4, HBV (confirmed); 2, other TTIs (HEV); 2, bacterial infections; 57, hypotensive reactions; 113, other TRs, and 9, UCT. The numbers and the proportion of these cases are shown in Figure 13.3.

The trends of the numbers of adverse reactions over the last three years are shown in Table 13.2 (2006–2008).[4]

Results of data utilization for prevention and evaluation

Overall transfusion safety has been extremely improved in recent years, but some residual issues remain to be addressed.

To decrease the incidence of transfusion of blood products with infectious agents, serum testing has been changed from agglutination methods to chemiluminescent enzyme immunoassay. NAT sensitivity was improved by implementing a new NAT testing instrument (Cobas s401/TaqScreen MPX, Roche) in 2008 for the detection of HBV, HCV, and HIV.

In an effort to decrease the incidence of anaphylactic reactions, we have been conducting a survey of the deficiency of several plasma proteins

Table 13.2 Trend of numbers of recipient adverse reaction cases in 2006–2008.

Adverse reaction	2006	2007	2008
AHTR	25	13	11
DHTR	7	7	11
DSTR	0	0	0
Allergic reaction	822	885	956
FNHTR	199	160	186
TACO	0	17	39
TRALI	57	43	32
TAD	123	94	152
HBV	6	13	4
HCV	1	1	0
HIV	0	0	0
Others (HEV)	2	0	2
Malaria	0	0	0
Other parasites	0	0	0
Bacteria	3	0	2
Hypotension	39	33	57
TA-GVHD	0	0	0
PTP	0	1	0
Hyperkalemia	0	2	0
Hypocalcemia	0	0	0
Other TRs	56	83	113
UCT	0	0	9

and anti-plasma protein antibodies in patient blood samples as a causal agent for transfusion-related anaphylaxis. We detected the IgG and IgE classes of anti-haptoglobin antibodies in the haptoglobin-deficient patients with anaphylactic shock following transfusion. Anaphylaxis caused by the IgA antibody is common among Caucasians, but less frequent among Asians. Other protein antibodies are sometimes detected in the patient blood samples, but the causal relationship between antibody and symptoms is rarely proven.

The male-predominant plasma strategy for reducing the incidence of TRALI has just started. The screening of parous and/or female donors for HLA antibodies is now under investigation.

Usefulness of data from our hemovigilance system

Transfusion-transmitted viral infections have long been a major problem in Japan, and the Safety

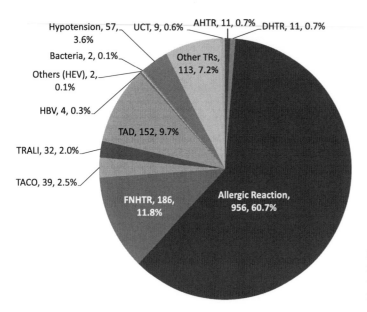

Figure 13.3 Numbers and proportion of recipient adverse reaction cases in 2008; total number of adverse event cases reported in 2008 was 1572.

Supervision Unit is apt to take strong measures against such infections. As shown in the above data, viral infections are very rare. However, the social impact of viral infections is much larger than that of other adverse events. The preventive measures for severe adverse events such as TRALI or anaphylaxis are one step behind those for viral infections. This is partly because the causal relationship between the causal agents and adverse events is not always proven compared with that between infectious agents and viral infections, where a viral nucleic acid sequence can be analyzed for the suspected cases using donor repository samples and patient samples and, if needed, a look-back study can be performed. Implementation of preventive measures for both infectious and noninfectious adverse events are equally important, and we are trying to develop more efficient measures.

Advantages and limitations of Japanese hemovigilance system

Hemovigilance conducted by the blood-product manufacturer has some advantages and limitations. Because donor care is the first priority for the blood service, donor vigilance has been performed for almost 30 years, and various preventive measures for safe donation have been implemented. Blood products can be traced from donors to patients; moreover since 1996, we have stored 6 ml of whole blood samples from each donation for 11 years in special refrigerated facilities with a computerized robotic system. By using these stored samples, we can perform look-back studies of infectious complications and also identify alloantibodies in TRALI cases when no other samples can be obtained. Thus, the product information is easily accessible through the computer-based system. Moreover, a detailed analysis of adverse events cannot be performed without sample collection from patients and associated donors.

There are some limitations, however, in this system. We usually do not know the final destination of blood products; that is, we do not know whether a particular product was used or destroyed. We do not have the power to control the usage of blood products in hospitals. Hence, full traceability has not been achieved. It is not an easy task to trace each blood product distributed to over 10,000 hospitals. Furthermore, the JRCS is not informed about transfusion errors and near-misses. We hope that our hemovigilance system will work harmoniously together with other error reporting systems in the near future.

Moving towards evidence-based hemovigilance

Although the safety of the patients who need transfusion has been extremely improved, there are still a number of problems left unsolved. Expanding the scope of hemovigilance to transfusion errors and near-misses is one necessary direction of hemovigilance, but reducing the discomfort of patients as far as possible is also an essential target.

References

1 Satake M, Taira R, Yugi H, Hino S, Kanemitsu K, Ikeda H, *et al.*, 2007, Infectivity of blood components with low hepatitis B virus DNA levels identified in a lookback program. *Transfusion* **47**(7): 1197–205.

2 JRCS, 2003, Haemovigilance Annual Reports 2001 and 1993–2001. Transfusion Information Department, Japanese Red Cross Central Blood Center. http://www.jrc.or.jp/vcms_lf/haemovigilanceannualreport1993-2001.pdf [accessed February 26, 2012].

3 JRCS, 2010, Haemovigilance by JRCS 2007, Safety Vigilance Division, Blood Service Headquarters, Japanese Red Cross Society. http://www.jrc.or.jp/vcms_lf/haemovigilance2007_en.pdf [accessed February 26, 2012].

4 JRCS, 2010, Haemovigilance by JRCS 2008, Safety Vigilance Division, Blood Service Headquarters, Japanese Red Cross Society. http://www.jrc.or.jp/vcms_lf/anzen_HVreport2008_en.pdf [accessed February 26, 2012].

CHAPTER 14

Setting up a National Hemovigilance System: SHOT

Hannah Cohen[1] and Lorna M. Williamson[2]
[1]Department of Haematology, University College London Hospitals and University College London, London, UK
[2]NHS Blood and Transplant, Watford, UK

The origins of Serious Hazards of Transfusion (SHOT)

In 1994, the Medical Directors of the National Blood Service in England and the Scottish National Blood Transfusion Service (Dr Angela Robinson and Professor John Cash) attended a meeting in Dublin to discuss the forthcoming European Union (EU) Blood Directive, which would set standards for the provision of national blood supplies. They had the foresight to realize that to achieve full compliance with the Directive, a national hemovigilance scheme was going to be required, and they asked one of us (LMW) to convene a working group to establish such a system for the whole UK.

The working group, consisting entirely of transfusion specialists, met for the first time later that year to undertake what seemed a highly daunting prospect. The EU Directive was not part of UK law (and would not become so until 2005). With no force of statute, no internationally agreed blueprint for setting up hemovigilance, no staff, and no agreed budget, the chances of success seemed low. At that time, the only other hemovigilance scheme in operation was in France, where a statutory system had been established following the HIV litigation of the early 1990s. It was required to report every adverse event, even loosely associated with transfusion. The French scheme was very detailed and resource-heavy, with a hemovigilance officer in every hospital. The working group quickly agreed that a scheme of this complexity would not work in the UK, and looked around for other models.

We eventually concluded that a system based on the UK Confidential Enquiry system might be the answer, because it had already been shown to be both feasible and acceptable to UK health professionals. Confidential Enquiries were schemes for the reporting of major healthcare events in specific areas such as maternal deaths in childbirth and deaths after surgery. We were particularly helped by the National Confidential Enquiry for Peri-operative Deaths (NCEPOD), who provided invaluable advice on legal and practical aspects of confidential reporting. Establishing SHOT was greatly helped by two other developments in UK transfusion practice. First, the National Blood Service of England had established a joint scheme with the Health Protection Agency (HPA) for collection and collation of data on viral positivity in donors and transfusion-transmitted infections, with 1995 being the first year of reporting. Second, Dr Brian McClelland of the Scottish National Blood Transfusion Service (SNBTS) had done ground-breaking work mapping the logistics of delivery of blood to the patient, and identifying "hotspots" where errors could occur. Publications on deaths due to ABO-incompatible transfusions were beginning to

Hemovigilance: An Effective Tool for Improving Transfusion Safety, First Edition. Edited by René R.P. De Vries and Jean-Claude Faber.
© 2012 John Wiley & Sons, Ltd. Published 2012 by John Wiley & Sons, Ltd.

appear in the literature, giving the group direction as to its priorities.

Getting SHOT started

Three key areas for the running of SHOT had to be decided:

- type of events to be reported;
- governance of the scheme;
- infrastructure and budget.

Table 14.1 summarizes the main characteristics of the SHOT scheme (www.shotuk.org).

Type of events to be reported

We agreed early on that we would have to start by focusing on the biggest threats to the patient, and therefore we would collect data only on incidents with potentially fatal consequences. So from the outset, the following have been included in SHOT reports:

- *Incorrect blood component transfused (IBCT):* This category was intended to capture incidents where blood intended for one patient was given to another, and also where specific requirements had been omitted, for example, for irradiated or CMV negative blood. We took the decision, which has stood the test of time, to collect all such incidents whether any harm came to the patient or not, because we believed that there was a great deal to be learnt from every such incident, and so it has proved.
- *Acute severe transfusion reactions,* whether hemolytic, febrile, allergic, or anaphylactic, but not mild fever alone.
- *Delayed hemolysis,* but not development of alloantibodies alone.
- *Post-transfusion purpura.*
- *Transfusion-related Acute Lung Injury.*
- *Transfusion-associated Graft-Versus-Host Disease.*
- *Transfusion-transmitted infection.*

The definitions of these categories were largely the creation of the working group, because no standard definitions existed at the time. More recently, SHOT definitions are generally based on those of the International Society for Blood Transfusion

(ISBT) Working Party on Hemovigilance.[1,2] The ISBT standard definitions are important because they will help hemovigilance organizations to generate data that will be comparable at an international level.

With some modifications, these still remain the core reporting categories of SHOT, and have since been supplemented by a number of additional categories, either as projects or as permanent features. These additional categories and the modifications to existing categories are detailed below and summarized in Table 14.1.

In the UK, the Medicines and Healthcare products Regulatory Agency (MHRA) was appointed as the competent authority to implement the EU Blood Directive[3] and Blood Safety and Quality Regulations (BSQR),[4] the UK transposition of the EU Directive. Since 8 November 2005, all suspected serious adverse events (SAEs) and serious adverse reactions (SARs) related to the quality and safety of blood and blood components must be reported to MHRA through the SABRE (Serious Adverse Blood Reactions and Events) online reporting system. Reporting to SHOT is via SABRE, and all events that are reportable to MHRA are now also collected by SHOT. In addition, SHOT collects a wider scope of data than required by the BSQR, extending into the professional and clinical areas of transfusion practice.

Additional SHOT reporting categories

Anti-D immunoglobulin (Ig)

Although not specifically sought at the outset, SHOT received reports of adverse events (errors) related to administration (or failure of administration) of anti-D and took a decision to include these, because the "Yellow Card" system in the UK does not cover these errors. Initially, these reports, from which many learning points emerged, were included in the IBCT chapter, and in the 2007 report, a separate chapter was established. The new SHOT online reporting system (see below) has also been collecting data from 2010 on the outcome of clinical follow-up and retesting in six months of patients in whom anti-D has been delayed or omitted. From the start of 2013 SHOT will seek

Table 14.1 Summary of main characteristics of the SHOT scheme.

Characteristic	SHOT
UK-wide hemovigilance	• SHOT is professionally led, with the SHOT Steering Group including representation from virtually all Royal Colleges and professional bodies • Effective hemovigilance: fall in serious outcomes (deaths and major morbidity) from 34% in 1996/7 to 6.9% in 2011
Hemovigilance: Serious Adverse Reactions (SARs)/Events (SAEs) recorded	• Patient SARs • Hospital SAEs including those in the clinical arena but currently not Blood Establishment SAEs • Includes highly clinically relevant additional plasma products and components: solvent-detergent FFP and anti-D immunoglobulin, MB-FFP, and cryoprecipitate (not covered by BSQR 2005) • Includes autologous transfusion (e.g., cell salvage) • Continual development: a) newer categories: TACO, TAD, under/delayed transfusion, inappropriate and unneccessary transfusion; b) category for unexpected new reactions/events ('previously uncategorized complications of transfusion'), which includes a mechanism to report on processes to reduce vCJD • Optional reporting categories: alloimmunization and hemosiderosis • Donor incidents (under development with UK Blood Services)
Web-based reporting platform	Dendrite
Funding	Via UK Blood Services
Reporting	Initially voluntary but now requirement of Clinical Pathology Accreditation, Health Service Circulars, and Healthcare Standards
Validation of all reports (including imputability)	• By SHOT Clinical and Laboratory Incidents Specialists and acknowledged national/international experts on the SHOT Working Expert Group (WEG) • TRALI: by expert panel assessment before investigation by Blood Services and followed by WEG specialist review • TTI: investigated by UK Blood Services and reported to NHSBT/HPA Epidemiology Unit
Use of data	• Evidence-based recommendations to improve patient safety—data informs policy in blood transfusion and supports guidelines • Feedback to reporters and stakeholders through 14 annual reports and symposia, website, newsletters, lectures, national/international scientific meetings, publications • SHOT monitors effects of implementation of recommendations (e.g., by SHOT-initiated UK Transfusion Laboratory Collaborative) • SHOT undertakes research, studies, and audit in the area of transfusion safety
Development	Responds to the strategy provided by the Steering Group

additional information about women who are found at booking, during pregnancy or at delivery to have developed a new anti-D.

Near-miss

Near-miss events are well recognized to be a good indicator of both strengths and weaknesses in many fields and industries. SHOT collected data on near-miss incidents in the transfusion process nationally since 2000/2001. The scheme was first piloted in 1998 in 25 hospitals over a 7-month period. A larger survey was carried out the following year, which provided very valuable data and a clear impetus to continue. In the 2008 and 2009 reports, data were reported on phase 1 and 2 of a pilot study, which demonstrated the need for training and adherence to policies for venepuncture. In 2010, the new web-based reporting system included near-miss reporting.

Transfusion Associated Circulatory Overload (TACO)

Cases of TACO were specifically requested in 2008, and detailed since then in a new chapter.

Transfusion Associated Dyspnea (TAD)

One reported case in 2008 was designated by SHOT as TAD and since then this category has been reported separately. This type of pulmonary transfusion complication is recognized by the ISBT and included in their definitions.[1]

Autologous transfusion

Autologous transfusion related to pre-deposit was covered by the initial reporting system. In the 2008 report a substantive separate chapter on autologous transfusion-related adverse incidents contained the reports related to a cell salvage adverse events pilot, a joint initiative between the UK Cell Salvage Action Group and SHOT. This chapter is now established to include all adverse events relating to cell salvage as well as any other autologous transfusion-related events.

Pediatrics

Since the 2008 report, SHOT has had a formal link with the National Health Service Blood and Transplant (NHSBT) Paediatric Transfusion Group, and as a result a more detailed analysis of pediatric SHOT reports is undertaken. Previously, short pediatric chapters appeared in 2003 and 2007. SHOT now analyzes pediatric cases systematically every year in detail, because it is clear that there are specific areas of risk affecting children. These relate in part to the small size and blood volume of pediatric patients, to the range of medical and surgical conditions affecting this age group (and the special transfusion requirements that ensue), and to difficulties of venous access, identification, and other practical issues.

Under/delayed transfusion

In recent years, there has been increasing interest in the literature in possible patient harm arising from undertransfusion or delayed transfusion. The 2008 report included one such case, and since then SHOT has actively sought these reports. Just as with other "new" categories, it is often reporter concern that results in a new type of report being collected.

Changes to IBCT chapter sections

The number of IBCT cases together with the total number of SHOT reports has increased year by year. The breakdown of IBCT cases has also changed over the years. In 1996–97, IBCT consisted only of phlebotomy errors, wrong blood in tube (WBIT), collection and administration (ward-based patient identification) errors, and laboratory errors resulting in wrong transfusion. Two additional categories, *handling and storage errors* and *inappropriate and unnecessary transfusion,* emerged around the year 2000, and these have increased in absolute numbers and also as a proportion of the IBCT category. In 2008, these became stand-alone categories with separate chapters.

The IBCT chapter now contains the following four categories:

- *Administration of wrong blood* where there was a collection error and/or failure of the bedside check.
- *Special requirements not met* where the patient's special requirements have not been met irrespective of the location of the error, that is, both laboratory and clinical will be included in the total.
- *WBIT* are those events that resulted in a transfusion irrespective of outcome.
- *Laboratory errors* where the primary error has occurred in the laboratory.

There is one further subsection that includes reports from all these categories: *IT errors* where the reporter has identified a specific problem that matched the categories from the 2007 SHOT report. These reports also appear in their primary category.

In addition there is a subsection entitled Right Blood Right Patient (RBRP) which includes incidents where a patient was transfused correctly despite one or more serious errors that in other circumstances might have led to an IBCT.

Handling and storage errors are related to the administration of expired components, excessive time to transfuse, and cold chain errors. Cases arise in clinical and laboratory settings, and in the transport of blood components.

Inappropriate and unnecessary transfusion comprise events in which a transfusion was given because of an incorrect result or poor knowledge or prescribing. Incorrect results may arise from verbal or written communication errors, or an error in the transfusion, hematology, or coagulation laboratory, or during point-of-care testing. Aside from this chapter, and some comments in the annual report regarding inappropriate use of fresh frozen plasma (FFP) rather than prothrombin complex concentrate for warfarin reversal,[5] the analysis of SHOT reports has not included any formal assessment of the appropriateness of the transfusions implicated in the cases. This is because the questionnaires do not request sufficient detail on this aspect, and many reporters are not in a position to pass comment because they are not directly clinically involved with the majority of cases they report.

Changes to acute and delayed reactions

Acute transfusion reactions now exclude those due to hemolytic reactions and include mild and moderate as well as severe reactions. Hemolytic transfusion reactions comprises a separate category that is split into two: acute and delayed.

Major morbidity has been defined from the outset to include the following:
- intensive care admission and/or ventilation;
- dialysis and/or renal impairment;
- major hemorrhage from transfusion-induced coagulopathy;
- evidence of intravascular hemolysis;
- potential risk of anti-D sensitization in a female of childbearing potential;*
- persistent viral infection;
- acute symptomatic confirmed infection.

More recently, two further categories have been incorporated within the definition of *major morbidity:*
- reaction resulting in a low or high hemoglobin level of a degree sufficient to cause risk to life without immediate medical intervention (2007);
- life-threatening acute reaction requiring immediate medical intervention (2009).

*This category was amended for 2010 as potential for major morbidity defined as:
- potential risk of D or K sensitization in a woman of childbearing potential.

Imputability

In the 1999/2000 annual report, SHOT introduced case analysis by *imputability,* that is, the likelihood that a serious adverse incident in a recipient can be attributed to the blood component transfused. Since the 2005 report, SHOT has followed the BSQR recommendation of a scale from 0 to 3[3] as follows:
- 0 = excluded/unlikely: the evidence is clearly in favour of attributing the reaction to other causes.
- 1 = possible: the evidence is indeterminate for attributing the reaction to the blood component or to alternative causes.
- 2 = likely/probable: the evidence is clearly in favour of attributing the adverse reaction to the blood component.
- 3 = certain: there is conclusive evidence beyond reasonable doubt attributing the adverse reaction to the blood component.

In sick patients with complex conditions, it may be difficult to ascribe imputability.

Scope and reporting system

From the outset, SHOT reporting has encompassed all labile blood components issued by the four UK Blood Transfusion Services (NHS Blood and Transplant, Scottish National Blood Transfusion Service, Welsh Blood Service, and Northern Ireland Blood Transfusion Service), the Ministry of Defence, and the Blood Services in the Crown Dependencies. Reactions and events related to all forms of autologous transfusion, including cell salvage, are included. Adverse reactions and events related to virus inactivated FFP (solvent detergent (SD-FFP) and methylene-blue treated (MB-FFP) are also included because these are recommended in specific situations rather than standard FFP.[6] In addition, adverse events (errors) related to administration (or failure of administration) of anti-D Ig are included, because the "Yellow Card" system does not cover these errors. New types of components regularly become available (e.g., MB-cryoprecipitate in 2008) and SHOT will collect adverse events on all or any of these that the Steering Group considers to be within the scope of SHOT.

We decided on a two-stage reporting scheme, with a short initial report being followed up with a detailed questionnaire specific to the type of event being reported. The reporting forms have evolved over the years, but have remained in the same basic format. Importantly, once all information had been received about a case, all hospital and patient identifiers were removed before it was entered into the database. This approach removed any possibility of SHOT information about a specific case being used for the purposes of litigation. SHOT questionnaires are reviewed annually with changes approved by the Steering Group and documented.

All cases are validated, if necessary by obtaining further information from reporters. and imputability is either confirmed or amended. As part of this process, SHOT works in close collaboration with the NHSBT/HPA Epidemiology Unit, which receives reports of cases of possible transfusion-transmitted infection (TTI) from blood services across England and Wales (to whom suspected cases of TTI are reported directly by hospitals), together with relevant information about the case.

Blood center involvement is essential to ensure rapid withdrawal of other implicated components and appropriate donor follow-up. The NHSBT/HPA unit subsequently receives final reports indicating whether the case was formally investigated and the final conclusion of the investigation. Cases from Scotland and Northern Ireland are collated with the English and Welsh cases by the Epidemiology Unit and an annual report prepared, which is published as part of the SHOT report. During preparation of the annual report all cases are reviewed in detail, if necessary with input from experts in virology or other transfusion-transmitted infection. Consequently, the conclusions are robust and take into account all the circumstances.

Cases of suspected transfusion-related acute lung injury (TRALI) are also initially reviewed by two intensive care specialists with specific interest and expertise in this field, together with a transfusion medicine expert, prior to laboratory investigation by NHSBT, and this system also prevails in Northern Ireland. The cases are reviewed for a second time taking into account the laboratory findings.

On January 4, 2010, the new SHOT web-based reporting system (developed with Dendrite, www.e-dendrite.com) went live, replacing the previous paper-based system. This system enables capture of all current reporting categories as well as a category for unexpected new reactions/events (designated "previously uncategorized complica-

tions of transfusion"), which includes a mechanism to report on processes to reduce vCJD. Dendrite has been evaluated by NHS Connecting for Health (CFH) as compliant with the terms and conditions of the CFH Information Governance Statement of Compliance (IGSoC). The IGSoC is the agreement between NHS CFH and any organizations with access, directly or indirectly, to NHS CFH services including the NHS Care Records Service (NHS CRS) and includes obligations to maintain the confidentiality, integrity, security, availability, and accuracy of personal data used in these services.

Information is the main asset of SHOT. Hospital-based reporters entrust information about adverse events relating to transfusion to SHOT and the protection of this information is fundamental to the reputation of SHOT within the transfusion community as well as a legal and professional obligation. In order to function, SHOT must maintain the confidentiality of the information it receives and ensure its availability to authorized users. In order to fulfill all these requirements, SHOT has developed an information governance policy that clearly delineates the responsibilities of all those involved in handling SHOT data from the SHOT office staff to the members of the Working Expert Group and the Steering Group.

Impact of the European Union (EU) Blood Directive on SHOT reporting

Hemovigilance reporting system

Since November 8, 2005, all suspected SAEs and SARs related to the quality and safety of blood and blood components must be reported to MHRA through the SABRE online reporting system. The annual SHOT report, which analyzes data collected each calendar year, is published in June or July to coincide with the requirement under the BSQR 2005 for annualized UK hemovigilance data to be sent to the EU Commission. The MHRA's Blood Consultative Committee (to date chaired by the SHOT Medical Director) conducts a reconciliation between SHOT and MHRA figures before the data for the EU are finally submitted.

Hemovigilance reporting: Statutory or voluntary?

Reporting to MHRA is statutory. In the past, reporting to SHOT was voluntary, however, in recent years a number of UK quality, safety, inspection, and accreditation organizations and government bodies have made it a requirement. These include the following:

- Clinical and Pathology Accreditation (CPA UK) standard H2;[7]
- the National Patient Safety Agency (NPSA) Safer Practice Notice 14 (SPN 14);[8,9]
- NPSA Rapid Response Report 2010/RRR017;[10]
- Health Service Circular (HSC) 2007/001 Better Blood Transfusion;[11]
- NHS Quality Improvement Scotland, Clinical Standards for Blood Transfusion, Standard 4b.3;[12]
- Welsh Assembly Government Healthcare standards for Wales, Standard 16.[13]

Participation

Since the 2008 annual report, there has been a chapter on participation in SHOT reporting, which shows the number of SHOT reports sent in by the four UK countries and by the ten English regions. There is also some analysis of the category of reports most often sent (i.e., errors, physiological reactions, and reports on anti-D).

In 2012 more detailed analysis has been undertaken, including on a trust by trust basis, allowing benchmarking between hospitals, trusts, and regions, which will provide the basis for sharing good practice and for learning opportunities. It is only by continuous monitoring, or audit, of transfusion practice and outcomes that patient care can undergo continuing improvement in quality and safety, with further risk reduction, as demonstrated during the years of SHOT reporting.

Governance

When the group that established SHOT was formed in 1994, we knew that the forthcoming EU Directive was likely to mandate national hemovigilance systems, and that laws would have to be passed within each EU member state to cover all the requirements of the Directive. However, the EU Blood Directives were not transposed into UK law as the Blood Safety and Quality Regulations until 2005. Thus, there was no possibility that SHOT would be operating in its early years under any specific legal umbrella. Therefore, we took the model of the UK Confidential Enquiries, which was to create hemovigilance as a voluntary professional activity, not governed by any external rules or regulations, and with no formal links to the Department of Health or any other part of government.

A number of other decisions were taken regarding the governance of SHOT. First, it was agreed that there was no specific role for the regulator that licensed Blood Centres, the Medicines and Healthcare Regulatory Agency. Blood components are not licensed medicinals in the UK, and there was concern that hospitals would be deterred from reporting if a regulator became involved. Second, we agreed that the management of SHOT needed to be separate from that of the Blood Services, again because we did not think that hospitals would be comfortable reporting their errors to their supplying Blood Centre. However, SHOT needed to be funded from somewhere, and have a physical location, and the Blood Services had indicated that they would be willing to provide both to get SHOT established.

To "square the circle," we eventually agreed that SHOT would be funded by the four UK Blood Services, and that it would be housed rent-free within the National Blood Service's Centre in Manchester, but that it would be governed and professionally led by a Steering Group consisting of representatives of all Royal Colleges and other professional bodies relevant to the handling and prescribing of blood. The UK Blood Services (through the UK Forum) would have one representative on this group (not the Chair), but would not otherwise attempt to influence overly SHOT's activities.

The Steering Group initially had representation from no fewer than eight Royal Colleges and six professional bodies. The final piece in the governance was to provide a professional home. We were fortunate that the Royal College of Pathologists' (RCPath) representative on the SHOT Steering Group at the time was a hematologist,

Professor John Lilleyman (subsequently President of the RCPath), who was highly sympathetic to the aims of SHOT. He advised that SHOT should apply to be an affiliated organization of the RCPath, which was subsequently achieved in November 1997, thus making it clear to hematologists in hospitals that SHOT was rooted in the world of healthcare professionals and not that of regulators or government.

SHOT was therefore established with a Steering Group chaired by the representative of the British Society for Haematology (HC), and a Standing Working Group chaired by LMW to run the scheme. The Steering Group provides professional ownership and strategic direction, monitors the performance of SHOT, and is accountable to the UK Forum through the Medical Director for the use of resources and management of the budget.

Membership of the Steering Group consists of nominated representatives of the Royal Colleges and other professional bodies. The Steering Group will always include the Medical Director, National Co-ordinator for Transfusion Transmitted Infections, the Operations Manager, and a representative from each of the following: Health Protection Agency; Transfusion Microbiology (a consultant specialist); British Committee for Standards in Haematology (BCSH) Transfusion Task Force; the Chief Medical Officer's National Blood Transfusion Committee (NBTC) and its counterparts in Scotland, Wales, and Northern Ireland; and the UK Forum (of the four UK Blood Services).

It is also desirable that membership of the Steering Group includes a representative of each of the following: the Institute of Biomedical Science; the NHS Confederation; Royal College of Anaesthetists; the Royal College of Pathologists, the British Society for Haematology; the Royal College of Obstetricians and Gynaecologists; the Royal College of Surgeons; the Royal College of Nursing and the Royal College of Midwives; the Intensive Care Society; the Royal College of Emergency Medicine; the British Society of Gastroenterology; the Faculty of Public Health; the Defence Medical Services; and a co-opted representative from the National Patient Safety Agency (NPSA) and MHRA. The Steering Group should also include a lay member.

The Standing Working Group has evolved into the Working Expert Group chaired by the SHOT Medical Director, who is also Secretary of the Steering Group.

Expert review of all cases reported by the Working Expert Group Expert Panel, who write the annual report and chapter-specific recommendations, as well as active Steering Group input into the main SHOT recommendations, are fundamental to SHOT's approach and have been key in the acceptance of SHOT's evidence-based recommendations by the UK transfusion community and policy-making organizations.

SHOT's relationship with other professional bodies

SHOT aims to work collaboratively with other bodies with responsibility for transfusion safety, for example, MHRA, NPSA, the NBTC and its counterparts in Scotland, Wales, and Northern Ireland, the four UK Blood Transfusion Services, and the Department of Health Blood Policy Unit. From the outset, SHOT highlighted the need for a national body with relevant expertise and resource to advise government of priorities for improvement in blood safety. We were therefore pleased that the Advisory Committee for the Microbiological Safety of Blood, Tissues and Organs (MSBTO) was formed in 2001, and subsequently in 2007 was replaced by the Advisory Committee on the Safety of Blood, Tissues and Organs (SaBTO), which had a wider remit and which included noninfectious as well as infectious complications of transfusion. SHOT, and other bodies such as NPSA, MHRA, the Spongiform Encephalopathy Advisory Committee (SEAC), and NBTC, are in attendance at SaBTO meetings as observers. The Competent Authority for the Blood Safety and Quality Regulations UK (2005) is MHRA.

SHOT aims to promote international hemovigilance by collaborative working within the International Hemovigilance Network, the International Society of Blood Transfusion (via its hemovigilance working party), and the European Commission via its Competent Authorities Haemovigilance Subcommittee. SHOT has reciprocal representation on the BCSH Transfusion Task Force.

Infrastructure and budget

We decided that SHOT needed a small team devoted to running the scheme. At the beginning, this consisted of a part-time Medical Co-ordinator, a scheme manager who doubled as IT manager, and a part-time administrator. NHSBT "hosts" SHOT and provides resources such as office space and services such as IT, human resources, and finance support. The initial budget from the four UK Blood Services, with funding from the Research and Development budgets, was only £20,000, an amount that now seems naïve, but which was in line with other Confidential Enquiries at the time.

In 2007, SHOT's budget was uplifted to support the implementation of web-based reporting and the current SHOT office staff complement, which comprises the Medical Director, operations manager, clinical incidents specialist, laboratory incidents specialist, transfusion liaison practitioner, research analyst, and two information officers. In addition, SHOT has a National Co-ordinator for Transfusion Transmitted Infections. The day-to-day management of SHOT is undertaken by the Medical Director and the Operations Manager (see Figure 14.1). The SHOT office team publishes a regular newsletter.

Accountability

The Medical Director of SHOT is employed by one of the UK Blood Services and is managerially accountable to the UK Forum. It is essential for SHOT to retain autonomy for professional accountability and that it is independent of the UK Blood Services. For that reason professional accountability of the Medical Director is to the Steering Group through its Chair. The National Co-ordinator for Transfusion Transmitted Infections is employed jointly by the HPA and the NHSBT and is managerially accountable to the Consultant in Epidemiology and Health Protection at the HPA.

The launch of SHOT

To ensure complete coverage of hospital transfusion laboratories, we obtained the participation list of hospitals taking part in the National External Quality Assurance Scheme (NEQAS). (Provision of such a list would probably be forbidden today on grounds of data protection.) All hematologists on this list were notified of the launch of SHOT, and invited to submit reports. We were highly aware of considerable nervousness among hematologists, at a point when   litigation against individuals by

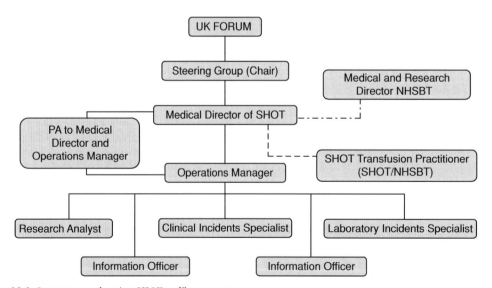

Figure 14.1 Organogram showing SHOT staffing structure.

patients with hemophilia was taking place. We took trade stands at the 1995 annual conferences of the British Society for Haematology and the British Blood Transfusion Society. We also provided a news item for the newsletters of all organizations represented on the Steering Group, and encouraged cascade from the professional representatives back to their members. We managed to persuade the *British Medical Journal* to run an editorial[14] on the importance of establishing UK hemovigilance.

The stated aims of the scheme were to
- inform policy with UK Blood Services;
- improve standards of hospital transfusion practice;
- aid production of clinical guidelines;
- educate users on transfusion hazards and their prevention.

Now all we needed was a title for the scheme. To emphasize the fact that we did not want to receive reports on every minor febrile reaction, the words Serious and Transfusion were essential, and a snappy acronym was agreed to be useful. For obvious reasons, the option of Serious Hazards in Transfusion was quickly rejected, and the Serious Hazards of Transfusion (SHOT) scheme went live on November 1, 1996.

The first year of SHOT, and the first report

Understandably, reporting was slow to take off, but by the end of the first year, we had a respectable 169 initial reports and 141 questionnaires from 94 hospitals to analyze. It would be fair to say that an electronic database of a professional standard had not been established by this point. Although an Access database was used for analysis of the largest category (Incorrect Blood Component Transfused), collation of data in the smaller immunological categories was done manually, requiring considerable checking. Despite the IT limitations, the first year's report, which was based on cases analyzed between October 1, 1996, and September 30, 1997, was published in March 1998. There was much discussion as to whether individual "vignettes" should be included, because of concerns that individual patients or hospitals would be identified. We went ahead and included them, and feedback over the

years has confirmed that they have been invaluable educational tools, as well as bringing a potentially dry report to life.

There was considerable trepidation as to how the first annual report would be received by the media, and so we hired a professional communications consultant for advice. It was agreed that we should take a highly proactive approach so that we would not be put in a defensive position. Therefore, the three senior doctors running SHOT had some rapid media training, and health correspondents of national newspapers and medical media were invited to a press launch at the Royal College of Pathologists. Press releases also went to radio and television stations, and we conducted many interviews with local and national stations in the 24 hours after the launch.

After the nervousness as to how the SHOT findings would be reported, we were pleasantly surprised at the moderate tone and balanced approach of most of the coverage. One or two reporters commented that they felt reassured by how safe transfusion now appeared to be, after the hepatitis and HIV problems of the previous decade.

Subsequent annual SHOT reports and SHOT recommendations

SHOT has now published 14 annual reports and summaries. The launch of the second annual report was a relatively quiet affair, which attracted only modest press attention. In the third year, we launched the report to an invited audience of senior national stakeholders in blood transfusion. In the fourth year, we established an annual educational symposium, which is well attended by healthcare professionals in transfusion, with the venue now alternating between the north (Manchester) and the south (London) to emphasize SHOT's UK-wide status.

Reports are circulated to members of the hospital transfusion team (all consultant hematologists with responsibility for transfusion, the transfusion laboratory manager, and the lead transfusion practitioner) and key individuals in stakeholder organizations, and summaries are sent to all chief executives and medical directors. All reports and summaries, additional data, and presentations from annual symposia are on the SHOT website. Summaries are also distributed at various professional meetings where SHOT is able to obtain a free stand and when SHOT team members give presentations at hospital or regional meetings.

SHOT recommendations are categorized as main recommendations and those specific to each chapter. It became clear that the impact of recommendations could be strengthened if they were targeted to specific professional/managerial groups or organizations, and this was implemented from the 2003 report onwards. Since 2006, the annual report has included a list of previous recommendations still active with a progress report on actions being undertaken and highlighting areas where more work is needed.

What would we have done differently?

SHOT was launched 18 years ago, at a time when the laws governing transfusion, public attitudes to risk, and the approach to governance in public life were all very different. Looking back, it seems extraordinary that we did not, for example, seek a formal legal opinion on any aspect of what we were doing. Equally, IT systems have moved apace and no national hemovigilance group would now choose to build a system using a Microsoft Access database, as we did. Having said that, our naivety was perhaps a strength, and if we had overconsidered some of the potential pitfalls, we might never have started at all. Instead, the foundations that we built have not only withstood the passage of time, but also allowed the development of a hemovigilance system that is now embedded in UK transfusion practice, and recognized internationally.

In 2010, SHOT received approximately 2500 reports, the annual launch is now an educational day attended by a wide cross-section of the transfusion community, and SHOT's evidence-based recommendations underpin transfusion safety initiatives in the UK. We remain grateful to the small group of enthusiasts who made it all possible.

References

1 ISBT, 2011, Proposed standard definitions for surveillance of non-infectious adverse transfusion reactions. http://www.isbtweb.org/fileadmin/user_upload/WP-on_Haemovigilance/ISBT_definitions_final_2011_4_.pdf [accessed February 27, 2012].

2 SHOT, 2009, Definitions of Current SHOT Categories and What to Report. http://www.shotuk.org/wp-content/uploads/2010/04/SHOT-Categories-2009.pdf [accessed February 14, 2012].

3 European Union, 2003, Directive 2002/98/EC of the European Parliament and of the Council of January 2003 setting standards of quality and safety for the collection, testing, processing, storage and distribution of human blood and blood components and amending Directive 2001/83/EC. *Official Journal of the European Union* 8.2.2003: L.33/30. http://eur-lex.europa.eu/LexUriServ/LexUriServ.do?uri=OJ:L:2003:033:0030:0040:EN:PDF [accessed February 14, 2012].

4 UK National Archives, 2005, The Blood Safety and Quality Regulations, No. 50. http://www.opsi.gov.uk/si/si2005/20050050.htm [accessed February 14, 2012].

5 Keeling D, Baglin T, Tait C, *et al.*; British Committee for Standards in Haematology, 2011, Guidelines on oral anticoagulation with warfarin, 4th edition. *British Journal of Haematology* **154**: 311–24. www.bcshguidelines.com

6 Department of Health, 2006, Availability of imported Fresh Frozen Plasma in England and North Wales. Gateway reference 5999. http://www.dh.gov.uk/prod_consum_dh/groups/dh_digitalassets/@dh/@en/documents/digitalasset/dh_4127680.pdf [accessed February 14, 2012].

7 Clinical Pathology Accreditation (UK) Ltd, 2009, Standards for the Medical Laboratory. http://www.cpa-uk.co.uk/files/PD-LAB-Standards_v2.01_Mar_09.pdf [accessed February 14, 2012].

8 NPSA, 2006, Safer Practice Notice 14, Right Blood Right Patient. http://www.nrls.npsa.nhs.uk/EasySiteWeb/getresource.axd?AssetID=60046&type=full&servicetype=Attachment. [accessed February 14, 2012].

9 NPSA, 2009, Safer Practice Notice 14 Right Blood Right Patient. Clarification to CEOs. http://www.info.doh.gov.uk/sar2/cmopatie.nsf/vwDiscussionAll/8011E0968997252880257420002A5711?OpenDocument [accessed February 14, 2012].

10 NPSA, 2010, Rapid Response Report 2010/RRR017. The transfusion of blood and blood components in

an emergency. DH Gateway reference 14960. www
.nrls.npsa.nhs.uk/alerts [accessed February 14, 2012].

11 Department of Health, 2007, Health Service Circular,
Better Blood Transfusion—Safe and Appropriate Use
of Blood. HSC 2007/001. http://www.dh.gov.uk/en/
Publicationsandstatistics/Lettersandcirculars/Healthser
vicecirculars/DH_080613 [accessed February 14, 2012].

12 Healthcare Improvement Scotland, 2006, NHS Quality
Improvement Scotland, Clinical Standards for Blood
Transfusion. http://www.healthcareimprovementscot

land.org/idoc.ashx?docid=8370be96-990f-4b06-be38-
825372a2a90b&version=-1 [accessed February 14,
2012].

13 Standards for Health Services in Wales: *Doing Well,
Doing Better*, 2010. Standard 17, Blood Management.
http://www.wales.nhs.uk/sites3/page.cfm?orgid=919
&pid=47620 [accessed April 2012].

14 Williamson LM, Heptonstall J, and Soldan K, 1996, A
SHOT in the arm for safer blood transfusion. *Br Med J*
313: 1221–2.

CHAPTER 15

The Dutch Hemovigilance System: Transfusion Reactions in Patients (TRIP)

Martin R. Schipperus, Johanna Wiersum-Osselton, Pauline Y. Zijlker-Jansen, and Anita J.W. van Tilborgh-de Jong

Dutch National Hemovigilance Office TRIP, The Hague, The Netherlands

Introduction

The Transfusion Reactions in Patients (TRIP) foundation was founded in 2001 by representatives of the various professional organizations involved in the field of blood transfusion. Since 2003, the TRIP National Hemovigilance Office has managed the national reporting system for transfusion reactions in collaboration with contact persons in the hospitals and the blood supply service Sanquin. Reporting to TRIP is anonymous and in principle voluntary. However, reporting to TRIP is considered the norm by the Healthcare Inspectorate (IGZ) and the Dutch Institute for Healthcare Improvement (CBO) Guidelines for Blood Transfusion.[1] The digital reporting system that came into use in 2006 was used actively by the majority of the hospitals in 2009.

Relevant findings of investigations and the degree of severity of the clinical symptoms need to be included in the report. An assessment is also given of the *imputability*, the extent of certainty with which a reaction can be attributed to an administered blood transfusion. If necessary, TRIP will ask the reporting party for further explanations or additional data. This allows the TRIP physicians to assess the coherence of the reports and to verify the reported category of (potentially) serious reports.

Reporting to TRIP is not directly linked to patient care and is also separate from any other non-voluntary reporting routes: to the IGZ in case of calamities, to the blood supply foundation Sanquin in the case of possible consequences for the safety of the blood component or related components, and within the hospital to the committee for the reporting of incidents in patient care. The criteria of the European directive[2] stipulate that there is an obligation to report serious undesirable adverse events and incidents that may be associated with the quality and/or safety of the blood components. TRIP ensures the analysis and reporting of these serious (grade 2 or higher) adverse events on behalf of the competent authority IGZ. At the end of 2008, the hospitals were informed in a combined circular from the inspectorate and TRIP about the option of making serious reports available to the IGZ and where relevant to the blood supply foundation Sanquin via the TRIP online reporting system.

An Expert Committee (EC), appointed from the TRIP Governing Board, assesses all submitted reports. After approval by the EC the reports are definitively included in the TRIP database.

Hemovigilance: An Effective Tool for Improving Transfusion Safety, First Edition. Edited by René R.P. De Vries and Jean-Claude Faber.
© 2012 John Wiley & Sons, Ltd. Published 2012 by John Wiley & Sons, Ltd.

Since August 2006, TRIP has also managed a national reporting system for serious undesirable adverse events and/or incidents associated with the use of human tissue and cells. TRIP tissue vigilance reports (available on www.tripnet.nl) describe this system and the findings.

Participation

Numbers of actively participating hospitals, their degree of participation, and the quality of information they submit determine the value of registering and evaluating transfusion reactions nationally. In 2009, 99 of the 103 (96%) of hospitals participated by reporting results. Of these, 92 hospitals reported transfusion reactions and 7 hospitals indicated that they had none to report. In addition, TRIP received information about blood use from all 99 hospitals. As in the past, it was the responsibility of those reporting to determine at which moment subsequent to a merger different locations became sufficiently comparable to proceed further under one reporting code. Every year, a several hospitals do not manage to send in data before the closing date: these hospitals have the status of "nonparticipants" in the TRIP report (see Figure 15.1).

Additionally, Sanquin's central departments made available to TRIP their summaries of seri-ous reports and of administered blood components for which, after administration, they determined positive bacterial-screen results. A number of reports came in as well from contact persons in Sanquin's regional blood-bank divisions. Annually, TRIP checks on double reports and combines these after discussing with reporters.

Reports received

A total of 2384 reports of transfusion reactions were collated in 2009. In 2008, the number was 2052, and so an increase of 16% occurred in 2009. The number of reports on serious reactions was 98, a slight decrease compared to the previous years (2006–2008) when the number of reports on serious events was 116 annually. Of the total number of reports, 2109 were on transfusion reactions and 275 on incidents. There are some non-serious categories that, until now, have been optional for reporting: mild febrile reactions, near-misses, and information from hospitals about positive bacterial screen and other component incidents. TRIP sees it as useful to register these, but does not necessarily need all hospitals to cooperate. Of all reports, 2019 were submitted digitally (85%, 71 hospitals).

After EC assessment, reporters received supplementary questions in a number of instances.

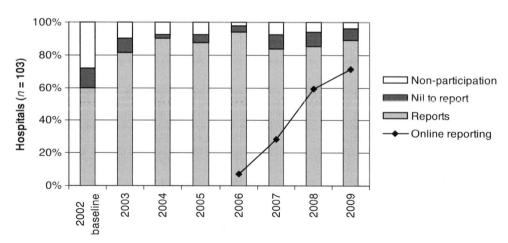

Figure 15.1 Degree of participation over the years from 2002 (the serial measurement) up to and including 2009, as of March 1, 2010.

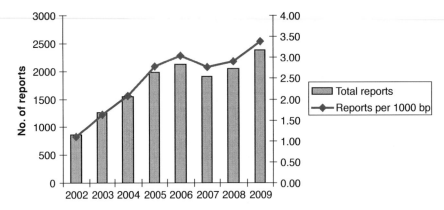

Figure 15.2 Number of reports to TRIP 2002–2009.

Discussions with the reporter led in a few cases to amending the reporting category. Reporters were able to give relevant, supplementary information in other cases to reach consensus or adjust the degree of severity or extent of imputability. Figure 15.2 shows the number of reports from 2002 until 2009.

All definitions can be found at www.tripnet.nl. At the beginning of 2008, TRIP distributed revised definitions, which came into force as of January 1, 2008.

Transfusion reactions and incidents from 2003 up to 2009

Table 15.1 shows the number of reports per category for the years 2002 up to and including 2009 and Table 15.2 shows numbers of incidents for the same period.

The increase in the number of reports in 2009 is mainly due to an increase in the number of reported febrile reactions, new red blood cell

Table 15.1 Transfusion reactions (TR)* reported to TRIP from 2003 up to and including 2009.

Reaction	2003	2004	2005	2006	2007	2008	2009	Degree 2 or higher[#]
NHTR	318	345	435	490	452	453	485	15
Mild febrile reaction	326	341	375	363	327	275	357	4
AHTR	8	14	9	17	11	18	18	6
DHTR	19	14	12	14	11	18	8	3
TRALI	7	9	17	25	31	21	12	10
Anaphylactic reaction	8	21	26	19	54	65	69	19
Other allergic reaction	132	171	219	222	202	171	180	0
Circulatory overload	7	6	27	34	31	39	41	14
Post-transfusion purpura	0	0	0	0	0	1	0	0
TA-GvHD	0	0	0	0	0	0	1	0
Hemosiderosis	0	0	3	5	3	5	2	0
New antibody production	244	428	571	607	600	607	753	2
Other reactions	54	64	67	61	55	101	132	15
Post-transfusion bacteremia/sepsis	9	5	10	7	19	37	50	0
Viral infection	5	7	8	7	7	7	2	0
Total TR	**1137**	**1425**	**1779**	**1871**	**1803**	**1818**	**2110**	**88**

*Imputability certain, probable, or possible.

Table 15.2 Incidents per year from 2003 up to and including 2009.

Incident	2003	2004	2005	2006	2007	2008	2009
Incorrect blood component	34	36	60	64	64	59	60
Near-miss	31	62	79	77	74	55	72
Other incident	5	12	51	86	100	83	110
Look-back (hospital to Trip)		2	2	1	4	9	6
Virally infected component					2	2	1
Positive bacterial screen	61	10	13	27	29	2	1
Bacterial contamination					5	23	22
Total	**131**	**122**	**205**	**255**	**278**	**233**	**272**

antibodies, and reports on other reactions and incidents. The category "other reactions" in Table 15.1 contains several reports on hypotensive reactions and reports on dyspnea, without other symptoms of Transfusion Related Acute Lung Injury (TRALI), for which no specific TRIP category exists.

Severity of transfusion reactions

Table 15.3 details the definitions of the severity of transfusion reactions.

The definition of severity relates to clinical symptoms observed in the patient; it is only meaningful for transfusion reactions. In the following, "clinical transfusion reaction" means all reports in the transfusion-reaction categories (2010 in 2009), plus reactions arising after reports in the incident category (25 in 2009). The degree of severity had been assigned to 2093 of the 2134 reports (98.1%) of

Table 15.3 Severity of transfusion reactions.

Severity	Definition
0	No morbidity
1	Limited morbidity, no threat to life
2	Medium to serious morbidity, with or without threat to life, or leading to hospitalization or prolongation of illness, or accompanied by chronic invalidity or disability
3	Serious morbidity, directly life-threatening
4	Mortality subsequent to the transfusion reaction

clinical transfusion reactions. Figure 15.3 shows the severity assigned to clinical transfusion reactions from 2003 up to and including 2009.

Figures reveal decreases in reports of degree of severity for incidents lacking clinical consequences,

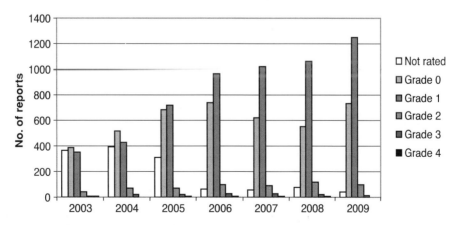

Figure 15.3 Number of reports and severity of the transfusion reaction.

and—even for clinical transfusion reactions—the continuance of two desired trends visible since 2005. First, TRIP has maintained continuously its standpoint that the report must assign a minimum degree of severity if clinical symptoms are present. Second, for incidents, reporting should include a subcategory if a reaction occurs. Reporting should include both the reaction's degree of severity and its imputability. Severity and imputability are irrelevant if events lack a clinical picture.

There were 113 (5.3% of total) reports of serious incidents (degree of severity 2 up to and including 4), which is a decrease compared to the previous years (with a mean of 130 in 2006–2008). Since the total number of reports has increased in 2009 this reduction of the number of serious transfusion reactions cannot be explained by a diminished "vigilance" of the reporters. It is too early, however, to draw any conclusions on this decrease of serious transfusion reactions.

Relationship to the blood transfusion (imputability)

The reports were also categorized according to imputability, a measure of probability that the reaction resulted from the transfusion (see Table 15.4). The reporting of imputability is also only relevant in cases of a transfusion reaction. Of the 2134 transfusion reactions reported in 2009, the imputability was listed for 2093 reports (98.1%). Of these, 330 (15.8%) were considered certainly related to the transfusion, 623 (29.8%) were probable, 975 (46,6%) were possible, 145 (6.9%) were unlikely, and 20 (1.0%) were excluded.

Variation among hospitals

The number of transfusion reactions per 1000 administrated blood components per hospital varies from 0 to 13.84 (the maximum in 2008 was 11.14, the maximum in 2007 was 9.5); the median is 3.18.

Various factors determine the variations between institutions:
- Differences due to factors outside the transfusion chain: for instance, differences in the patient population and differences in the proportions of platelet components.
- Differences arising from working techniques in the blood-transfusion chain, which can indicate differences in quality of blood-transfusion practice or safety.
- Differences in reporting cultures among the hospitals.

Factors within an institution, such as the availability of education and training and the reporting

Table 15.4 Relationship to the blood transfusion (imputability).

Imputability	Definition (imputability solely applies to clinical transfusion reactions)	Definition details
Certain	Clinical symptoms present, and	• clear course of incidents • temporarily related to the transfusion • accompanying laboratory findings • other causes excluded
Probable	Clinical symptoms present, but	• no clear course of incidents • not temporarily related to the transfusion • no accompanying laboratory findings • possible presence of other cause(s)
Possible	Clinical symptoms present, but	• not temporarily related to the transfusion • no accompanying laboratory findings • possible presence of other cause
Unlikely	Clinical symptoms present, but	• not temporarily related to the transfusion • no accompanying laboratory findings • other more probable explanation present
Excluded	Clearly demonstrable other cause(s)	

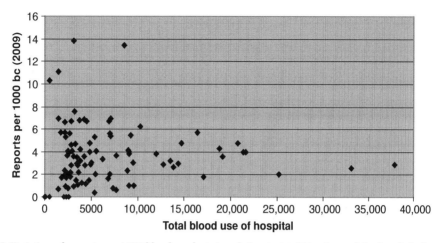

Figure 15.4 Variation of reports per 1000 blood products in relation to total blood use of the hospitals (bc = blood components).

culture, probably largely determine report numbers. TRIP's ultimate goal in registering reports is to acquire more insight into the occurrence of transfusion reactions and incidents and to recommend ways of improving the safety of blood transfusion. TRIP uses the registered data, both individual reports and the indicators they suggest, to achieve this aim. Further research is needed into the factors influencing numbers of reports and how numbers of reports reflect the level of safety of an institution's blood-transfusion practices (see Figure 15.4).

Numbers of transfusion reactions in relationship to numbers of supplied blood components

In 2009, Sanquin supplied the Dutch hospitals with a total of 699,720 blood components; this number does not include special components such as lymphocytes and granulocytes. The total number of reports for 2009 is 2384. On average, that is 3.4 reports per 1000 components (in 2007: 2.7 and in 2008: 2.9). Table 15.5 shows the relationship between supplied blood components and numbers of reports.

Table 15.5 Reports in 2008 and 2009, per type of blood component (RBC = red blood cells; NR = numbers not reported).

Blood component type	2008 reports	2008 blood components issued	2008 reports per 1000	2009 reports	2009 blood components issued	2009 reports per 1000
RBC concentrate	1518	559,372	2.71	1812	559,976	3.24
Platelet concentrate	262	50,584	5.16	302	49,354	6.12
Fresh frozen plasma (FFP)	81	96,622	0.84	99	90,390	1.10
Autologous (RBCs, predeposit)	1	110 (donations)		1	NR (donations)	
Cell-saver and drainblood	24			32		
Other components	4			0	0	
Combinations	95			70	NR	
Not indicated	79			68	NR	
Total/Average	**2064**	**706,688**	**2.9**	**2384**	**699,720**	**3.49**

Table 15.6 Numbers and imputability of reports of degree 2 and higher in 2007 and 2008.

Type of reaction	Serious reports		Possible		Probable		Certain	
	2008	2009	2008	2009	2008	2009	2008	2009
Acute hemolytic TR	10	11	1	3	4	1	5	7
Delayed hemolytic TR	4	3	0	0	1	1	3	2
TRALI	18	12	6	5	9	5	3	2
Anaphylactic reaction	29	19	10	7	15	11	4	1
Other allergic reaction	5	0	4	0	0	0	1	0
Circulatory overload	17	15	9	5	6	7	2	3
Post-transfusion bacteremia*	4	1	3	0	0	1	1	0
Post-transfusion viral infection	2	1	1	0	1	1	0	0
Post-transfusion purpura	0	0	0	0	0	0	0	0
TA-GvHD	0	0	0	0	0	0	0	0
Other severe reactions	42	36	18	22	18	13	6	1
Total	131	98	52	42	54	40	25	16

*This category includes "bacterial contamination" under 2007 definitions; 2008 has one report of severity-2 bacterial contamination of blood component.

Obligatory reports of serious adverse events in the transfusion chain

According to the European directives 2002/98/EG and 2005/61/EG and conforming to the common approach the European Committee set up in spring of 2009, this overview includes only reports with possible, probable, or certain imputability. The relevant category includes other incidents and reactions to incorrect blood component transfused. Table 15.6 shows data for 2008 and 2009.

Comments on some categories of transfusion reactions and incidents

Transfusion Related Acute Lung Injury (TRALI) and the Dutch "male-only plasma" measure

Definition: Dyspnea and hypoxia within six hours of transfusion; chest X-ray shows bilateral pulmonary infiltrates. There are negative investigations (biochemical or blood-group serological) for hemolysis, bacteriology is negative, and no other explanation exists.

In 2009, 12 reports of TRALI came in, a decrease compared with the previous years (21 in 2008, 31 in 2007, and 25 in 2006). TRALI report numbers rose from 2003 to 2007, probably due to increased national and international attention for this transfusion reaction (see Figure 15.5).

At the end of 2006, the Dutch Sanquin Blood Supply Foundation introduced the measure of using solely plasma from male, never-transfused donors to prepare quarantined fresh frozen plasma (FFP) for transfusion. After all, female plasma more often contains HLA-antibodies and parties observed that some TRALIs subsequent to transfusion of plasma-containing blood components show these antibodies that target HLA markers (Class I or II) or other antigens on the receiver's leucocytes. Due to the quarantine period, the measure was effective

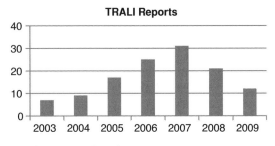

Figure 15.5 Number of TRALI reports 2003–2009.

from mid-2007. From that time TRIP observed a decrease in the number of TRALI reports. An additional analysis of the TRALI data revealed that the "male-only plasma" measure has resulted in a 30% reduction of the total number of TRALI cases yearly.[3]

Anaphylactic transfusion reaction

Definition: Rapidly developing reaction occurring within a few seconds to minutes after the start of transfusion with features such as obstruction, in- and expiratory stridor, fall in blood pressure of 20 mm Hg or more (diastolic or systolic); nausea, vomiting, or diarrhea, possibly with skin rash.

Anaphylaxis is one of the most important categories of serious reports. Of the reports, 11 were associated with the administration of red blood cells, 22 with plasma, and 31 with platelet concentrates. The risk of an anaphylactic reaction is greatest for a unit of platelets concentrate. The total number of reports of anaphylactic reaction is slightly higher than in 2008, but fewer of these reported were serious ones. After the introduction of the "male-only plasma" measure there is no indication of a decrease in the number of reports of anaphylactic transfusion reaction.

Other allergic reactions

Definition: Allergic phenomena such as itching, redness, or urticaria but without respiratory, cardiovascular, or gastrointestinal features, arising from a few minutes of starting transfusion until a few hours after its completion. Hemolysis testing and bacteriology negative if performed.

The number of reports of other allergic reactions in 2009 is similar to the final total of 2008 (180 compared to 171 in 2008), but slightly lower than the average number of 210 for 2005–2007. The "missing" reports were probably reported in the category of anaphylactic reaction in accordance with the request by TRIP to categorize allergic reactions with more than just skin symptoms in this category. In 2009, there were no reports of serious (grade 2 or more) other allergic reactions, in contrast to the previous five years.

Transfusion Associated Circulatory Overload (TACO)

Definition: Dyspnea, orthopnea, cyanosis, tachycardia >100/min, or elevated central venous pressure (one or more of these signs) within six hours of transfusion, usually in a patient with compromised cardiac function. Chest X-ray consistent.

The number of reports of TACO in 2009 was 39, which is consistent with the number of reports in the previous years. Two reports were grade 3 and thirteen were grade 2, also comparable with the previous years. Over two thirds (69%) of the reports of circulatory overload involved the administration of red blood only.

The majority of the patients were female. There were some relatively young patients of 40 years or younger. TACO is frequently associated with renal failure, but also in post-partum patients.

A number of reports of circulatory overload were initially thought to be a TRALI. The clinical distinction between TACO and TRALI remains difficult, even when a chest X-ray is present. TRIP always tries to verify the diagnosis of TACO. The correct diagnosis is based on the patient's history, the clinical observations (including chest X-ray and fluid balance), and the patient's response on diuretics.

Incidents in the transfusion chain

Incorrect blood component transfused

Definition: All cases where a patient received a transfusion with a blood component that did not fulfill all requirements to be suitable for the relevant patient or that was intended for another patient.

Since 2005, numbers of reports in this category have fluctuated at around 60 per year. The number of cases of incorrect blood component transfused where clinical symptoms are observed shows greater variation: 4 in 2007; the highest number until now is 16 in 2005. For the 60 incidences of incorrect blood component transfused collated in 2009, there are 9 cases of clinical symptoms observed in the patient.

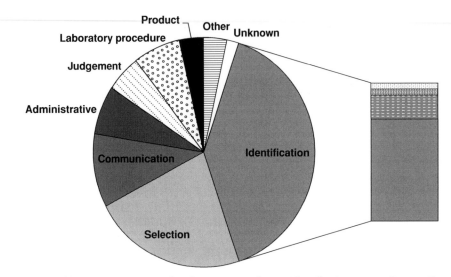

Figure 15.6 Incorrect blood component transfused 2009: Type of error, identification error split according to step in the chain.

For the reports of incorrect blood component transfused, 30 (50%) were evaluated as ABO risk; the components that were administered for the incidents with ABO risk were RBCs 25x, platelets twice, and plasma three times.

For the 30 reports of incorrect blood component transfused with ABO risk, there were 23 cases of identification error as a first error, with this identification error taking place in the last check (bedside check) before administration of the blood component 17 times. In two cases a selection error resulted in a potential ABO risk. The other reports of incorrect blood component transfused (28) this year were mainly selection (11) and communication (6) errors. An overview of the type of risk per first error is provided in Figure 15.6.

Other incidents

Definition: Errors or incidents in the transfusion chain that do not fit into any of the above categories, for instance patient transfused whereas the intention was to keep the blood component in reserve, or transfusing unnecessarily on the basis of an incorrect Hb result or avoidable wastage of a blood component.

There is a marked increase in the number of reports of other incidents in the years 2008 and

2009: 83 in 2008 and 110 in 2009. Symptoms were observed in the patient in seven of these reports. There were also three reports of transfusion reactions (NHTR, new antibody formation, and other reaction once each) for which the additional category of other incident was reported.

Near-misses

Definition: Any error that, if undetected, could have led to a wrong blood group result or issue or administration of an incorrect blood component, and which was detected before transfusion. Please indicate where the error arose, any further errors or failed checks, and how the error was discovered.

In comparison to the previous reporting year, there were over 30% more near-miss incidents (72) reported in 2009 by 16 hospitals, varying from 1 to 10 reports, a marked difference from 2008 when nearly half of the reports (24 out of 53) in this category were received from one hospital. The first error in over 75% of the cases was made in the steps of transfusion request (12) or pre-transfusion testing (42) and 41 of these 54 errors involved an error in identification of the patient, blood sample, and/or request form. In 19 cases, blood group discrepancy was the reason that an identification error was discovered in a timely manner.

Checks and vigilance by employees of the blood transfusion laboratory were responsible for preventing more serious incidents in the majority of these near accidents. However, there appears to be an increase in the number of reported near-misses (19%) in which an error was discovered by nurses or other staff from clinical areas by checking at issue or checking prior to transfusion on the ward or in the operating room. This could be related to the arising of an improved reporting culture in hospital departments. Two of these 14 reports also indicated that training about blood transfusion had taken place recently.

It is noteworthy that the first errors in the reports of a near-misses—the errors that were discovered in a timely manner—were mainly identification errors (65%), and communication and selection errors account for less than 10% of the near-miss reports. Comparing this to the first errors in reports of an incorrect blood component being transfused reveals a greater percentage of identification errors in 2009 than in 2008 (41% versus 23%). The percentage of reported communication errors for incorrect blood component transfused (10%) is significantly lower than in 2008 (23%), while the percentage of selection errors (22%) has increased since 2008 (16%). An overview of the types of errors in near-misses is shown in Figure 15.7.

General considerations and conclusions

After seven reporting years, we see a more or less stable number of reports, both for serious and non-serious events. Although after the introduction of "male-only plasma" an interesting decrease of the number of TRALI cases was observed, this does not explain the decrease in the total number of reports on serious events in 2009. Still we can state that national reporting has produced "knowledge of the nature and extent of the transfusion reactions." Thanks in part to the role of hemovigilance employees, in the Netherlands levels of use of RBC concentrates are among the lowest in European countries and there is a well-developed blood supply.

TRIP will continue the way it began, providing the hospitals with benchmark information that mirrors the status of their own reports versus the number of reports received nationally. The availability of this information can be a trigger for hospitals and research groups to initiate research into clarifications and factors relevant to the safety of blood transfusion in the Netherlands.

Concurrently, TRIP has to admit to the limitations of a system of this type. First, even extensive research and discussions with experts can fail to

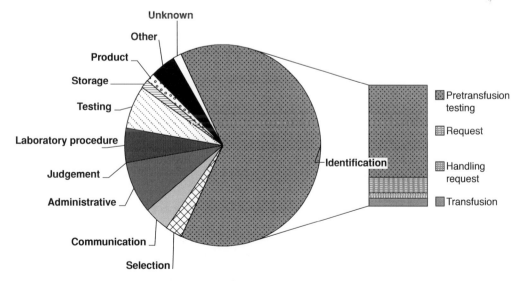

Figure 15.7 Near-misses 2009: Type of error, identification error split according to step in the chain.

produce consensus as to the diagnosis (category) or even the degree of severity of a transfusion reaction. Second, spontaneous reports are not a good way of measuring incidents. For some time, TRIP has been indicating the likeliness of too little reporting of incorrect blood component transfused. Continuing TRIP registration has made clear that reporting behaviors of the different hospitals vary considerably, thus influencing national figures. National hemovigilance registration is not an aim in itself, but an instrument, necessary but not perfect.

The variation in categorization of reports from year to year needs study and clarification. It is necessary to seek the relationship between numbers of reports and other indicators and the safety and quality of blood transfusion. In addition to fundamental laboratory work, this requirement demands randomized clinical trials, post-marketing surveillance studies, and practically oriented research into the transfusion chain. TRIP hopes that hospitals and other research groups will use TRIP reports to trigger research and to support their own efforts at hemovigilance.

For references for the TRIP annual reports 2003–2009 and TRIP publications see www.tripnet.nl.

References

1 Dutch Institute for Healthcare Improvement (CBO), 2011, Guidelines for Blood Transfusion. http://www.cbo.nl/thema/Richtlijnen/Overzicht-Richtlijnen/Bloedtransfusie and http://www.cbo.nl/en/Guidelines [in English] [accessed February 25, 2012].

2 European Union, 2003, Directive 2002/98/EC of the European Parliament and of the Council of January 2003 setting standards of quality and safety for the collection, testing, processing, storage and distribution of human blood and blood components and amending Directive 2001/83/EC. *Official Journal of the European Union* 8.2.2003: L33/30.

3 Wiersum-Osselton JC, Middelburg RA, Beckers EA, van Tilborgh AJ, Zijlker-Jansen PY, *et al.*, 2011, Male-only fresh-frozen plasma for transfusion-related acute lung injury prevention: Before-and-after comparative cohort study. *Transfusion* **51**(6): 1278–83.

CHAPTER 16

Regulatory, Public Health, and International Aspects of Hemovigilance in Canada

Peter R. Ganz[1] and Jun Wu[2]

[1]Centre for Blood and Tissues Evaluation, Biologics and Genetic Therapies Directorate, Ottawa, Ontario, Canada
[2]Blood Safety Surveillance and Health Care Acquired Infection Division, Public Health Agency of Canada, Ottawa, Ontario, Canada

Introduction

Overview of hemovigilance in Canada

Hemovigilance comprises a set of organized surveillance protocols or procedures relating to the cataloging of serious adverse or unexpected events or reactions in blood donors and recipients. It is characterized by an epidemiological investigation following these unintended events.

Hemovigilance has been recognized as an integral aspect of the safety of blood systems. National Regulatory Authorities (NRAs) have for many years understood that reporting of serious adverse events (SAEs) related to transfusion of blood components represents an important element of blood safety surveillance.[1,2] Such a serious adverse event is defined as an untoward occurrence associated with blood collection, testing, processing, storage, and distribution of blood components that might lead to morbidity or life-threatening or incapacitating conditions for recipients or which may result in prolonging hospitalization. For blood products marketed in Canada, there is also a regulatory requirement to report SAEs as part of Canada's broader pharmacovigilance surveillance system.[3]

Public health authorities as well as regulatory authorities are also concerned with adverse transfusion events (ATEs), which are defined as an unintended response in a donor or a patient associated with the collection or transfusion of blood components that is fatal, life-threatening, disabling, or incapacitating. Many countries have in place a regulatory requirement to report SAEs such as death within 24 hours.[4] This allows both the blood center and regulatory agencies to investigate promptly and carry out a root cause analysis so that if there are issues identified with the blood component in question, there would be opportunities to remove other components from distribution or perhaps quarantine units depending on the circumstance.

Within Canada, the scope of surveillance activities is fairly broad. It includes collecting data regarding donor safety or donor vigilance such as syncope and untoward effects of donation on donor health. Regarding assessments of safety of blood components prepared within blood centers in Canada, there is also collection of data regarding incidence of positive test results for various infectious agents and prevalence of same in the donor population. The latter areas are important in look-back investigations. Within hospitals, transfusion services monitor adverse effects of transfusion in recipients including identification of transmission of infections, which is a key ingredient for

Hemovigilance: An Effective Tool for Improving Transfusion Safety, First Edition. Edited by René R.P. De Vries and Jean-Claude Faber.
© 2012 John Wiley & Sons, Ltd. Published 2012 by John Wiley & Sons, Ltd.

traceability. Also, near-misses are also tracked by transfusion services.

Canada's blood system: The importance of hemovigilance

There are over 800 hospitals serving approximately 33 million people in Canada. Every year, over 1 million units of blood, which is subsequently processed into red cells, plasma, and platelets, are collected and distributed to hospitals by Canada's two blood operators, Canadian Blood Services (CBS) and Héma Québec (HQ). Even with the introduction of the best available screening technologies to test donated blood and blood products, blood transfusion, like other medical procedures, still poses a certain level of risk to recipients and so transfusion is not a zero-risk medical intervention. Therefore, it is imperative that an effective hemovigilance system be in place to monitor adverse events in recipients of blood and blood products.

Hemovigilance allows an assessment of the magnitude and trending of new and emerging/re-emerging infectious agents and reactions in recipients. Outcomes of an effective hemovigilance system provide information for developing strategies or policies for regulatory and public health authorities in order to mitigate risks, evaluate the effectiveness of actions taken to reduce the risks, and thus improve clinical practice and patient safety as the ultimate goal.

Increasing blood safety is of major importance in Canada. Improvements to blood system safety were precipitated following the tainted blood "tragedy" in the 1980s in which approximately 1000 Canadians acquired human immunodeficiency virus (HIV) and another 25,000 were infected with the hepatitis C virus (HCV) through the transfusion of tainted blood in large measure because Canada's blood system "did not respond to the HIV/AIDS challenge as quickly as it might have."[5] Blood safety enhancements became a necessity in the country following the recommendations of the Commission of Inquiry on the Blood System in Canada by Justice Horace Krever.

The final report of the Krever Inquiry, which was released in November 1997, emphasized the importance of hemovigilance and the roles of the regulator and public health authorities at the federal level, and blood operators in the blood system in Canada.[5]

Hemovigilance in Canada: Key elements

The Canadian hemovigilance system is an important component of Canada's blood system. As for any licensed medicinal, collection of surveillance data regarding SAEs is both necessary and beneficial for ensuring overall safety and optimal clinical use of the drug. For blood and blood components this situation is identical since the goal of hemovigilance is to monitor transfusion safety through the collection of surveillance data that can then be analyzed and used to make improvements in the quality and safety of transfused components. Operationally, the goals of the hemovigilance system within Canada's public health system are as follows:

• To partner with Provinces/Territories (P/Ts) to establish and maintain an independent national hemovigilance system for adverse events (e.g., infectious diseases and noninfectious adverse events) related to blood and blood product transfusion.

• To carry out targeted research in order to provide information for risk assessment to further mitigate the risks associated with blood and blood products transfusion in Canada.

One of the concerns of the Krever Commission was that a fragmented blood system would not allow an integrated approach for blood safety.[5] For this reason the blueprint for future development focused on the establishment of key roles and responsibilities for each of the principal stakeholders in the blood system and their coordinated roles in a national system. For example, within Canada's blood system, the regulatory authority (Health Canada) has the key responsibility for the following:

• regulation of the blood system;

• developing and updating standards and policy on blood safety as new evidence becomes available;

• maintaining laboratory capacity within the federal government to support the regulations and standards development for the blood system;

- evaluation of test kits and medical devices for use in the blood system;
- responsibility for post-market surveillance, compliance, and enforcement activities.

The public health authority within the federal government, the Public Health Agency of Canada (PHAC) is responsible for

- surveillance of known infectious agents (e.g., HBV, HCV, HIV, WNv, vCJD prion) and potential emerging blood-borne pathogens (e.g., Xenotrophic Murine Leukemia Virus Related Virus) in the population;
- outbreak and field investigations for blood-borne diseases;
- targeted studies to support risk assessment and management.

Finally, CBS and HQ are responsible for recruiting and screening donors, and collection, processing, testing, storage, and issuance of all blood components. Both operators exert considerable effort toward compliance with regulations concerning good manufacturing processes and related activities within their Health Canada-licensed facilities. However, responsibility for clinical practice of transfusion medicine rests with hospitals and clinicians.

Although transfusion-associated SAEs are required to be reported to Health Canada, participation in more comprehensive and rigorous hemovigilance is voluntary. All blood surveillance systems supported by the PHAC are voluntary systems, which were established to collect more comprehensive data on adverse events and reactions required to be reported to Health Canada. Therefore, participating sites use the same reporting forms to collect data for the purposes of both regulatory requirements and public health needs. These surveillance systems supported by the PHAC are not intended to replace those managed by the regulatory authority.

Health Canada's Blood-borne Pathogens Division (transferred to PHAC) was created to carry out the surveillance aspects of the blood safety programs. In order to develop the infrastructure for Canada's hemovigilance system, the federal government, through Health Canada, allocated approximately CN$4 million annually, including approximately CN$1.9 million of grants and contributions to provincial and territorial governments, and CN$1.6 million in salaries, operations, and maintenance. Partners include not-for-profit organizations, blood operators, healthcare organizations for high-risk patients as well as the regulator. Funding to support activities related to blood-safety surveillance was originally provided by Health Canada at that time prior to the creation of PHAC in 2004.

An important aspect of the hemovigilance system is to develop data linkages with public health, regulators, and healthcare providers so that the statistical integration of PHAC's databases with other databases of blood operators and P/Ts can be conducted in order to strengthen public health responses to known and emerging blood-borne pathogen threats. Currently, the Canadian hemovigilance system has five components: Transfusion Transmitted Injuries Surveillance System (TTISS); Transfusion Errors Surveillance System (TESS); Cells, Tissues, and Organs Surveillance System (CTOSS); targeted surveillance/research for high-risk populations; and target surveillance for emerging pathogens. These separately established but linked elements will be examined in detail in the later sections "Evolution of Canada's hemovigilance system", "Further enhancement of TTISS, TESS surveillance systems", and "Building on the hemovigilance system within Canada's National Health Care System: Biovigilance."

Scope and governance of the hemovigilance system in Canada

Responsibility for hemovigilance rests in a number of arenas in Canada and spans local, regional, and national activities. At the national level, Canada's blood system operators, which include CBS and HQ, are licensed by Health Canada and legislation exists under Canada's Food and Drugs Act and Regulations requiring the collection of data regarding SAEs. Data regarding errors and accidents concerning manufacturing processes for blood components are also tracked by CBS and HQ and are risk managed by Health Canada through its annual inspection and compliance activities of all licensed blood centers. All blood centers in Canada are inspected annually. PHAC is responsible for the

TTISS, TESS, and targeted blood safety surveillance elements as well as CTOSS.

The Canadian model for governance of hemovigilance is thus a blend of mandatory reporting for SAEs as monitored by Health Canada and a voluntary reporting system for ATE through PHAC. Both government agencies cooperate through established communication links and both are represented in the national data analyses committee. Some of the advantages to this model are that it is centralized, which allows dissemination of national policies and employs uniform standards for definitions and reporting. In addition, a centralized model facilitates data collection and analyses and provides the opportunity to have a single point of contact for international coordination (see the later section "International linkages and Canada's roles"). The linkage between Health Canada with responsibility for regulatory activities and PHAC for public health surveillance with strong linkages to P/Ts allows for coordination between manufacturers and transfusion services within Canada's regions. (Other governance models for hemovigilance as operationalized in other countries are explored in other chapters of this book.)

Non-governmental organizations (NGOs) as well as professional bodies operating at the national level also have a role in promoting education and communicating the importance of hemovigilance activities. Within Canada, the Canadian Society for Transfusion Medicine sponsors annual meetings often in conjunction with the blood operators as a forum for discussing the latest science and data concerning hemovigilance.

At the regional level, Canada's P/Ts have seen hospitals with active transfusion services usually at tertiary care hospitals form regional transfusion services offering operational support to one another and standardizing activities. This has allowed the sharing of information about transfusion practices and provides a centralized point of contact regarding adverse events.

Recognizing the importance of hemovigilance within public health, the province of Québec has promulgated an act[6] that outlines the requirement to establish a hemovigilance committee, its linkage to HQ, membership, and its roles and responsibilities within the provincial public health context.

Evolution of Canada's hemovigilance system

Hemovigilance systems are dynamic and responsive to feedback mechanisms generated by data gathered or by experience gained through surveillance activities.[7]

In the next few sections, we examine the various surveillance systems in place and their interconnections.

Transfusion Transmitted Injuries Surveillance System (TTISS)

In March 1998, the Surveillance and Epidemiology of Transfusion (SET) Working Group within the Blood-borne Pathogens Division was formed to be responsible for planning and establishing pilot sites for the national blood surveillance system. The initial sites chosen were the provinces of British Columbia, Québec, Prince Edward Island, and Nova Scotia, which provided pilot data for analysis for the period 1999–2002. The SET Working Group consisted of various experts from different stakeholders including public health officials and regulators within the federal government, clinicians, epidemiologists, and researchers from blood operators and provincial and territorial governments.

Although the SET Working Group provided expertise during the formative stages of establishing hemovigilance in Canada, there was a need to have ongoing stakeholder participation in the TTISS initiative. Thus, TTISS is currently supported through the National Working Group for TTISS (NWGTTISS). The Working Group is comprised of 20 members, including all participant data collection sites, blood operators, regulators, and public health officials from the PHAC. The goal of this Working Group is to identify and address technical issues raised by the members to improve the TTISS through upgrading the manual, reporting forms, case definitions, and protocol. Unexpected or unusual adverse events are usually identified by

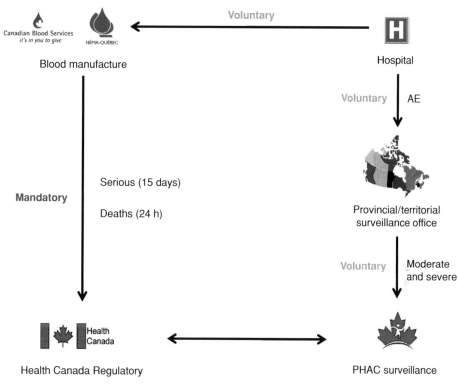

Figure 16.1 Reporting mechanism for transfusion adverse events.

this Working Group during routine practice of the surveillance.

Within Canada's hemovigilance system, the standard user's manual, reporting forms and protocol, and data-sharing agreements were developed and agreed upon by all the participated sites. Adverse events that meet standard case definitions are reported from hospitals to the P/Ts, and then to the PHAC. The dataflow from hospitals to P/Ts and to PHAC is described in Figure 16.1. All non-nominal data are kept in a database developed and maintained by the PHAC. The PHAC also provides ongoing IT support to all participated sites. Annual reports are prepared by the PHAC in collaboration with all participant sites.

At the end of 2007, Canada's national hemovigilance system, TTISS, was extended to cover approximately 83% of the transfusion activities in the country (see Table 16.1). A total of 495 validated ATEs were included for the final analysis,

of which 430 cases were related to blood components and 65 related to plasma derivatives and recombinant clotting factor products. A total of 104 cases were excluded from the final analysis due to the fact that they were classed as minor events, for example, febrile reactions, post-IVIG headache, minor allergic or delayed serological reactions, or did not meet the standard case definitions. The overall quality of the data, including completeness, cases with missing information, and the proportion of "qualified" cases for the final analysis, significantly improved from 2004–2007 (as Table 16.1 shows).

The total incidence of ATEs in 2007 was reported as 1:3147 units transfused (see Table 16.2). Of these, Transfusion Associated Circulatory Overload (TACO) was the most frequent adverse event with 188 reported to the TTISS at a ratio of 1:6545. This rate is much higher (about 6-fold) than that reported by the French Hemovigilance System

Table 16.1 Adverse transfusion events (ATEs) reported through TTISS and other sources, 2004–2007.

Year	ATEs reported to TTISS	Excluded ATEs and reasons for exclusion								Included ATEs from TTISS		CBS	Health Canada— Santé Canada	Total cases
		Non-reportable minor event		Incomplete/ missing information		Not meeting standard definition								
		N	%[1]	N	%[1]	N	%[1]			N	%[2]	N	N	
2007	540	84	80.8	0	–	20	19.2			436	80.7	39	20	495
2006	612	113	65.3	50	28.9	10	5.8			439	71.7	23	35	497
2005	569	176	85.4	25	12.1	5	2.4			363	63.8	21	27	411
2004	489	106	53.3	74	37.2	19	9.5			290	59.3	22	39	351

[1]Proportion within excluded events; [2]proportion of ATEs reported to TTISS.

between 2004 and 2007 (ratio 1:42,322).[8] Possible explanations may be related to variations in case definitions and reporting of TACO or different transfusion practices; for example, more systematic use of diuretics in France. Given the high incidence of TACO and its contribution to overall mortalities in Canadian transfusion medicine, efforts need to be taken to improve fluid management during transfusion practices.

The second most frequent reaction reported to the TTISS in 2007 was severe allergic or anaphylactic reactions (SAAR) with 62 cases, representing an incidence of 1:19,845 units (as shown in Table 16.2). The overall incidence of Transfusion Related Acute Lung Injury (TRALI) that meet the complete case definition was 1:55,927 units transfused. However, the TTISS has also captured data where not all the criteria for TRALI have been met. These have been categorized as "possible TRALI." If possible TRALI reports are also included in the analyses; the incidence rate becomes 1:36,188 units (see Table 16.2). Most of the TRALI cases reported to the TTISS were related to RBC transfusion. In Canada the data show that transfusion respiratory complications—including TACO, TRALI, possible TRALI, and Transfusion Associated Dyspnea (TAD)—were the leading cause for transfusion-related fatalities in 2007 (13 out of 14 deaths). The incidence of bacterial contamination as shown in Table 16.2 is very low with a ratio of 1:1,230,398

units. The incidence of hypertensive reactions was analyzed to be 2.6 per 100,000 in 2007, dropping from 4.2 per 100,000 in 2006. The contributing factor for this result may be the introduction of a more restrictive case definition in 2006.

National Working Party for Data Review (NWPDR)

Within Canada's hemovigilance system, a National Working Party for Data Review (NWPDR) was also created and housed within the blood safety program at the PHAC to support all elements of the program. Serving as the steering committee function, this Working Party consists of a group of experts, including hematologists, epidemiologists, infectious disease specialists and ex-officio representatives from PHAC, Health Canada, CBS, and HQ. This Working Party reports to the Blood Safety Surveillance and Health Care Acquired Infection Division at the PHAC. The goals of this Working Party are to
• investigate unexpected or unusual adverse events identified by the NWGTTISS;
• review the data collected in the databases within the PHAC hemovigilance system;
• make recommendations to the PHAC concerning research questions and hypotheses for targeted studies to address emerging blood safety issues.

With regard to the surveillance datasets for the TTISS, currently it collects 125 variables from all

Table 16.2 Incidence of adverse transfusion events reported in 2007 (blood components).

| Event diagnosis | Red blood cells (741,349) | | Apheresis platelets (42,906) | | Whole blood derived platelets | | | | Plasma (195,380) | | Other[2] (49,219) | | All components (1,230,3980) | |
| | | | | | Units (210,544) | | Pools[1] (45,749) | | | | | | | |
	N	Incidence	N	Incidence	N	Incidence	N	Incidence	N	Incidence	N	Incidence	N	Incidence
SAAR	24	1:30,890	8	1:5363	10	1:21,054	10	1:4575	19	1:10,283	1	1:49,219	62	1:19,845
AHTR	20	1:37,067			1	1:210,544	1	1:45,749	1	1:195,380			22	1:55,927
DHTR	37	1:20,036											37	1:33,254
TACO	152	1:4877	1	1:42,906	8	1:26,318	8	1:5719	27	1:7,236			188	1:6545
All TRALI	26	1:28,513			2	1:105,272	2	1:22,875	5	1:39,076	1	1:49,219	34	1:36,188
TRALI	16	1:46,334			1	1:210,544	1	1:45,749	4	1:48,845	1	1:49,219	22	1:55,927
Possible TRALI	10	1:74,135			1	1:210,544	1	1:45,749	1	1:195,380			12	1:102,533
TAD	7	1:105,907			2	1:105,272	2	1:22,875	2	1:97,690			11	1:111,854
Bacterial contamination[3]	1	1:741,349											1	1:1,230,398
Hypotensive reaction	22	1:33,698			3	1:70,181	3	1:15,250	7	1:27,911			32	1:38,450
PTP	1	1:741,349											1	1:1,230,398
Other[4]	2	1:370,675							1	1:195,380			3	1:410,133
Total	292	1:2539	9	1:4767	26	1:8098	26	1:1760	62	1:3151	2	1:24,610	391	1:3147

[1]Not included in total for "All components"; [2]cryoprecipitate and others; [3]two cases reported to CBS only not included in rate calculations; [4]hypertensive reactions.

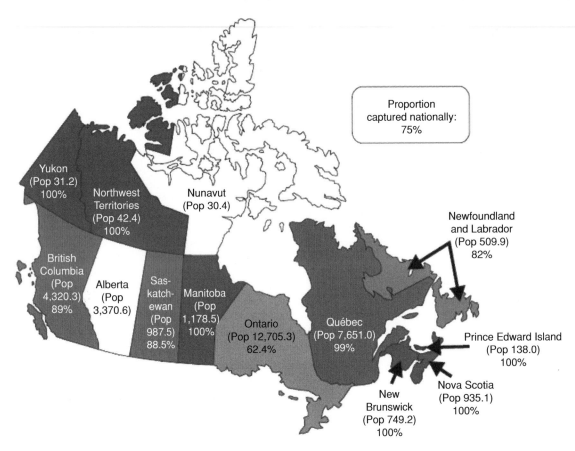

NOTE: Population estimates (in thousands) from Statistics Canada. Canadian Population Census, 2007.

Figure 16.2 Proportion of Canadian RBC transfusion activity captured by hospitals participating in TTISS as of December 31, 2007.

P/Ts. Overall hospitals participating in the TTISS represented 83% of the transfusion activity in Canada. As of December 31, 2007, the proportion of Canadian RBC transfusion activity captured by hospitals participating in the TTISS is 75%, as shown in Figure 16.2.

Transfusion Errors Surveillance System (TESS)

During the operation of the TTISS, it was evident that some events identified do not always meet the case definitions or necessarily lead to an "event" that can comfortably be reported in the TTISS. Specifically, these represent errors or near-misses

that occur associated with transfusion. For a list of the type of events captured in both the clinical and laboratory settings, please refer to Table 16.3. There is great value in capturing these types of errors because it allows incidence data to drive changes in improving transfusion practice.

As a result, the TESS was "spun-off" from the TTISS to capture these types of incidents. The TESS was initiated in 2004 starting with 11 hospitals from four provinces as pilot sites (British Columbia, Nova Scotia, Ontario, and Québec). The types of events captured in the TESS are not related to quality problems with the products themselves, but rather the errors associated with the use of

Table 16.3 TESS: Rates by type of events (2005–2007).

Type of events (general codes)	Denominators	N	Rates per 100,000 (10^5)	Rates
Clinical:				
Product/test request	544,755	1495	274.4	1:364
Request for pick-up	544,755	435	79.9	1:1252
Sample collection	454,890	9402	2066.9	1:48
Sample handling	454,890	2497	548.9	1:182
Unit transfusion	614,543	4969	808.6	1:124
Laboratory:				
Donor codes	672,430	448	66.6	1:1501
Product check-in	672,430	1903	283.0	1:353
Sample receipt	454,890	1361	299.2	1:334
Sample testing	1,492,673	4014	268.9	1:372
Unit selection	641,606	101	15.7	1:6353
Unit manipulation	641,606	623	97.1	1:1030
Unit issue	614,543	1848	300.7	1:333
Unit storage	672,430	1593	236.9	1:422

Table 16.4 Errors reported in TESS by type.

	N	%
Actual—Harm	23	0.1
Actual—No harm	919	2.9
Near-miss—Unplanned recovery	742	2.3
Near-miss—Planned recovery	30,305	94.7
Total	31,989	100.0

these products and potential untoward events of transfusion. TESS data also include near-misses. As with the TTISS, the TESS is based on the use of a standards manual, reporting forms, case definitions, and a data-sharing agreement developed and agreed upon by all parties. Currently, the TESS is collecting 61 variables from 14 pilot sites in Canada, which represents approximately 10% of the transfusion activity across the country.

The incidence of errors collected through the TESS are presented in Table 16.3 and categorized into laboratory and clinical areas, reflecting the location of reporting the errors. Errors are most likely to occur at the sample collection step within the transfusion chain, which has the highest rate of 1:48.

Sample collection errors in crossmatching scenarios include mislabeling, sample size errors, or poor sample tracking. With such a high rate and occurring at such a key step, it may pose a major safety issue to blood recipients due to the possibility of ABO-incompatible blood transfusion. Data

collected through the TESS indicate that the highest rates of sample mis-collection occurred in the Emergency Room, the Intensive Care Unit, and the Operating Room, where patients may suffer from critical conditions. This phenomenon has also reported elsewhere in the literature.[9–12]

Therefore, measures need to be in place to target these areas to ensure that the right patient receives the right blood product, especially the right ABO type. As shown in Table 16.4, a total of 31,989 errors were reported to the TESS from 11 hospitals in four provinces between 2005 and 2007. On review of the data, 0.1% represented the incidences for actual harm events such as newly acquired infections. Other no-harm events, for example, mislabeled units not transfused, accounted for a rate of 2.9%. Of these errors, 3% (0.1% plus 2.9%, see Table 16.4) led to "events" and 97% (2.3% plus 94.7%) were categorized as near-misses.

Apart from sample mis-collection, the TESS data also indicate that high severity error rates seemed more common in hospitals with lower transfusion volumes. Although data collected only from limited pilot sites are insufficient to support such a conclusion, some factors have been speculated, for example that hospitals with lower transfusion volume have a less robust inventory system or lack human resources to oversee each step of the transfusion chain. The ultimate goal of the TESS is to implement a standardized system for all institutions in the country that would allow a benchmarking and a more appropriate comparison between jurisdictions.

During the pilot phase of the TESS, it was difficult to determine the severity of the 23 harm events caused by errors, because the "consequent" codes for several sites were uninterruptible (see Table 16.4). It also appears that errors from clinical services (2%) may be under-reported compared to that reported from laboratory services (98%). Clinicians should certainly be encouraged to report errors and near-misses to improve this situation.

In the 11 hospitals participating in the TESS with a transfusion volume of approximately 615,000 units of components, a total of 1,600 RBC units were discarded. While statistical representativeness was not reached, it could translate into approximately 18,000 RBC units not being transfused in Canada every year as a result of errors within the transfusion chain. Clearly, this signals that efforts extended to improving practices, and preventing or reducing errors and wastage, would be well placed.

Similar to the role of the NWGTTISS, the TESS is supported by the National Working Group for Transfusion Error Surveillance System (NWGT-ESS), which was created to identify and address technical issues raised by the participant sites in order to ensure the quality of the data collected in the TESS database. This Working Group (WG) is also responsible for making recommendations to PHAC for future direction of the TESS and informing the NWGTTISS of progress of the TESS. The WG is comprised of 13 members drawn from all participant sites, blood operators, PHAC, and Health Canada. The long-term goal is to integrate the TESS into the TTISS as a web-based, national adverse event reporting system.

Targeted surveillance/research for high-risk populations and emerging pathogens

Targeted surveillance systems are important components of a wide ranging hemovigilance system. Two types of targeted surveillance are carried out in Canada. One is focused on a defined series of pathogens while the other addresses the need for surveillance of targeted patient groups. the next two sections feature examples of these types of surveillance.

Targeted pathogens: CJD Surveillance System (CJDSS)

The Canadian risk-management approach to regulatory and public health decision-making is predicated on evidence-based decision-making. Thus, data from surveillance, clinical, and scientific studies, epidemiology, as well as statistical modeling, are considered essential to this process. In response to the epidemic of bovine spongiform encephalopathy (BSE) in the UK in the 1990s, it became evident that there would be value in establishing surveillance for Creutzfeldt-Jakob Disease, particularly the variant form (vCJD), to assess incidence and prevalence rates owing to the potential risk posed by vCJD to Canadians and the potential for transmission via the blood system. Thus, in April 1998, Health Canada launched the CJDSS to monitor for all forms of CJD, in the event of any cases appearing in Canada.

This comprehensive surveillance system relies on the reporting of Canadian specialists, such as neurologists, neurosurgeons, neuropathologists, infection-control practitioners, and infectious-disease physicians. Within the CJDSS, all specialists involved in the care of suspected cases of CJD are asked to notify the CJDSS to assist in performing a thorough case follow-up and in using and completing a standard questionnaire. This involves the collection of a blood sample from the patients for a series of testing, and medical information gained through a review of the medical records and an in-depth interview. The PHAC also maintains a reference center at the National Microbiology Laboratory in Winnipeg, which provides state-of-the-art neuropathology diagnostic service.

The CJDSS is the only CJD surveillance system in Canada to inform regulatory and public health policy. Each year, the CJDSS routinely investigates around 80–100 reports of suspected classical CJD and a few reports of suspected vCJD. On average, about 30–35 cases of classical CJD are diagnosed each year in Canada. Many reports of initially suspected classical CJD are later diagnosed as Alzheimer's disease or other neurological disorders. Data collected in the CJDSS thus far indicate that the incidence rate for classical CJD in Canada is comparable with international figures of approximately 1 case per million of the population per year.

Targeted "at-risk" patient population: Hemophilia surveillance

One of the key Justice Krever recommendations concerned preventing recurrence of the transmission of blood-borne pathogens through improved tracking of blood products and surveillance for transmission-transmitted injuries. To respond to Krever's recommendations, Health Canada (now the PHAC), in collaboration with the Association Hemophilia Clinic Directors of Canada, developed the Blood-borne Pathogens Surveillance Project (BBPSP) to archive samples collected from the hemophiliac population. The main goal of this project is to provide a resource to be used not only for tracking known blood-borne pathogens, but also for the monitoring of emerging pathogens. A multidisciplinary committee oversees the project. The oversight committee is comprised of the Canadian Hemophilia Society, CBS, HQ, and PHAC.

The BBPSP is a secure archive of plasma, DNA, RNA, and cell samples managed with a robust data management/inventory system linked to the Canadian Hemophilia Registry. All archived samples are consented for emerging blood-borne pathogens testing, when needed. To date, the BBPSP has archived samples from 23 centers across Canada. It will continue to collect samples from bleeding disorder patients and continues to expand the collection to patients with other rare blood disorders who receive blood products in the treatment of their conditions that put them at a higher risk of acquiring blood-borne infections.

Further enhancement of TTISS, TESS surveillance systems

More than a decade after the release of Krever's recommendations, the reform of the Canadian blood system has been regarded as very successful.[13] The current blood system has regained public confidence and the development of a national hemovigilance system allows for a measure of performance evaluation as the system evolves.

As future goals, it is expected that TTISS will continue to expand by continuing to collect and analyze annual data so as to provide types and trends in adverse event reporting. An ongoing need is to identify strategies for increased reporting. The goal is to reach a capture rate of 98% for Canada as against the current rate of 83%.

Efforts to build on successes with the TESS are first to expand the sentinel system with the addition of 11 sites to a total of 25, allowing for the provision of the highest level of representative data for all Canada. Second, data analyses are planned to identify trends in transfusion errors for parameters such as comparisons of errors reported during work weeks versus weekends, taking into account variables such as staffing. A key aim is to merge the TTISS and TESS systems for the benefit of establishing a single national reporting system.

International linkages and Canada's roles

There are many advantages to international collaboration in the area of blood safety and transfusion medicine. Global hemovigilance activities provide a source of rich data that can be mined for trend analyses or benchmarking. However, these efforts would be of benefit only if methodologies are standardized for data reporting. To work toward exchanging information and to standardize data elements, the International Society of Blood Transfusion (ISBT) established a Working Party on Hemovigilance encompassing over 30 countries including Canada. Experience with development and implementation of the TTISS has allowed Canada to validate many of the reporting parameters through discussions within the ISBT Working Party.

Recently, the International Hemovigilance Network (IHN) evolved from the inaugural European Hemovigilance Network and has been functioning actively since the 1990s. It is composed of over 23 countries and aims to function not only as a forum for data exchange, but also to foster cooperation in the area of hemovigilance and to serve as an early warning system for members. Canada contributes actively to the work of the IHN and has shared data collected through its hemovigilance system with international partners.

In 2007, the WHO's Global Collaboration for Blood Safety identified the importance and need to support developing countries in implementing hemovigilance systems to support blood and transfusion safety. To this end a new committee, the Global Steering Committee on Hemovigilance (GloSCH), was formed. It is comprised of a multilateral group of stakeholders including representation from the WHO, IHN, ISBT, as well as representatives from the Canadian Government and the US Department of Health and Human Services. At a strategic level, GloSCH is working as an international forum to provide advice, exchange information, and promote hemovigilance globally. A recent project involves the development of a Guidance document under the WHO umbrella that identifies the advantages of establishing hemovigilance systems and provides detailed guidance on establishing reporting and analyses of hemovigilance data. It is felt that these efforts will enhance blood safety globally.

Most recently, in 2010, the 63rd WHO World Health Assembly endorsed a resolution (WHA63.12) that urges member states "to ensure the reliability of mechanisms for reporting serious or unexpected adverse reactions to blood and plasma-derived medicinal products, including transmissions of pathogens." The resolution further outlines the adoption of quality systems in blood programs of which hemovigilance is an accepted component.[14]

Building on the hemovigilance system within Canada's National Health Care System: Biovigilance

To the authors' knowledge, no formalized cost benefit analyses have been carried out or published to ascertain whether hemovigilance efforts are cost effective in increasing the safety and quality of blood transfusion. However, it seems intuitive that these benefits may manifest only over the course of many years. Nevertheless, the investments made in both information management reporting systems and human resources can be justified as part of the broader surveillance systems for infectious diseases and as part of the quality control systems for blood safety. Additionally, Canada's view is that the investment in several of the key elements developed as part of hemovigilance systems can serve as a basis for building a broader surveillance function notably in the area of cells, tissues, and organs. Many of the activities that fall within the scope of hemovigilance are also central to a surveillance system for safety of cell, tissues, and organs used in transplantation. These include such areas as donor vigilance and screening, some testing for infectious agents, processing controls, distribution, and tracking functions. These integrated surveillance systems have been referred to as a *biovigilance system.*

Given the advantages of economies of scale as above, Canada has embarked on developing a broader surveillance network to include cells, tissues and, organs used for transplantation. This surveillance system, defined as the Cell, Tissues, and Organs Surveillance System (CTOSS), is now under development. Although there is currently no data collection, efforts have been devoted to the development of a manual, reporting forms and protocols, case definitions, and data-sharing agreements, which are being implemented as part of the CTOSS system. Key partners in CTOSS involve all participating pilot sites, PHAC, Health Canada, as well as transplant centers.

Starting in 2011/2012, five pilot sites will begin collecting 106 variables from tissue transplantation programs. The future plan is to expand the aforementioned pilot to include all organ and cell transplant centers across Canada. The important goals are to conduct yearly analysis on the data to determine the incidence of transplantation adverse events in Canada and determine the subsequent rates. It is planned to develop a three-year progress report with lessons learned and the impact of developing the system. As for hemovigilance systems, surveillance and subsequent data analyses of adverse events in the area of transplantation afford opportunities to modify policies and practices to improve transplantation outcomes.

Acknowledgements

The authors appreciate helpful comments from staff of the Centre for Blood and Tissues Evaluation and the Blood Safety Surveillance and Health Care Acquired Infection Division. We thank Dr F. Agbanyo, Dr W. Stevens, Ms C. Hyson, and Dr S. Elsaadany for review of the manuscript.

References

1 de Vries RRP, Faber J-C, and Strengers PFW, 2011, Haemovigilance: An effective tool for improving transfusion practice. *Vox Sang* **100**: 60–7.

2 Epstein J, Seitz R, Ganz PR, *et al.*, 2009, Role of regulatory agencies. *Biologicals* **37**(2): 94–102.

3 Health Canada, 2011, Adverse Reaction Database, http://www.hc-sc.gc.ca/dhp-mps/medeff/databasdon/index-eng.php [accessed February 15, 2012].

4 Faber J-C, 2004, Worldwide overview of existing haemovigilance systems. *Transfus Apher Sci.* **31**(2): 95–8.

5 Krever H, 1997, Commission of Inquiry on the Blood System in Canada. Final Report. Minister of Public Works and Government Services, Ottawa, Canada.

6 Canadian Legal Information Institute, 2011, An Act respecting Héma-Québec and the haemovigilance committee, RSQ, c H-1.1, http://www.canlii.org/en/qc/laws/stat/rsq-c-h-1.1/latest/rsq-c-h-1.1.html [accessed February 15, 2012].

7 Public Health Agency of Canada, 2009, Summative Evaluation of the Blood Safety Contribution Program—Final Report, http://www.phac-aspc.gc.ca/about_apropos/reports/2008-09/blood-sang/app-c-eng.php [accessed February 15, 2012].

8 AFSSAPS, 2008, Annual Haemovigilance Report, http://www.afssaps.fr/var/afssaps_site/storage/original/application/1f44f2c686fe6d3dd4b22a0f20d6c.pdf [accessed February 15, 2012].

9 Rothschild JM, Landrigan CP, Cronin JW, *et al.*, 2005, The Critical Care Safety Study: The incidence and nature of adverse events and serious medical errors in intensive care. *Crit Care Med* **33**: 1694–517.

10 Brennan TA, Leape LL, Laird NM, *et al.*, 2004, Harvard Medical Practice Study I. Incidence of adverse events and negligence in hospitalized patients: Results of the Harvard Medical Practice Study I, 1991. *Qual Saf Health Care* **13**: 145–51.

11 Gawande AA, Thomas EJ, Zinner MJ, *et al.*, 1999, The incidence and nature of surgical adverse events in Colorado and Utah in 1992. *Surgery* **126**: 66–75.

12 Baker GR, Norton PG, Flintoft V, *et al.*, 2004, The Canadian Adverse Events Study: The incidence of adverse events among hospital patients in Canada. *CMAJ* **170**: 1678–86.

13 Wilson K, 2007, The Krever Commission—10 years later. *Can Med Assoc J.* **177**(11): 1387–9.

14 WHO, 2010, WHA63/2010/REC/1, http://apps.who.int/gb/or/e/e_wha63r1.html [accessed February 15, 2012].

CHAPTER 17

Setting up and Implementation of the National Hemovigilance System in Italy

Giuliano Grazzini and Simonetta Pupella
Centro Nazionale Sangue, Istituto Superiore di Sanità, Rome, Italy

Introduction

In Italy, a national hemovigilance system (HVS) has been implemented since 2008 in compliance with the transposition of Directive 2005/61/EC[1] into a national legislative decree,[2] which defines the procedures of notification, recording, and monitoring of serious adverse reactions (SARs) in transfused patients and serious adverse events (SAEs) potentially affecting quality and safety of blood and blood components (BCs). Notification of SARs in blood donors has also been included in the HVS since the issue of the national legislative decree,[3] which at the end of 2007 updated the first transposition[4] of Directive 2002/98/EC,[5] specifically adding this requirement. Furthermore, surveillance of transfusion transmissible infections (TTIs) in blood donors is part of the new HVS. Compliance with the HVS's regulation is mandatory nationwide.

Before the institution of the National Blood Center (NBC)—the national blood competent authority on behalf of the Ministry of Health (MoH), which became operational in August 2007—hemovigilance (HV) data collection was coordinated by the National Institute of Health (ISS), to which the Regional Blood Centers/Authorities (RCs) used to report HV data on a voluntary basis according to a specific database.[6] The data-reporting coverage of this system proved to be rather low and the tools provided to collect and forward data were technologically poor. The first and last HV report carried out according to the preexisting system was released by the ISS in 2007,[7] reporting 2004–2005 data covering less than 50% transfused BCs.

In 2008, the NBC and the MoH promoted and managed the implementation of a new HVS, as part of the newly established national blood information system (SISTRA: *Sistema Informativo dei Servizi Trasfusionali*).[8] The latter is managed by the NBC in cooperation with the Health Information System Directorate (HISD) of the MoH. The NBC is by law in charge of coordinating and supervising data collection, analysis, and reporting, and is also appointed to report on HV to the European competent authorities. Beyond the need to comply with the European Directives, the decision to implement a totally new HVS was very much influenced by the demand for an effective and advanced system that could efficiently contribute to the monitoring and continuous improvement of transfusion practices and provide reliable data to wider (European/international) HVSs.

The HVS framework was designed by a national working party coordinated by the NBC, composed of representatives from the 21 RCs, from the four nationally accredited blood donor associations and the MoH. The technological platform was projected by the information technology (IT) company appointed by the MoH to build the whole IT platform of SISTRA. The HV project was validated by the HISD of the MoH within the SISTRA project. SISTRA is actually a part of the comprehensive national health information system and its design and implementation were funded with 6.5 million € starting from 2005; its maintenance and evolution, including the HVS, are sustained by an annual fund of about 1 million €.

The national HV working party defined the type of information to be collected by the HVS following the criterion to comply strictly with the mandatory provisions envisaged by the national legislation transposing Directives 2005/61/EC and 2002/98/EC. Therefore, data reporting concerns adverse reactions and events that are defined as "serious," that is, whenever they reveal life-threatening effects, produce severe inability, or cause death to transfused patients or blood donors. Near-miss reporting is also included, being specifically envisaged in the legislative decree transposing Directive 2005/61/EC. The type of information to be reported was officially approved by the RCs and the MoH.

Governance

In Italy, blood establishments are exclusively public hospital-based blood transfusion centers (BTCs), mostly organized in transfusion medicine departments and regionally coordinated by the RCs. The NBC coordinates and supervises the 21 RCs. The notification system is based on a local-to-regional-to-national reporting network. Any blood user experiencing a SAR or a SAE must report to the competent local BTC, which is in charge of collecting all pertinent information from its own operative environment and of the final definition of the grade of severity and imputability of reactions/events.

In each hospital/health trust a specific procedure regulating this process must be in place and periodically assessed. The BTCs must report to the competent RCs, which in turn report to the NBC after regional data validation. Each BTC and RC must have a physician responsible for HV. At the NBC, the HVS is under the responsibility of a senior physician, who is in charge of analyzing and vali-

dating national data, assessing the system's performance, collecting comments and requests from the regional HV officers, and managing selected cases in cooperation with them. Each BTC must produce a complete annual HV report to be notified to the relevant RC. BTC annual reports must be validated at the regional level by the RCs, which in turn produce validated regional annual reports within the month of February. The NBC assembles the regional reports, analyzes the data, and produces annual national reports. The denominators necessary to evaluate the incidence of each type of SAR or SAE as well as the prevalence and incidence of TTIs are automatically provided by SISTRA, being figures routinely collected by the overall blood information system.

Use of a computerized system

All notifications and reports are forwarded exclusively through the SISTRA IT system The latter is fully web-based and allows direct authorized access and data input, as well as authorized "extensible markup language" (XML) file transmission; data protection is in compliance with the relevant national and international regulation. Each SAR and SAE notification is identified by a univocal code tracing the region's code, the BTC code, and the notification's progressive number, in order to guarantee full traceability of the reported reaction/event. Moreover, the system has been designed so as to allow the prompt notification of all grade 3-4 severity and grade 2-3 imputability SARs and SAEs. For this purpose it can manage a real-time reporting function by means of a rapid alert utility to be activated in case of very serious reactions/events.

The new HVS tools have facilitated the standardization of definitions and procedures and are proving to be user-friendly and technologically advanced, as well as versatile compared to the data-collection and reporting procedures already in place in some regions and readily usable in regions where no specific procedures had ever been implemented. Nevertheless, optimal development of all regional blood IT resources, which is still to be fully achieved, will contribute to maximally exploit the national system's potentialities (e.g., XML file transmission). However, since the implementation of the new HVS during 2008, the BTCs' participation has been very significant to the extent that 90% participation was recorded in 2011, and data related to 3.4 million BCs transfused was collected and analyzed. Furthermore, data collected in 2009 seems to be comparable to HV data reported by other EU member states.[9,10]

Framework

The Italian HVS includes the following four sections:
- SARs in transfused patients (and transfusion errors, including near-misses);
- SAEs;
- TTI surveillance in blood donors;
- ARs (adverse reactions) in blood donors.

SARs

According to Directive 2005/61/EC[1] and the relevant national decree,[2] SARs are classified as follows:
- *symptomatic,* characterized by recognizable clinical signs and symptoms occurring during transfusion or in the short period after;
- *asymptomatic,* characterized by absence of clinical signs or by delayed clinical consequences.

SARs in transfused patients must be notified by any clinical area where transfusion therapy is administered. Clinical units practicing blood transfusion must have written procedures in place in order to guarantee systematic notification of SARs to the competent BTC. In the same section of the HVS, transfusion errors and near-misses are included. They are classified as errors/near-misses possibly occurring due to
- wrong recipient identification;
- wrong recipient sample;
- wrong product type.

Monitoring SARs in transfused patients and transfusion errors and near-misses represents a fundamental tool to report deviations in transfusion practices, to implement preventive and corrective actions, and to provide epidemiological evidence upon which local and national safety guidelines may be based.

SAEs

This section is dedicated to the collection of information on the events that may occur throughout the whole transfusion process affecting quality and safety of blood and BCs. SAEs are classified as follows:
- product defect;
- equipment failure;
- human errors;
- other events.

The adverse events may occur during different phases of the transfusion process: whole blood collection, apheresis collection, donation testing, processing, labeling, storage, and distribution. For this type of events the system allows rapid notification, beyond envisaging the usual annual report. A rapid alert function is triggered by any SAE occurring in a single BTC but also possibly occurring in others (e.g., a serious product defect or equipment failure). It allows the prompt notification of all RCs and consequently all BTCs about the detected event, in order to prevent its replication.

TTI surveillance in blood donors

This section is dedicated to the collection of information concerning HCV, HIV, HBV, and syphilis positive cases in blood donors/donations. The notification of positive cases must include
- identification of the notifying BTC;
- anonymous identification of blood donors;
- results of testing;
- methods used for screening and confirmatory testing;
- risk factors and risk behaviors in the positive donors' histories.

Systematic monitoring of blood donors/donations for the main TTIs is a major goal for the national blood system as it allows the creation of a dynamic epidemiological vision aimed at the continuous assessment of blood safety. Moreover, it may provide useful information to improve or modify testing procedures, as well as collecting data on emerging issues such as occult hepatitis B.[11]

Annually, the NBC reports data concerning HCV, HIV, HBV, and syphilis prevalence and incidence in blood donors. Importantly, since the implementation of the new HVS, stratification of data by region and single BTC/transfusion medicine department has become available as a ready-to-use utility, which is very useful for carrying out national and local TTI assessments and residual risk evaluations, epidemiological comparisons among regions, as well as complying with the European "plasma master file" (PMF)[12] requirements concerning TTIs.

ARs in blood donors

Adverse reactions in blood donors may occur during or after whole blood/apheresis collection procedures. Information concerning SARs in blood donors must be collected and recorded applying a classification derived from the one proposed by ISBT-EHN.[13] Systematic monitoring of SARs in blood donors is an important tool for the assessment and continuous improvement of safety, effectiveness, and appropriateness of donor selection and whole blood/apheresis collection procedures.

Aims and responsibilities

As already described, in the organizational framework of the Italian blood system, hospital-based BTCs are entrusted with collecting, recording, and reporting information concerning HV. For this purpose, BTCs must define standard operative procedures (SOPs). As regards SARs and transfusion errors and near-misses, specific HV SOPs must be in place in all hospitals/health trusts performing transfusion therapy. As regards ARs in blood donors, specific SOPs must be in place in all BTCs and external blood collection sites and mobile units.

In order to facilitate and standardize data collection, the HVS allows direct download of standard forms to record information concerning SARs and SAEs. Another available tool is represented by an online guide that can be consulted while drawing up the notification forms. The online guide proposes all the relevant definitions applicable for

the classification of reactions, events, transfusion errors, and near-misses. Whenever applicable, the HVS allows the selection of standardized answers from drop-down lists when filling in the notification forms, in order to simplify data input and obtain a higher degree of homogeneity of information. However, the system also allows the reporting of additional information through free-text input and/or the upload of attached files, where reactions or events can be more extensively described. This important function is routinely used by the SHOT system[10,14] but is not yet similarly applied by the Italian HVS users, and so represents a goal to be pursued.

The Italian HVS provides tools for continuous monitoring of the system itself. Through the online web-based consultation RCs can check every single notification recorded by BTCs, identify incorrect information or mistakes, and perform appropriate corrective and preventive actions, and the NBC can in turn check all data/information collected and reported by each RC. As with any advanced information system, several useful data processing tasks can be carried out and all required reports produced, both at the regional and national level. Furthermore, basic statistical functions are available and any useful stratification criteria can be implemented to support the statistical evaluation of HV data.

All the above mentioned tools aim at improving the overall quality of HV data collection and reporting and are progressively proving to be effective. Nevertheless, periodical training dedicated to the HV reference persons, possibly including e-learning tools, shall become a systematic commitment both at the regional and national level, in order continuously to improve the quality of data collection and reporting.

Systematic communication of local, regional, and national HV results to both institutional and scientific stakeholders, such as hospitals, hospital transfusion committees, health trusts, regional and national health authorities, scientific societies, professional associations, and so on, is currently being implemented. The aim is to obtain positive feedback on transfusion practices, as well as to increase healthcare providers' and operators' awareness on the need for appropriate and safe procedures and behaviors throughout the whole transfusion chain.

References

1 European Union, 2005, Commission Directive 2005/61/EC of 30 September 2005 implementing Directive 2002/98/EC of the European Parliament and of the Council as regards traceability requirements and notification of serious adverse reactions and events. *Official Journal of the European Union* L256, October, 1.

2 Italian Government, 2007, Decreto Legislativo 9 novembre 2007, n. 207. Attuazione della direttiva 2005/61/CE che applica la direttiva 2002/98/CE per quanto riguarda la prescrizione in tema di rintracciabilità del sangue e degli emocomponenti destinati a trasfusioni e la notifica di effetti indesiderati ed incidenti gravi. *Gazzetta Ufficiale della Repubblica Italiana* [Official Gazette of the Italian Republic] **261:** November 9, Supplemento Ordinario n. 288.

3 Italian Government, 2008, Decreto Legislativo 20 dicembre 2007, n. 261. Revisione del decreto legislativo 19 agosto 2005, n. 191, recante attuazione della direttiva 2002/98/CE che stabilisce norme di qualità e di sicurezza per la raccolta, il controllo, la lavorazione, la conservazione e la distribuzione del sangue umano e dei suoi componenti. *Gazzetta Ufficiale della Repubblica Italiana* [Official Gazette of the Italian Republic] **19:** January 23.

4 Italian Government, 2005, Decreto Legislativo 19 agosto 2005, n. 191. Attuazione della direttiva 2002/98/CE che stabilisce norme di qualità e di sicurezza per la raccolta, il controllo, la lavorazione, la conservazione e la distribuzione del sangue umano e dei suoi componenti. *Gazzetta Ufficiale della Repubblica Italiana* [Official Gazette of the Italian Republic] **221:** September 22.

5 European Union, 2003, Directive 2002/98/EC of the European Parliament and of the Council of 27 January 2003 setting standards of quality and safety for the collection, testing, processing, storage and distribution of human blood and blood components and amending Directive 2001/83/EC. *Official Journal of the European Union* L33, February 8.

6 Grazzini G, Hassan JH, Aprili G, and International Forum, 2006, Haemovigilance. *Vox Sang* **90**: 207–41.

7 Giampaolo A, Piccinini V, Catalano L, Abbonizio F, Vulcano F, Hassan HJ, 2007, Primo Programma di emovigilanza sulle reazioni avverse e gli errori trasfusionali in Italia: dati 2004–2005. Rapporti ISTISAN 07/22. http://www.iss.it/binary/publ/cont/07-22.1189418036.pdf [accessed February 16, 2012].

8 Italian Government, 2008, Decreto del Ministero della Salute 21 dicembre 2007. Istituzione del sistema informativo dei servizi trasfusionali. *Gazzetta Ufficiale della Repubblica Italiana* [Official Gazette of the Italian Republic] **13:** January 16.

9 Pupella S, Piccinini V, Catalano L, and Grazzini G, 2010, Primi dati del sistema informativo dei servizi trasfusionali (SISTRA). Proceedings of the 39th National Congress of the Italian Society of Transfusion Medicine and Immunohaematology. *Blood Transfus* **8**(Suppl 2): s43–44

10 Taylor CPF, 2010, A comparison of the haemovigilance data in the UK and in Italy. Proceedings of the 39th National Congress of the Italian Society of Transfusion Medicine and Immunohaematology. *Blood Transfus* **8**(Suppl 2): s44–45.

11 Allain JP, Candotti D, 2008, Diagnostic algorithm for HBV safe transfusion. *Blood Transfus* **4**: 24–7.

12 European Medicines Agency, 2003, Plasma Master File. http://www.ema.europa.eu/ema/index.jsp?curl=pages/regulation/general/general_content_000069.jsp&jsenabled=true [accessed February 16, 2012].

13 International Society of Blood Transfusion and European Haemovigilance Network, 2007, Complications related to blood donation. Version 2007. http://www.isbt-web.org/members_only/files/society/DOCO%20Standard%202007%20%20List%20and%20Descriptions%20FINAL.pdf [accessed February 16, 2012].

14 SHOT—Serious Hazards Of Transfusion. Available from: http://www.shotuk.org/ [accessed February 16, 2012].

CHAPTER 18

The Australian Hemovigilance System

Erica M. Wood[1,2], Lisa J. Stevenson[1], Simon A. Brown[3], and Christopher J. Hogan[4]

[1]Blood Matters Program, Department of Health and Australian Red Cross Blood Service, Melbourne, Australia
[2]Monash University, Melbourne, Australia
[3]Queensland Blood Management Program, Brisbane, Australia
[4]National Blood Authority, Canberra, Australia

Introduction

Australia has one of the safest blood supplies in the world thanks to major investments in its blood sector over recent decades. With this system in place, there has been a growing understanding of the importance of reducing other transfusion hazards.

Reviews of Australian transfusion practice from the 1990s onward[1–3] highlighted evidence of variation in use and inappropriate use, procedural risks, the importance of considering alternatives to transfusion, the role of institutional transfusion committees, the potential for hospital accreditation to drive practice improvements, patient-informed consent and participation in decision-making, and the potential for reduction in avoidable blood wastage. The Stephen review summarized experiences from pilot projects prior to 2001 and recommended the

> establishment of a national, voluntary, confidential scheme to monitor untoward transfusion events and outcomes in hospitals…and to provide data that places Australian transfusion risks in perspective. Efforts in this area should be a component of adverse events monitoring in Australian hospitals and part of a national approach to improve patient safety.[2]

In recommending the establishment of a hemovigilance program, the review noted international experiences, including resource requirements to create effective and sustainable systems.

The blood sector and context for hemovigilance programs in Australia

Structures, responsibilities, and activities of some of the main parties in the Australian blood sector with respect to hemovigilance are described below.

Australia is a federation of states and territories. Health ministers, through the Commonwealth Department of Health and Ageing and state/territory health departments, set policies and their supporting legal and funding frameworks, and ensure compliance with international obligations. In line with its commitment to the 1975 World Health Assembly resolution, Australia is self-sufficient in fresh components (except for some rare units sourced under international exchange programs), and largely self-sufficient in plasma-derived products.

Australia has a national health system. State/territory health departments operate most public hospital services. A large private sector also provides inpatient hospital care and pathology services, including autologous transfusion. In many cases, private and public hospitals coexist and are supported by the same pathology providers (either publicly or privately operated).

Hemovigilance: An Effective Tool for Improving Transfusion Safety, First Edition. Edited by René R.P. De Vries and Jean-Claude Faber.
© 2012 John Wiley & Sons, Ltd. Published 2012 by John Wiley & Sons, Ltd.

The National Blood Agreement sets out policy objectives and the role of governments in blood sector governance and funding. The National Blood Authority (NBA) was established under this agreement as a statutory agency, to enhance the management of the Australian blood sector at a national level. The NBA has responsibility for support and coordination of hemovigilance through its safety, quality, and risk-management mandates, and has established a national structure and Hemovigilance Advisory Committee (HAC), endorsed by Commonwealth and state/territory governments, as outlined below.

The Therapeutic Goods Administration (TGA) is the national regulatory authority for blood components, fractionated plasma and recombinant products, medicines, and devices. It sets standards for good manufacturing practice for the Blood Service and other suppliers (including international companies for fractionated and recombinant products). Defined product-related and clinical events require notification to the TGA, which also oversees product recalls where necessary. The TGA does not regulate clinical transfusion activities in hospitals or pathology services. Pathology laboratory accreditation is overseen by the National Association of Testing Authorities and the Royal College of Pathologists of Australasia (RCPA).

The Australian Red Cross Blood Service is Australia's national blood service. Funding for its blood sector work is administered by the NBA on behalf of governments. Allogeneic components and plasma for fractionation are provided from voluntary non-remunerated donors, along with autologous collections, reference testing, and clinical and other services. Blood Service manufacturing activities are subject to TGA licensure.

Professional societies, such as the Australian and New Zealand Society of Blood Transfusion (ANZSBT), and specialist colleges, such as RCPA, promote transfusion best practice as part of the national safety and quality agenda, formulate guidelines, provide undergraduate and postgraduate education and training, as well as expert advice. The RCPA Key Incident Monitoring and Management (KIMMS) system aims to establish a national pathology dataset to measure and monitor incidents, set standards and benchmarks for practice, exchange information on methods to reduce errors, raise awareness of practices that will reduce errors, and increase patient safety.[4] ANZSBT develops and promulgates national guidelines on areas of transfusion practice, such as pre-transfusion patient identification, sample labeling, laboratory practice, bedside administration and monitoring,[5] and contributes to development of national standards in these areas.

In the past decade, transfusion collaboratives have transformed Australian clinical practice. Although these programs have their own emphases and structures to meet local needs and arrangements, they share important goals:

• promoting practice improvement;
• strengthening clinical governance in hospitals, including transfusion committees;
• developing and implementing evidence-based clinical guidelines;
• reducing unnecessary transfusions through comprehensive patient blood-management activities;
• developing a competent clinical workforce, through training and support of specialist transfusion practitioners and other clinical staff;
• providing data to guide practice (for example, clinical audit results);
• monitoring incidents and reactions through development of hemovigilance systems.

Examples of these programs, and their main supporting institutions, include the following:

• Appropriate Use of Blood Reference Group (Australian Capital Territory, ACT Health);
• Blood Matters (Department of Health Victoria and Blood Service, with participation from Tasmania, Northern Territory (NT) and ACT);
• BloodSafe (South Australia Health and Blood Service);
• Blood Watch (New South Wales (NSW) Clinical Excellence Commission and NSW Health);
• Northern Territory Transfusion Safety program (NT Department of Health and Families);
• Queensland Blood Management Program (Queensland Health);
• Western Australia (WA) Patient Blood Management Program (WA Department of Health).

Input from a broad range of stakeholders, including patients, and strong jurisdictional health department support, have been important in the success of these programs. More information on their wider activities is beyond the scope of this chapter and is available via the program websites.

The Australian Commission for Safety and Quality in Health Care (ACSHQC) was established by health ministers to develop a national healthcare safety and quality framework. ACSQHC identifies priority policy areas, leads development of national standards, advises on data requirements, and reports to the community. A new standard for hospital transfusion practice has been published,[6] addressing areas from staff training and competency assessment, to blood storage and handling, and documentation of transfusion outcomes, including adverse event monitoring and reporting. It is anticipated that this will be implemented in the future as the national standard for transfusion clinical practice.

Examples from Australian regional hemovigilance systems

This section outlines the major existing Australian regional hemovigilance programs. Typically they are relatively recently established, voluntary (except for defined sentinel events), focused on fresh components, and based on the UK Serious Hazards of Transfusion (SHOT) scheme, with modifications to reflect jurisdictional interests or identified problems.

Serious Transfusion Incident Reporting (STIR) system

Blood Matters commenced in 2002 as a project of the Department of Human Services Victoria, and the Blood Service, with the intention of improving transfusion practice in Victorian hospitals. Among its original aims was establishment of a hemovigilance system for Victoria. STIR is a voluntary reporting program for adverse events and near-misses, aiming to identify hazards in clinical prac-

tice and develop strategies to improve transfusion safety.

STIR operates through the Blood Matters program, with administrative and clinical support from the program secretariat and Blood Service. STIR links with the Victorian sentinel event system. ABO-incompatible transfusions must be reported directly to the health department and other transfusion-related events with severe, or potentially severe, clinical consequences can also be reported under the "other, catastrophic" category. A multidisciplinary expert group with representation from all reporting jurisdictions reviews cases and assigns final diagnoses and imputability and severity ratings. Feedback is provided to Victorian health services on sentinel events following review of their reports and root-cause analyses.

STIR commenced with preparatory work in 2005 and a pilot in 2006 involving 15 metropolitan and regional hospitals. The program expanded to additional major public and private centers in Victoria and Tasmania in 2007, and subsequently to smaller metropolitan and regional health services, and institutions in ACT and NT. Tasmania, ACT, and NT had all participated in Blood Matters, and it was anticipated that this arrangement would provide immediate access to an established system without the costs and complexities of setting up new structures, and that events from these smaller jurisdictions would be able to be managed within STIR's resources. In its most recent report, events had been reported to STIR from 64 hospitals or pathology services.[7] For non-reporting institutions, it is not assumed that no events occurred, but simply that none were reported.

STIR captures clinical adverse reactions and procedural events. Categories are based on those used by the SHOT and New Zealand programs, and include the following:

- incorrect blood component transfused (IBCT);
- acute transfusion reaction (including anaphylaxis);
- delayed transfusion reaction;
- transfusion-associated graft-versus-host disease (TA-GVHD);
- transfusion-related acute lung injury (TRALI);

- transfusion-associated circulatory overload (TACO);
- post-transfusion purpura (PTP);
- post-transfusion viral infection;
- transfusion-transmitted bacterial infection;
- wrong blood in tube (WBIT);
- other "near-miss" events.

Hospitals report incidents on an initial event notification form and then further information using a form provided by STIR according to the type of event. All reporting is now web-based and reports are automatically transferred to the STIR database. Institutions are expected to perform data validation and case review prior to submission, using their established clinical governance frameworks. Data validation is also performed by STIR and more information may be sought from institutions prior to assignment for expert review. Feedback and final diagnoses are reviewed at expert group meetings. No information identifying reporting institutions, staff, or patients is retained in the database.

STIR received a total of 989 reports between the 2006 pilot and March 2012. Acute reactions are the most numerous reported clinical reactions (50% of all reports); many were not serious. Procedural events include IBCT, WBIT, and near-misses: these currently account for 42% of all reports, with WBIT the largest at 24%. Nine sentinel events, mostly ABO-incompatible transfusions, have been reported since 2007. Event rates are not calculated because transfusion episode denominators are not known, and numbers of participating institutions have increased over time; however, reporting hospitals currently reflect utilization of about 68% of red cells issued in Victoria by the Blood Service. Assuming most units were transfused, this suggests approximately one event reported to STIR per 3300 red cells issued.

STIR reports quarterly to the Blood Matters Advisory Committee. Data and analysis are presented in reports distributed widely throughout public and private sectors, available through the program website,[8] and by presentations to transfusion committees, educational meetings, and scientific conferences.

Queensland Incidents in Transfusion (QiiT)

The Queensland Blood Management Program (QBMP) was established by Queensland Health in 2005. One of its main objectives is promotion and development of quality and safety programs, with aims to promote appropriate blood use, reduce adverse events, and improve patient outcomes. QiiT is QBMP's hemovigilance program and an integral part of its safety and quality activities.

QiiT is a voluntary reporting scheme that harnesses existing incident management systems within Queensland's private and public health systems. It collects de-identified information on events related to allogeneic and autologous components, and cell salvage/post-operative reinfusion devices. Reporting categories are based on SHOT, and include hemolytic (ABO-related, acute non-ABO and delayed) reactions, febrile non-hemolytic and severe allergic reactions, and anaphylaxis. Other events are as for STIR, above, except that bacterial contamination of fresh components without clinical consequence is included under transfusion-transmitted infections. ABO-incompatible hemolytic reactions are reportable sentinel events, and although QiiT does not substitute for those reporting pathways, it provides a safety net through recognition of cases. Limited data on "near-miss" events are collected from some participating hospitals.

Initial notification of an event to QiiT occurs automatically via electronic feeds from hospitals and pathology providers using Queensland Health's PRIME incident management system; all others use paper-based reporting. Events are logged into a database that generates unique case numbers. These are entered onto follow-up forms issued to reporting hospitals for collection of further relevant information. Data from follow-up forms allow central validation of events, and confirmation or revision of hospital-assigned diagnoses, severity, and imputability scores. To facilitate collection of de-identified data, hospital hemovigilance coordinators orchestrate completion of follow-up forms.

A six-month pilot was conducted at four sites in 2007, to test development of a proposed system that would be user-friendly and acceptable to public and private health services, and to assess its robustness in clinical settings and its ability to collect and validate reports and communicate results. Fourteen events were reported, including one IBCT.[8] An evaluation of content and process aspects of the pilot showed increased awareness over time at participating institutions. Supporting materials such as booklets, information sheets, and reaction charts were considered useful resources, and some materials were revised following feedback. Currently, 109 public and private hospitals across Queensland participate in QiiT, and over 377 events, excluding "near-miss" events, have been reported up to September 2010.

The QBMP team and QiiT working group are responsible for program management, data validation, and incident analysis. A Haemovigilance Committee meets bi-annually and provides program oversight. An annual report is prepared for the Queensland Blood Board (QBB). Performance indicators for all major activities including communications are reviewed by the Haemovigilance Committee and QBB. Feedback is provided to hospitals through newsletters, a bi-annual audit report, an annual report, and the activities of institutional hemovigilance coordinators.

South Australia: BloodSafe

The South Australian (SA) BloodSafe program has implemented a number of activities to improve transfusion practice and capture errors and adverse events. Transfusion nurses provide support across major public, private, and regional health services, including management and reporting of adverse reactions, and monitoring of practice through clinical audit. Statewide transfusion test request, adverse event investigation, and reporting forms are being developed. SA is moving to a single public sector laboratory information system, which will support consistent diagnostic and transfusion record-keeping, improve access to information, and reduce the potential for errors and omissions.

Hemovigilance reporting in SA is voluntary, except for ABO-incompatible hemolytic reactions, which are sentinel events and must be reported by all heath services to the Department of Health and Ageing. In the public sector, incidents and adverse events were previously captured via the Advanced Incident Management System (AIMS, iSOFT Group Ltd), using a transfusion/hemovigilance module developed by BloodSafe and the Australian Patient Safety Foundation and piloted in 2004. A new web-based incident management and reporting system (Safety Learning System, Datix Ltd) was introduced across the public sector in 2011. Although this dataset is closely is aligned to the national dataset, it requires some manual review and reclassification prior to reporting.

The BloodSafe e-learning module has been widely promulgated throughout SA health services and adopted nationally.[9] It provides online training for clinical staff and others (for example, hospital porters) involved in transfusion and includes a section dedicated to the management, reporting, and prevention of adverse reactions.

New South Wales Blood Watch

The New South Wales (NSW) Blood Watch program was established as a partnership between the Clinical Excellence Commission and NSW Health. One of the program's first activities was an analysis of incidents reported in NSW health services between July 2005 and June 2006 using the Incident Information Management System. Of 680 entries reviewed, mislabeled specimens were the most frequently reported event. Blood storage and handling issues were also common. However, more than half the cases coded under "blood" issues were potentially not transfusion-related. The program's clinical audit and data linkage projects will provide valuable information for future hemovigilance activities. Further information is available at: http://www.cec.health.nsw .gov.au/programs/blood-watch.html.

Australian national hemovigilance arrangements

The NBA established a working group and then a national Hemovigilance Advisory Committee (HAC) composed of relevant clinical experts, with representatives from the private sector, epidemiology, jurisdictional health departments, NBA, TGA, ACSQHC, the Blood Service, and Australian Institute of Health and Welfare (AIHW) to oversee development of national hemovigilance arrangements.

The national system relies on reporting, capture, and analysis of transfusion-related adverse events by jurisdictional hemovigilance programs, according to the following agreed framework:

- national minimum dataset and data dictionary defined by HAC (currently fresh blood components only);
- individual adverse events reviewed at institutional and jurisdictional/regional levels;
- regional programs submit validated, aggregate, de-identified data with causation/imputability/severity scores.

Adverse events presently in the national dataset are IBCT, other acute and delayed hemolytic reactions, severe febrile non-hemolytic and allergic reactions, anaphylaxis, TACO, TRALI, TTI, TA-GVHD, and PTP. Currently, near-miss events are not reported nationally, although these are captured in some jurisdictional systems.

The HAC produced an initial national report in 2008 and a second report in 2010. The 2010 report provides data from all Australian states and territories except Western Australia according to agreed event definitions and requirements for data validation, severity, and imputability scoring.[10] Most cases were severe febrile non-hemolytic transfusion and allergic reactions, followed by IBCT.

The 2010 report recommended the following:

- *Data:* Jurisdictions should continue to improve their data capture and validation systems; programs should be implemented at national, state, and institutional levels to improve recognition of TRALI and TACO; jurisdictions should develop systems to enable the total number of products transfused to be known; HAC should consider inclusion of near-miss events in the national dataset.
- *Capacity:* Jurisdictions should improve timeliness and completeness of reporting.
- *Prescribing:* The National Health & Medical Research Council (NHMRC) and relevant professional bodies, colleges, and societies should

continue to develop and publish patient blood-management guidelines.

- *Procedural errors:* Transfusion facilities should reduce procedural errors through training, application of standards, proficiency testing, and accreditation; jurisdictions and the NBA should encourage research into the application of technological adjuncts to reduce the scope for error.
- *National blood safety and quality initiatives:* Hemovigilance should be included in hospital accreditation requirements; the NBA, JBC, and HAC should continue to engage with ACSQHC in the development of relevant indicators and standards.

Australian Red Cross blood service data

Adverse events reported to the Blood Service with product, donor management, component testing, and/or recall implications are used to monitor product safety and evaluate introduction of measures such as changes in donor selection criteria and manufacturing processes. Certain events are reportable to the TGA.

The Blood Service received reports of 612 reactions nationally between January 2006 and June 2009,[11] including 114 cases of suspected TRALI, 30% of which met the TRALI consensus definition.[12] Introduction of "male-predominant" plasma supplied for transfusion in mid-2007 appears to have contributed to reduced TRALI notifications. Other reports included febrile and allergic/anaphylactic reactions, TACO, ABO-incompatible transfusions, and suspected TTIs. There were no deaths. Where the Blood Service receives adverse event information, reporters are encouraged to notify institutional and jurisdictional hemovigilance systems. Additional work remains to be done to ensure full integration of these cases with reports to jurisdictional and national programs.

The Blood Service has introduced measures to reduce bacterial contamination of blood components, including routine platelet pre-release screening. No high-probability or confirmed cases of sepsis were reported from active follow-up of over 260,000 screened platelets from April 2008 to June 2010, compared with three serious reactions in

2006 and two in 2007, including one death in each of those years. One septic event was reported in 2009 from red cells contaminated with *Pseudomonas putida;* the patient recovered. Positive bacterial contamination screening results in platelets issued and transfused are monitored by QiiT but not by the other programs; this information is not presently included in the national dataset.

The Blood Service monitors donor incidents and adverse events, and captures data on blood component discards through an online reporting system. These are not presently included in the national hemovigilance dataset.

Data from other sources

Manufacturers/sponsors of fractionated and recombinant products are required to monitor and respond to defined clinical adverse events, and notify the TGA. Serious reactions are reviewed by the Advisory Committee on the Safety of Medicines. These reports are not presently included in the national hemovigilance dataset.

AIHW hospital sector information may be helpful in establishing transfusion episode data and demonstrating changes in practice over time.[13] For example, trends to increasing outpatient therapy may have implications for hemovigilance, such as in identification and management of transfusion reactions where outpatients are not immediately assessable by trained staff, or for capture of events where these are managed outside hospitals. Potential weaknesses in AIHW data include limitations of hospital-assigned coding, which may underestimate or misclassify procedures.

Patient identification and specimen labeling results from RCPA KIMMS[4] will, in time, provide useful data for inter-laboratory comparison and practice improvement.

Communication/reporting

The main aim of hemovigilance reporting is to provide analysis and recommendations to improve practice. Information from regional and national activities is disseminated widely through the following:

- *Reports and newsletters:* Most of these are available online for broad access and distributed to clinicians and health service executives for awareness and action. Case studies have been useful in engaging readers, highlighting types of events reported, and emphasizing consequences for patients. Program recommendations and messages regarding accountabilities for clinical and executive staff are clearly outlined.
- *Feedback:* Provided to reporting hospitals on sentinel events and root-cause analyses following review by jurisdictional programs.
- *Presentations:* To hospitals, conferences, jurisdictional Blood User Groups, and other interested parties.
- *Educational programs:* Outcomes from hemovigilance programs have been incorporated into training for clinical and laboratory staff, such as through specialist college training programs and resources from transfusion practice collaboratives, including the Blood Matters/University of Melbourne Graduate Certificate in Transfusion Practice and BloodSafe e-learning modules.

Lessons learned from implementing hemovigilance in Australia

Table 18.1 summarizes some important lessons from the implementation of hemovigilance programs in Australia, divided into "process-related" reflections on experiences from the introduction of various activities (the "how") and "content-related" lessons about the types of events and outcomes reported (the "what"). Naturally, there is some overlap.

Research opportunities in hemovigilance

Many events relate to staff knowledge or awareness, and/or failure to follow procedures, check, or communicate. Frequently there are also

Table 18.1 Important lessons from the implementation of hemovigilance programs in Australia.

Lesson	Example
Process-related	**Value of a pilot program** • Helps understand hospital culture and practical issues that may be barriers to participation • On-site meetings and education promote awareness and engage clinical, laboratory, and executive staff • Enables refinement of structures, processes, and supporting materials prior to large-scale implementation **Data management issues** *Health service data:* • Different computerized and paper-based systems in various clinical and laboratory settings • Challenges in access to relevant information, weak search and analysis functions, poor interoperability and integration, including limited linkage of incident-reporting systems with clinical files and/or laboratory data *Hemovigilance system data:* Finding the balance between amount and quality of data—more is not necessarily better and may even be a barrier to reporting *Dataset:* Early agreement on intended data elements and precise definitions informs program and materials design and implementation *Reporting tools:* • Paper-based tools may be simple, inexpensive, and faster to implement initially, but require manual data entry by hemovigilance program staff; online reporting tools are desirable for reasons including data integrity, security, and timeliness of reporting • Consider document control, traceability, confidentiality and completeness of data, and staff training *Data validation:* Validation by hospitals prior to submission, including transfusion committee review, improves completeness and accuracy, identifies the nature of problems occurring within an institution, provides teaching opportunities, and improves overall system efficiency *Databases:* Electronic investigation phase tools with automated import into databases facilitate validation and analytic processes **Resources** *Specialist transfusion practitioners in hospitals* link clinical and laboratory areas, blood services, and hemovigilance programs, providing support for incident identification and management, assistance in reporting problems and identifying/implementing solutions *Hemovigilance program staff:* • **Transfusion nurses/coordinators** assist in case assessments, reporting, program awareness, education, and troubleshooting • **Expert programmers and data managers** support IT systems, simplifying notifications, assessments, coding, review, and analysis • **Multidisciplinary expert group review** is very valuable prior to assignment of final diagnoses and imputability/severity *Educational materials* such as program guides, reports, and web pages are helpful for staff, patients, and other stakeholders **Program monitoring and evaluation** Regular review of progress by oversight committee and other stakeholders enables program monitoring and development
Content-related	**Staff training** • More staff training required in basic elements of transfusion safety (patient identification, specimen labeling, storage/handling, management/investigation of transfusion reactions) • Ongoing education about program activities required due to staff turnover **Collection of blood for transfusion** • Collection of red cells from blood refrigerators outside the transfusion laboratory is prone to error • Requirements for off-site storage should be reviewed and justified • "Smart" equipment may reduce some hazards

(continued)

Table 18.1 Important lessons from the implementation of hemovigilance programs in Australia (*Continued*).

Lesson	Example
	Out of hours transfusions
	• Out of hours incidents appear over-represented in reports
	• Staff numbers, opportunities for patient observation, on-site support, and advice for managing adverse events are limited after hours
	Communication issues
	• Communication between members of clinical teams, and clinical and laboratory staff, is frequently poor; examples include failure to identify patients properly at time of sample collection or transfusion, and communication of special requirements
	• Lack of integration between databases limits access to results from different laboratories, with consequences for meeting special requirements
	Severity and imputability scoring
	• Most reported cases are not serious or life-threatening, and many not be confirmed on review, creating challenges in balancing general awareness and encouragement of reporting, with reviewing and responding to numbers of reports
	• For WBIT, assignment of severity grading is problematic; by definition, these events did not result in incompatible transfusion, yet potential for serious outcome exists

organizational cultural and practical issues such as high-stress environments, fatigue, and multiple interruptions during critical tasks. Understanding the human factors involved during the transfusion process may help determine appropriate interventions to reduce hazards at the bedside or in laboratories.

A study by the Centre for Research Excellence in Patient Safety, Australian Centre for Health Innovation and the Transfusion Outcomes Research Collaborative, used direct observations, surveys, and interviews in three hospital emergency departments, and failure modes effects analysis, to identify factors relating to the environment, culture, staff and patients, equipment, and procedures with potential to contribute to significant adverse outcomes. STIR provided background material to the project. Recommendations provided to the Victorian Managed Insurance Agency (which insures Victorian public hospitals and funded the study), health departments, and hospitals will serve as the basis for further studies of potential interventions.[14]

Many other areas are suitable for future hemovigilance research, including gaps in system performance identified by clinical audit and jurisdictional and national hemovigilance data. Where interventions are introduced to reduce risks, they should be conceived with an awareness of the range of human factors contributing to transfusion errors, and formally evaluated to determine whether they are successful in achieving their aims. Development and roll-out of national blood ordering software systems and arrangements, along with clinical data-linkage capacities, will improve background and denominator data for hemovigilance analysis, reporting, and education.

Conclusions/future directions

Australia has relatively new hemovigilance structures, based on regional programs providing data for national review and reporting. Adverse event reporting and participation in all established regional programs is voluntary, except for a few defined sentinel events. There is expanding hospital participation, reflecting growing recognition of actual and potential problems related to transfusion, and in line with expectations from governments and professional bodies. Although further work is required before Australia's system is embedded and robust, available data already highlight where attention should be directed to improve transfusion safety. Australia's experience to date is broadly similar to that of other hemovigilance programs, in that the majority of serious events are related to human error and therefore potentially preventable. Availability of more robust program and research data, and development of a national dataset over time, will show whether, and if so how, Australian hemovigilance programs lead to improved transfusion outcomes.

Future aims include the following:

- increasing participation, especially from smaller and regional institutions and the private sector;
- incorporation of hemovigilance programs into jurisdictional incident management systems;
- more automation to simplify reporting and analysis;
- improved correlation of patient events with cases reported to the Blood Service or other suppliers;
- inclusion of donor-related adverse events;
- more high-quality research on causes and prevention of adverse events;
- inclusion of events related to fractionated plasma products;
- development and incorporation of better denominator data on transfusion rates and practices.

To achieve these aims, resources will be required, such as greater availability of transfusion practitioners in hospitals, with training and responsibility for investigation and follow-up of incidents and adverse reactions, and input from transfusion medicine experts and others for analysis and design of interventions.

In relation to the 2010 national hemovigilance report recommendation on development of clinical guidelines, the NHMRC and ANZSBT, supported by the NBA, are developing national patient blood management scenario-based guidelines, which will update and replace the 2001 product-based guidelines and underpin transfusion practice and related hemovigilance initiatives in Australia.

Acknowledgments

The authors thank Dr Kathryn Robinson (BloodSafe Program) and Ms Rachel Allden (SA Department of Health) for contributions to the section on South Australia. Dr Marija Borosak kindly provided results of platelet bacterial screening and data on adverse events reported to the Australian Red Cross Blood Service. Drs Louise Phillips and Shelly Jeffcott (Monash University) shared research information. Dr Michael Gilbertson and Ms Sally Nailon provided helpful comments on the manuscript.

References

1 McKay B, and Wells R, 1995, Commonwealth Review of Australian Blood and Blood Product System. Commonwealth Department of Human Services and Health, Canberra.

2 Commonwealth Department of Health and Ageing, 2001, Review of the Australian Blood Banking and Plasma Product Sector. Commonwealth Department of Health and Ageing, Canberra.

3 Boyce N, and Brooks C, 2005, Towards better, safer blood transfusion—A report for the Australian Council for Safety and Quality in Health Care, Commonwealth of Australia 2005. http://www.safetyandquality .gov.au/wp-content/uploads/2012/01/bloodrept05.pdf [accessed April 5, 2012].

4 Royal College of Pathologists of Australasia, 2006, Key Incident Monitoring and Management (KIMMS) program. http://www.rcpaqap.com.au/kimms [accessed October 24, 2010].

5 Australian and New Zealand Society of Blood Transfusion, 2007, Guidelines for pre-transfusion laboratory practice http://www.anzsbt.org.au/publications /documents/PLP_Guidelines_Mar07.pdf; and, 2011, Guidelines for administration of blood products http:// www.anzsbt.org.au/publications/documents/ANZSBT _Guidelines_Administration_Blood_Products_2ndEd_De c_2011_Hyperlinks.pdf [both accessed February 16, 2012].

6 Australian Commission for Safety and Quality in Health Care, 2011, National Safety and Quality Health Service Standards. http://www.safetyandquality.gov .au/wp-content/uploads/2011/01/NSQHS-Standards-Sept2011.pdf [accessed April 5, 2012].

7 Blood Matters Program, Department of Health and Australian Red Cross Blood Service, 2011, Serious Transfusion Incident Report 2008–9. http://docs .health.vic.gov.au/docs/doc/Serious-Transfusion-Incident-Report-2008-2009- [accessed April 5, 2012].

8 QiiT, Queensland Blood Management Program: Queensland Incidents in Transfusion report of pilot project. http://www.health.qld.gov.au/qhcss/qbmp/ qiit.asp (report available on request to QiiT).

9 Blood Safe program, South Australia Department of Health and Australian Red Cross Blood Service, 2011, BloodSafe e-learning. https://www.bloodsafelearning .org.au [accessed February 16, 2012].

10 National Blood Authority, 2010, Australian Haemovigilance Report 2010, and data dictionary. http://www.nba.gov.au/haemovigilance/pdf/nba_hem report10.pdf [accessed February 16, 2012].

11 Borosak M, Dennington P, Bryant S, *et al.*, 2010, Adverse transfusion reaction reporting to the Australian Red Cross Blood Service; January 2006–June 2009. 12th International Haemovigilance Seminar, February 17–19, 2010, Dubrovnik, Croatia.

12 Kleinman S, Caulfield T, Chan P, *et al.*, 2004, Toward an understanding of transfusion-related acute lung injury: Statement of a consensus panel. *Transfusion* **44**: 1774–89.

13 Australian Institute of Health and Welfare, 2011, Australian Hospital Statistics 2009–10, Health services series no. 40. http://www.aihw.gov.au/publication-detail/?id=10737418863 [accessed April 5, 2012].

14 Jeffcott S, and Phillips LE, 2010, Reducing harm in blood transfusion: Investigating the human factors behind 'wrong blood in tube' (WBIT) events in the emergency department. Report prepared for the Victorian Managed Insurance Authority, Melbourne, Victoria, Australia. http://www.vmia.vic.gov.au/Risk-Management/Risk-partnership-programs/A-Z/Reducing-patient-harm-from-wrong-blood-in-tube .aspx [accessed April 5, 2012].

CHAPTER 19

Biovigilance in the United States

*D. Michael Strong[1], Barbee Whitaker[2], Matthew J. Kuehnert[3],
and Jerry A. Holmberg[4]*

[1]Department of Orthopaedics and Sports Medicine, University of Washington School of Medicine, Seattle, WA, USA
[2]Data and Special Programs, AABB, Bethesda, MD, USA
[3]Division of Healthcare Quality Promotion, Centers for Disease Control and Prevention (CDC), Atlanta, GA, USA
[4]US Department of Health and Human Services, Washington DC, USA

History of biovigilance development

Hemovigilance systems have been implemented in most developed countries to monitor the adverse reactions and events associated with blood donations and transfusion. *Biovigilance* extends this term to other biologics, in addition to blood, to incorporate monitoring of adverse reactions and events associated with tissue, organs, and cellular components.

In the US, several voluntary and mandatory reporting requirements currently serve as a patchwork for biovigilance, although no integrated national system currently exists. For example, at the clinical level, most hospitals have a transfusion reaction reporting system that reports into the hospital transfusion service and a transfusion committee with various department representatives, such that data can be aggregated and compared.[1] One example is the Medical Event Reporting System for Transfusion Medicine (MERS-TM) developed at Columbia University in New York for hospitals to submit reports anonymously to a central database, allowing analysis of an individual hospital's data and comparisons to that of aggregate data.[2]

Blood professional association and industry trade organizations have also engaged in gathering safety data for assessing risks. These organizations include the AABB (formerly the American Association of Blood Banks), of which nearly all blood-collection and manufacturing establishments are members; America's Blood Centers (ABC), which includes collaboration among independent, community-based blood programs; and the American Red Cross (ARC). The AABB, through funding from the Department of Health and Human Services (HHS) of the US government, conducts nationwide surveys to assess the amount of blood collected and transfused in the US and to provide data to assist the HHS in validating its Blood Availability and Safety Information System.

The 35 ARC regional blood centers, as well as independent centers, actively solicit reports of infectious and noninfectious complications in recipients of blood components. When reactions are reported, investigations are carried out to determine the likelihood that such reactions are caused by the transfusion. Outcomes from hospitals served by ARC are compiled and entered into the ARC's Donor and Recipient Complications Program (DRCP) database. This provides the ability to track and analyze trends in complications at each region and across the ARC system to provide opportunities for process improvement. Specific outcomes are also published periodically in peer-reviewed journals.[3]

Mandatory reporting to the federal government is through the US Food and Drug Administration (FDA) and is required for blood and blood components when a fatal adverse event occurs related to donation or transfusion. Mandatory reporting requirements for state government and private nonprofit member organizations also exist. Since 1989, the New York State Department of Health has required the reporting of all transfusion-associated incidents in the state that pose a significant risk to the donor or to the recipient, whether or not an incident results in an adverse outcome.[4] In 1996, The Joint Commission (TJC), an organization responsible for the accreditation of hospitals in the US, established a sentinel event reporting system, including transfusion related events, in support of its mission to improve the safety and quality of health care.[5] Finally, crude baseline rates of adverse reactions associated with blood donors and transfusion recipients, and adverse events in tissue recipients, have been derived from the Department of Health and Human Services National Blood Collection and Utilization Report (NCBUS).

This patchwork of reporting systems in the US, although providing valuable information, falls short of the advances being made in other countries. A need has been recognized for the collection of data for outcomes improvement and public health, in addition to regulatory reporting, for blood, organs, tissues, and cells, that is, biovigilance. In the US, these gaps led the AABB to incorporate an initiative into its strategic plan, in 2006, to go beyond hemovigilance and develop a Biovigilance Network. In cooperation with other interested stakeholder agencies, a plan was developed to incorporate transfusion and transplantation adverse event and incident reporting including donor and recipient outcomes.[6] Concurrently, the Advisory Committee on Blood Safety and Availability (ACBSA) of the Department of Health and Human Services (DHHS) recommended that the HHS Secretary coordinate federal actions and programs to support and facilitate biovigilance in partnership with private-sector initiatives.

Due to the multiplicity of both public and private organizations with a potential stake in such a network, an AABB Biovigilance Inter-organizational Task Force, composed of representatives from both the public and private sectors, was created to provide input into the process. From this AABB task force, an AABB steering committee was created with representatives from the private sector AABB, ABC, ARC, TJC, United Blood Services (UBS), and the College of American Pathology (CAP). Representation from government included Public Health Service agencies within HHS, including FDA, National Institutes for Health (NIH), Centers for Disease Control and Prevention (CDC), and Health Resources and Services Administration (HRSA). The steering committee defined the vision, mission, purpose, and charges and four surveillance activities were identified for development:

- blood transfusion;
- blood donation;
- tissue and organ transplantation; and
- cell therapy transplantation.

Initially, task-force working groups were identified to propose system infrastructure and content for blood transfusion and blood donation outcome surveillance. The working groups consisted of individuals with expertise in various operational aspects of transfusion services and blood collection, and both groups included corresponding members internationally to provide guidance and experience from other systems.

Currently the organizational and governance structure is being studied to determine the best structure for the public–private partnership. Until this is resolved, the task force and steering committee approach is still being used as the systems develop.

Transfusion recipient surveillance

After a review of potential infrastructures that could be used to collect transfusion safety data, the AABB Biovigilance Task Force recommended a public–private partnership building upon CDC's National Healthcare Safety Network (NHSN) as the surveillance system that could most closely meet the data requirements for a national surveillance system for blood-transfusion adverse events. NHSN is a secure, Internet-based surveillance system that collects data from participating healthcare facilities in the US to estimate the magnitude of adverse events among patients and healthcare personnel as well as adherence to best practices for prevention of such adverse events (www.cdc.gov/nhsn). A primary purpose of this surveillance system is to assist participating facilities in developing reporting and analysis methods that permit timely recognition of patient adverse events and prompt intervention with appropriate measures.

The creation of the recipient hemovigilance system was accomplished through collaboration between CDC and the AABB Biovigilance Inter-organizational Task Force. Data elements and case definitions were developed by a working group of transfusion medicine professionals under the AABB Inter-organizational Task Force and were developed into a functioning system as the Hemovigilance Module of the Biovigilance Component of NHSN by CDC. Data elements were defined to capture both patient adverse events (i.e., transfusion reactions) and quality-control incidents (i.e., errors and accidents. Data elements were patterned after existing systems in the US and other countries to ensure collection of useful and reliable information. Adverse-reactions definitions were harmonized with those created by the Hemovigilance Working Party of the International Society of Blood Transfusion (ISBT), including severity and imputability criteria, and Canada's Transfusion Transmitted Injuries Surveillance System (TTISS), while incident reports were harmonized with the classification scheme of MERS-TM and streamlined to collect data that most lends itself to developing purposeful interventions.

NHSN provides sophisticated data-analysis features for facilities to use to review their own data. In addition, the Hemovigilance Module data will be analyzed and published nationally in an anonymous, aggregate format and incorporated into the NHSN Hemovigilance Module for benchmarking purposes, as has been routine for data collected in the Patient Safety Component of NHSN. Participants can prepare tabular or graphic reports of their own data and will be able to compare to aggregate performance benchmarks from all participating facilities in an anonymous fashion. This information will facilitate their own data analyses,

discussion within their local transfusion committees, and improvement of local practices.

Perceived, as key to the success of recipient hemovigilance is the ability for transfusion safety experts to review and analyze data that has been reported to NHSN and recommend improvements in transfusion practice, while keeping data confidential and protected. When hospitals report to the CDC's system, their data are protected through confidentiality protections afforded by the US Public Health Act and are not shared with external partners. Data that are voluntarily submitted to NHSN, including all hemovigilance data, are not reported by CDC in a way that identifies any individual or institution. However, the NHSN Group function allows participating facilities to share their data directly with external partners of their choosing. An important caveat is that data stored in an external partner database are no longer protected by CDC's Assurance of Confidentiality (see Figure 19.1).

Some NHSN Groups offer additional protections through the Patient Safety Act of 2005, which allows entities identified as Patient Safety Organizations (PSOs) to protect data that have been shared with them. AABB has established a PSO, AABB's Patient and Donor Safety Center (PDSC), and has also established a Group in NHSN. Sharing hemovigilance data with AABB's PSO allows the review of facility data in a protected environment to develop interventions in transfusion practice and ultimately improve patient safety.

Reporting and analysis of hemovigilance data by participating facilities began in 2010. Aggregate analyses and public reporting of data will await sufficient participation to provide statistical confidence and to assure anonymity of participating facilities. It is anticipated that data sufficient for national aggregate analysis will be available in CDC's National Healthcare Safety Network Hemovigilance Module in 2012.

As this public–private collaboration in transfusion recipient hemovigilance is unique, each participating organization has its own appropriate role in support of the system. CDC operates and maintains the NHSN Hemovigilance Module and will generate public-health analyses of the data, including national statistics and performance benchmarks,

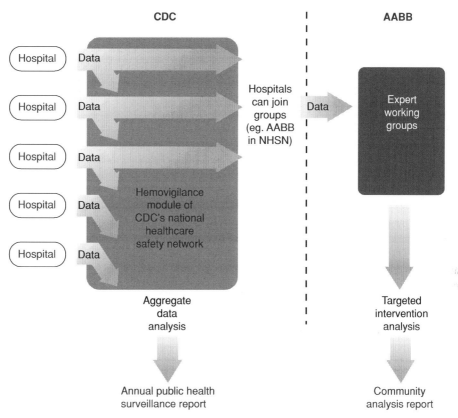

Figure 19.1 Use of the National Healthcare Safety Network Group Function to Enable Hemovigilance Reporting to Expert Working Groups.

and offer public-health recommendations based upon these data. It is anticipated that there will be regular reporting of aggregate data analyses through public-health reports and peer-reviewed journals.

The private sector's primary goal is the development of improvements to patient safety relating to transfusion. The private sector is involved in recruiting participants to the NHSN Hemovigilance Module and educating participants and nonparticipants alike on the value of hemovigilance. Through PSOs, such as AABB's PDSC, transfusion expert groups will assist with data validation and provide contextual analysis of findings and trends in the data shared with them by facilities reporting to NHSN. The private sector seeks to encourage practice improvement and will develop targeted interventions, based on data reported, to drive improvements in patient care.

Blood donation surveillance

The Donor Hemovigilance System was conceived to collect and analyze data on donor reactions to improve the outcomes for blood donors. The Donor System development is being funded by grants from HHS and the Department of Defense (DoD). The AABB Inter-organizational Task Force on Biovigilance established a Donor Working Group (DWG) consisting of representatives from the ARC, ABC, DoD, Plasma Protein Therapeutics Association, Canadian Blood Services, and the Mayo Clinic to establish the data requirements and support the system with analyses.

The DWG developed definitions for donor adverse reactions using a combination of the ISBT, ABC, and ARC definitions and those used locally in many blood centers. The resulting definitions differ from those used in any individual blood center in the US; hence almost all centers will be required to make some limited changes to harmonize with the system and participate. The US donor hemovigilance system differs from other countries in that denominator data will be collected. Stratified rates of reactions will be the basic data used for analysis. The group developed definitions that would capture the detailed information about a donor's reaction in order to meet the analytical and interventional needs to improve donor health and safety. Definitions (both nationally and within-organization) are translatable globally for comparison.

Data elements necessary to capture information about the donor, donation, and reaction were identified. These data elements from reactions identified with donors will be analyzed and compared with denominator data. It was recognized that many blood centers would not be able to provide complete data early in the process. It has been agreed, however, that blood centers should participate initially by submitting current data and that they should
• modify definitions to harmonize with system standards;
• change software to capture system data elements and definitions;
• change procedures to ensure that data are accurately captured; and
• develop the capacity to transfer denominator files electronically as soon as possible.

It is anticipated that although an electronic screen entry option will be available, most participants will seek an electronic interface to upload data from donor management systems already in use. Appropriate requirements for interfaces are being assembled now. The screen-based user interface was tested in December 2008; the file based-upload interface for denominator data in January 2009; and report and analysis options in April 2009. After incorporating improvements, final launch of the system was accomplished at the end of 2010.

Expert representatives from participating centers, who will design and implement routine and focused analyses of the donor reaction data, will oversee analyses of data from the system. The group will consider and select interventions to improve outcomes and will design systems to monitor the success or failure of the interventions. It is anticipated that there will be regular reporting of aggregated data, including de-identified data and its analysis to the HHS and its agencies (CDC, NIH, FDA, and HRSA). Official publications of the aggregate data analyses and journal reporting are also anticipated.

Transplantation Transmission Sentinel Network (TTSN)

Following a number of high-profile investigations of disease transmission events associated with transplantation, including transmission of West Nile virus, rabies, and lymphocytic choriomeningitis virus, CDC sponsored an organ and tissue safety workshop in 2005 to promote a better network within and between the organ and tissue communities.[7] The workshop identified a number of safety gaps and priorities for intervention. These priorities included the development of an electronic communication system involving transplant clinicians and other health professionals. The proposed system would have a clear mechanism for adverse event reporting by healthcare facilities, a unique donor identification system linking organs and tissues, and a notification algorithm for trace-back and trace-forward tracking. A pilot system to address these priorities, called the Transplantation Transmission Sentinel Network (TTSN), was developed by the United Network for Organ Sharing (UNOS) in a cooperative agreement with CDC.

The purpose of the pilot was to provide a system for detecting emerging infections among allograft donors and recipients and help healthcare personnel in detecting, communicating, tracking, and preventing the transmission of infections.

The TTSN was developed with input from an advisory committee of key stakeholders from the organ and tissue transplant community. The TTSN advisory committee identified five key areas for development, which were used to build the prototype system:
• registration or search for donors (Part A);
• registration of recipients (Part B);
• reporting of adverse events (Part C);

- dissemination of information to appropriate regulatory and public health agencies (Part D); and
- education within the community (Part E).

UNOS has overseen the software development that has been completed for Parts A–C. Pilot testing of TTSN was carried out in 2008. Participating institutions included eye, organ, and tissue recovery agencies, tissue processing and distribution agencies, and hospital allograft users.

For the pilot, data were entered for over 1800 donor events and over 900 transplant events. Since there were no adverse events identified during this time period, test cases were created in order to stress the system given the lack of reported events. Donations included combinations of organs, tissues, eyes, and multiple tissue types. Implant events included organs, eyes, musculoskeletal tissue, skin, and cardiovascular tissue.

A number of key challenges remain after completion of pilot testing for implementation of a full national system, including resources for system maintenance, data analysis, and interoperability with existing systems. Nevertheless, the pilot demonstration has proven successful as a prototype. When implemented nationally, the system will allow healthcare providers to recognize disease transmission more expeditiously, help the community to learn from these events, and assist facilities meet reporting requirements.[8]

The future of biovigilance in the US

Biovigilance in the US is in the early stages of development, and has evolved differently depending on the biologic (e.g., blood, organ, tissue) and population (i.e., donor or recipient) under surveillance. For systems that have been developed, such as for blood donors and transfusion recipients, it will take time for systems to build a sufficient base of participation for calculation of aggregate rates and comparison between facilities. Alternate sources, such as NCBUS data, may be useful in comparing to results from existing systems with consistent, regular reporting using common case definitions.

It is expected that as participation in the recipient and donor hemovigilance systems becomes more prevalent and data collection more robust, "data summits" with participation by the transfusion and transplant communities would assist with comparative analysis of reported data and collaborative discussion of identified trends that affect patient safety. For organ, tissue, and cellular product transplantation, comprehensive surveillance systems have yet to be built to monitor adverse events.

Acknowledgement

We would like to thank Alexis R. Harvey, MSPH, for her careful review of the manuscript.

References

1 Menitove JE, 1998, Hemovigilance in the United States of America. *Vox Sang* **74**(Suppl 2): 447–55.

2 Kaplan HS, Battles JB, Van der Schaaf TW, Shea CE, and Mercer SQ, 1998, Identification and classification of the causes of events in transfusion medicine. *Transfusion* **38**(11–12): 1071–81.

3 Eder AF, Kennedy JM, Dy BA, Notari EP, Weiss JW, Fang CT, et al., 2007, Bacterial screening of apheresis platelets and the residual risk of septic transfusion reactions: The American Red Cross experience (2004–2006). *Transfusion* **47**(7): 1134–42.

4 Linden JV, Wagner K, Voytovich AE, and Sheehan J, 2000, Transfusion errors in New York State: An analysis of 10 years' experience. *Transfusion* **40**(10): 1207–13.

5 Chang A, Schyve PM, Croteau RJ, O'Leary DS, and Loeb JM, 2005, The JCAHO patient safety event taxonomy: A standardized terminology and classification schema for near misses and adverse events. *Int J Qual Health Care* **17**(2): 95–105.

6 AuBuchon JP, and Whitaker BI, 2007, America finds hemovigilance! *Transfusion* **47**(10): 1937–42.

7 Fishman JA, Strong DM, and Kuehnert MJ, 2009, Organ and tissue safety workshop 2007: Advances and challenges. *Cell Tissue Bank* **10**(3): 27–80.

8 Strong DM, Seem D, Taylor G, Parker J, Stewart D, and Kuehnert MJ, 2010, Development of a sentinel network to improve safety and traceability of organ and tissue transplants: The need for common identifiers. *Cell Tissue Bank* **11**(4): 335–43.

CHAPTER 20

Arab Hemovigilance Network

Salwa Hindawi[1], Magdy Elekiaby[2], and Gamal Gabra[3]
[1]Blood Transfusion Services, King Abdalaziz University Hospital, Jeddah, Saudi Arabia
[2]Blood Transfusion Center, Shabrawishi Hospital, Giza, Egypt
[3]Birmingham Blood Transfusion Center, Birmingham, UK

Introduction

Hemovigilance is a safety concept referring to the use of a measurement system to record unwanted outcomes of the transfusion chain. It involves a continuous surveillance of all the procedures in the transfusion chain (from the blood donor to the recipient of the blood components) in order to improve the safety of both parties. The intention is to collect and evaluate information on unexpected or undesirable events and the aim is to prevent the risk and/or to reduce severity.

In each country setting up a hemovigilance system, a clear plan and proposal should be submitted to an official local body responsible for transfusion services to get approval and support. The proposal should include the aim and objective of having such system, a written policy and standard to be followed, a working group or committee to be responsible for the process of implementation, funds to cover the system requirements, and the running cost of the system. The decision must be taken to apply the hemovigilance system as a voluntary or mandatory process according to the needs of the country.

Training, education, and increased awareness among workers in blood transfusion facilities will facilitate the development and establishment of the hemovigilance system in all developing countries.

A decision was made by a group of professionals from the Arab-countries region to start a simple system for monitoring adverse events and incidents that occur throughout the transfusion chain. We describe that system—the Arab Hemovigilance Network—in this chapter.

Over two years the ISBT-ATMC (Transfusion Medicine Course for Arabic speaking countries) Hemovigilance Working Group worked hard to develop a system for the surveillance of hazards of transfusion practice, to be used on voluntary basis by facilities and transfusion medicine specialists as a confidential anonymous region-wide reporting system run by an independent professional group.

This scheme was launched as part of the ISBT Educational Transfusion Medicine initiative for the Arabic-speaking countries in North Africa and the Middle East. It aims to encourage and raise the awareness about self-regulation and thinking hemovigilance in a region of 21 countries where facilities and transfusion medicine specialists are starting to catch up with the safety measures that are proposed in other parts of the world, in order to increase safety and quality of the blood transfusion process that involves voluntary donors and giving blood to support patients who are in need of blood and components.

The Working Group has a Steering Committee (SC) of volunteer ISBT-ATMC professionals and a Core Scientific Team (CST) to manage the activities of the newly established Arab Hemovigilance Network (AHN). This includes registration and analysis of the reports of donor and patients' reactions,

Hemovigilance: An Effective Tool for Improving Transfusion Safety, First Edition. Edited by René R.P. De Vries and Jean-Claude Faber.
© 2012 John Wiley & Sons, Ltd. Published 2012 by John Wiley & Sons, Ltd.

incidents, and transfusion-transmitted infections. These are recorded online, collated, and reported anonymously on a regular basis providing medical and scientific analysis of adverse reaction reports in order to develop new policies for safe transfusion practice and improve standards of hospital transfusion practice.

Introducing the Arab Hemovigilance Network

Planning for the introduction of the AHN was through the following:
• Organizing educational activities to increase awareness on the importance of hemovigilance among all professionals involved in the transfusion chain.
• Encouraging the culture of reporting of errors and near-misses in a blame-free environment.
• Facilitating networking between the National Hemovigilance Unit, the blood establishments, and hospital blood banks.

The requirements and standards for a national or regional hemovigilance system are as follows:
• The National Authority for blood transfusion shall set quality and safety standards for 'vein-to-vein' traceability from the collection, testing, processing, storage, and distribution of blood and blood components, when these are intended for transfusion.
• Certain definitions related to hemovigilance and adverse events shall be put in place by the National Authority according to national and international guidelines and definitions of such events (e.g., IHN, WHO, AHN).
• The person responsible for the management of a hospital blood bank or the assigned hemovigilance officer shall notify the hospital transfusion committee with any serious adverse events related to the testing, storage, and distribution of blood or blood components by the hospital blood bank that may have an influence on their quality and safety.
• All hospitals shall have in place a Transfusion Committee (HTC), which will be responsible for

reviewing of all hemovigilance reports received from the hemovigilance officer and develop recommendations for future prevention of such incidents or events and for improvement of safety and quality of the transfusion chain.
• Blood establishments shall notify the National Hemovigilance Office (NHO) with any serious adverse events related to the collection, testing, processing, storage, and distribution of blood or blood components by the blood establishment, which may have an influence on their quality and safety.
• A professional scientific advisory group shall be available and assigned through the National Authority to be responsible for the NHO and developing the national recommendations and policies to improve the overall quality and safety of blood transfusion in the country.

Hemovigilance policies

The AHN system policies are as follows:
• All adverse events related to the transfusion chain should be collected, documented, and reported manually or electronically to the hemovigilance officer who has the responsibility to report to the HTC after analysis and investigation is completed by the blood bank for such events.
• Monthly reports of all events will be reviewed by the HTC and recommendations put in place for improvement of safety and quality of transfusion chain.
• Any serious adverse events should be reported by hemovigilance officer to the NHO in due time and annual hemovigilance reports should be submitted by all hospitals to the NHO.
• A professional advisory group should analyze, advise, and recommend guidelines for better practice in a confidential report to the participating hospitals.
• An annual anonymous report is to be prepared by the advisory group for all participant hospitals, to encourage reporting and improvement of practice through general recommendations.

Basic clinical and organizational guidelines and requirements for effective hemovigilance in all hospitals

Specific tasks are necessary for the implementation of the surveillance of transfusion therapy in hospitals and clinical departments including, primarily, definition of basic laboratory and clinical indications for the transfusion of blood products.

It is also essential to have in place systems for the following:[1–3]

• Ordering blood products and standardized forms for their request and forms that accompany them. This system must define labels that have to be put on blood products, which have been prepared for the transfusion of a defined patient, and labels that have to be put on withdrawn or recalled blood products.

• Unique identification system for the patient, blood product, and laboratory results.

• Collection of patient blood samples and their labeling.

• Transport of requests and blood samples to the Blood Bank, and a system for the transport of blood products from the Blood Bank to the clinical departments.

• Temporary storage of blood products in the required conditions in the clinical departments until they are transfused, or if they are not used until they are returned to the Blood Bank, and responsibility for the products.

• Identification of the patient and blood product immediately before the transfusion, and comparison of the data obtained from the patient with the data on the blood product and with the results of laboratory testing that are written in the form accompanying the blood product.

• Monitoring the transfusion process: Long-term monitoring of the transfused patient would provide more information about the outcome of transfusion therapy.

• Documentation of transfusion and its outcome in the patient's medical file.

• Reporting of the outcome of each transfused unit and of the monitoring of each transfusion event.

• Return of every empty blood product bag after the completion of every transfusion or of every nontransfused blood product to the Blood Bank.

• Monitoring documentation of patients' state and vital signs before and after the end of transfusion, or regularly at defined times during transfusion therapy.

• Documentation of the blood product.

• Documentation of the medical person, who performed the procedure and was responsible for it, in the patient's file.

• Documentation of each adverse event that occurred during or after the transfusion therapy in the patient's file.

• Collection of data on adverse reactions, and analysis by the HTC.[1–3]

The alert system involves information about any new threat to safety of blood transfusion, and recording the occurring of adverse events, measuring their prevalence and characteristics, notifying the Blood Bank (and with its assistance withdrawal or recall of all blood products produced from the same donor), and notifying other institutions that are mandatory or necessary for the prevention of adverse reactions in other patients.

Establishing a regional system (the AHN)

The current situation is that hospitals in the region in question are largely unaware of the extent to which serious errors and near-miss events occur in blood transfusion. Even among hospitals that have identified problems, there are no established benchmarks for performance. Hence the decision was made to create the AHN.

The AHN's aim is to increase safety and quality of the blood transfusion process for patients in need of labile blood components as well as donors and staff. A major part of the system is education, training, and support in relation to best transfusion practice at hospital level.

The AHN involves a set of organized surveillance procedures, from the collection of blood and its components, to the follow-up of recipients to

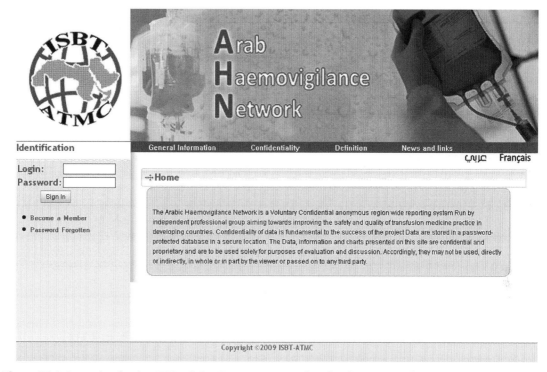

Figure 20.1 Screenshot for the AHN website: Home page (Reproduced with permission from ISBT–ATMC).

collect and assess information on unexpected effects or serious adverse events in recipients resulting from the therapeutic use of labile blood products, and to prevent their occurrence or recurrence.

The AHN has a website designed for easy reporting of adverse reaction or incidents by registered members (see Figures 20.1, 20.2, and 20.3). The report form is in three parts to report patient reaction, donor reactions, and near-miss events or incidents.

The software was developed with the assistance of Med-info, France, and allows the following:

• online access of forms for reporting incidents and adverse reactions;

• password protected anonymous database and reporting system;

• analysis of the incidents;

• preparation of an annual cumulative report that can be accessed by participants;

• online access of cumulative anonymous reports.

It is expected that the system will be fully functional in 2012.

Scope and procedure

Events include reactions (adverse events) and incidents including near-miss reports for donors, staff, and patients.

A *serious adverse event* means any untoward occurrence associated with the collection, testing, processing, storage, and distribution of blood and blood components that might lead to death or life-threatening, disabling, or incapacitating conditions for patients, or which results in, or prolongs, hospitalization or morbidity.

The process includes the following steps:

1 Registration form to be completed and sent confidentially to the AHN.

2 Hospital reports adverse events to the hemovigilance officer.

3 Hemovigilance officer reports to the HTC and to AHN.

4 AHN sends monthly advice to members.

5 AHN prepares an annual report of adverse events statistics, which includes recommendations.

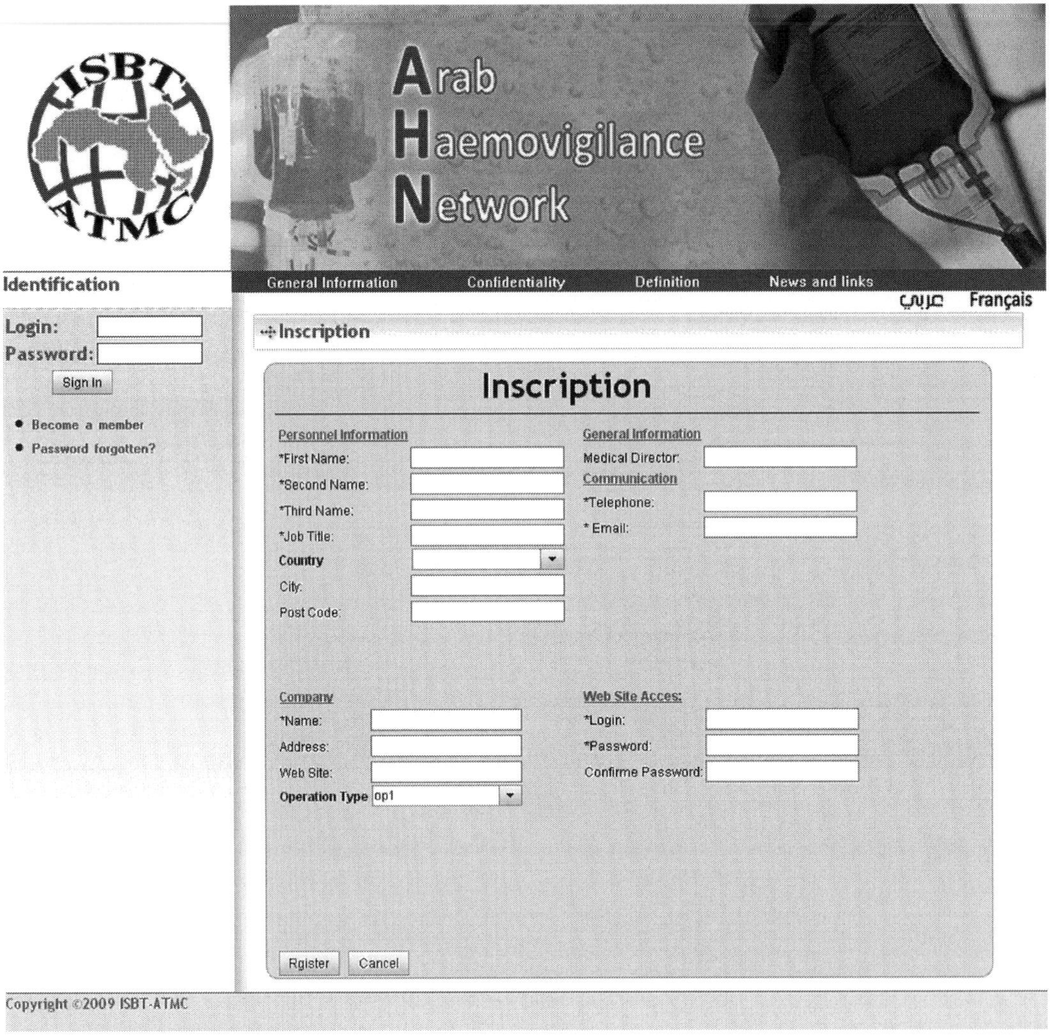

Figure 20.2 Screenshot for the AHN website: Inscription page (Reproduced with permission from ISBT–ATMC).

The Rapid Alert System will be activated and sent to all members at once if any new emerging hazards or incidence are reported to the AHN that may affect other members.

Auditing and updating for the system is done on a regular basis, once or twice yearly according to need.

Objectives of the program

The objectives of the AHN are as follows:[4]

• Receive and follow-up reports from hospitals and collection facilities of events or adverse reactions of donors or patients, and to provide feedback information to reporters as appropriate.

• Advise on the follow-up action necessary, particularly with regard to suspected hazards.

• Support the training of hospital-based transfusion surveillance officers under the hemovigilance program.

• Provide medical and scientific analysis of adverse reaction reports.

• Advise on improvements to the safety of transfusion practice based on the data made available by hospitals.

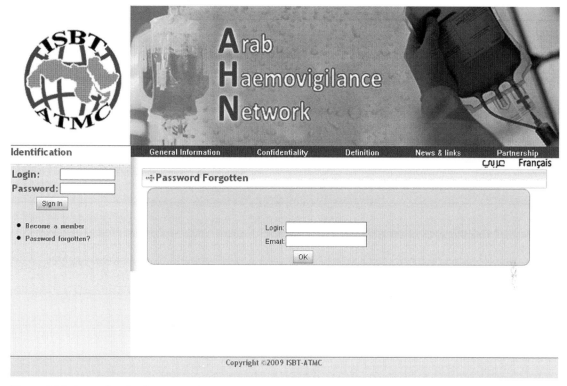

Figure 20.3 Screenshot for the AHN website: A help screen (Reproduced with permission from ISBT–ATMC).

- Help in the production of standard operating procedures.
- Help in the preparation of clinical guidelines.

Reporting process of the program

The AHN's reporting procedure involves the following:
- adverse event form;
- hospital transfusion medicine specialist/consultant;
- confidential anonymous electronic report to AHN, using confidential password;
- detailed formatted questionnaire to reporting person to help analysis of an incident;
- questionnaire returned confirming details;
- AHN formatting of incident and inclusion in the anonymous database;

- updating of website with formatted anonymous information;
- updating of website with cumulative formatted incidents;
- access to cumulative information using confidential password;
- annual report posted on website for confidential access and circulated to participants;
- annual report discussed at annual Steering Committee meeting.

In summary, Figure 20.4 contains a flowchart showing the following:
- Reporting of incidence or reaction to hemovigilance officer and/or HTC at hospital by the clinical staff/transfusion specialist.
- Collecting data and results of required investigations by the hemovigilance officer and sending it to the AHN via the specific website.

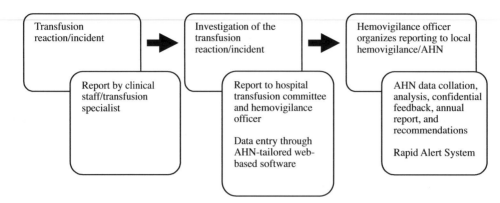

Figure 20.4 Summary of the AHN's processes.

• Confidential analysis by the AHN of the received forms and response to the hospital with advice required.
• Production of an annual report for member hospitals with recommendations for improvement.

Conclusion

This AHN will provide evidence-based knowledge for the improvement of safety and quality of blood transfusion services in the region. The hope is that it will also encourage countries in the region to establish their own national hemovigilance systems.

References

1 Grgičević D, Rašović G, Brubnjak-Jevtič V, Begovi-Dolničar M, and Rossi U, 2002, Ideas and proposals to meet basic clinical and organisational requirements for implementing an effective haemovigilance in South-Eastern Europe. In: Rossi U., Aprili G. (eds), Present and future problems of Transfusion Medicine in South-Eastern Europe. Proceedings of the SIMTI-ESTM Meeting, Lecce (Italy), June 5–6, 2002; pp. 249–63. Edizioni SIMTI, Milan, Italy.

2 Rossi U, 2002, Basic clinical and organizational requirements for an effective haemovigilance. In: Lukič L, Brubnjak-Jevtič V, Primozič J, Benedik-Dolničar M, Rossi U (eds), *Blood therapy in Neonatology and Paediatrics.* Haemovigilance. Proceedings Slovenian/ESTM residential course (5th Postgraduate course on "Blood safety and surgery"), Portorož, Slovenia, December 12–14; pp. 120–37. Blood Transfusion Centre of Slovenia, Ljubljana, Slovenia.

3 Strengers PFW, Love EM, Politis C, and Lissitchkov T (eds), 2002, Basic clinical and organisational requirements for an effective haemovigilance. *Proceedings of the ESTM residential course*, Sofia, Bulgaria), November 28–30. ESTM, Milan, Italy.

4 Hindawi S, 2010, Establishment of haemovigilance system in developing countries (Arab Haemovigilance Network), *Blood Transfusion, 12th International Haemovigilance seminar*, February 17–19, 2010; pp. s5–s7.

PART 4
Hemovigilance at the International Level

CHAPTER 21

Hemovigilance in the European Community

Jean-Claude Faber

Blood Transfusion Service of the Luxembourg Red Cross, Luxembourg

Introduction

In the European Union (EU), hemovigilance (HV) displays many different facets,[1,2] reflecting (i) the structural and organizational diversity of HV at different levels (institutional/local, regional, national, Community-wide) and (ii) the complexity of the European construction itself.

Even the term "Europe" can cause confusion and, as a political conglomerate, one needs to explain the difference between the European Union (EU) and the Council of Europe (CoE) when it comes to HV.

Council of Europe

The Council of Europe is an intergovernmental organization, founded in 1949 and headquartered in Strasbourg, with 44 member states at the moment.

In the context of blood transfusion, the CoE has a long tradition, going back to the 1960s, when a special group was set up to deal with blood transfusion and technical details surrounding blood grouping and transfusion practices. Later on this group was formalized and named SP-HM *(Santé Publique-Hématologie)*, working under the CDSP *(Comité Directeur-Santé Publique)*. Recently, this group came under the Partial Agreement, was renamed as the European Committee on Blood Transfusion (CD-P-TS) and is today attached to the EDQM (European Directorate for the Quality of Medicines and HealthCare).

The CoE has issued a great deal of documents, guidelines, recommendations, and agreements in the field of blood transfusion. One of the best known publications is Rec. No. R (95) 15 "on the preparation, use and quality assurance of blood components", better known as "the Guide", which is updated regularly (now: biennial revisions).[3]

Concerning HV, no specific targeted work has been undertaken by the CoE, but in several documents the importance of HV has been underlined. For quite a while, the CoE advocated in favour of surveillance of the blood chain, even before the term hemovigilance was coined. Hemovigilance as such made its official appearance in Rec. (95) 15 in the 9th edition. As the reference already indicates, the Guide is a recommendation and it is not legally binding to the Member States of the CoE. It is implicit that the CoE or the EDQM do not have regulatory authority over their Member States.

European Union

The European Union was set up with the aim of ending the frequent and bloody wars between neighbors, which culminated in the Second World War. As of 1950, the European Coal and Steel Community (CECA) began to unite European countries economically and politically in order to secure lasting peace. The six founders were France, Germany, Italy, and the three Benelux countries

---

Hemovigilance: An Effective Tool for Improving Transfusion Safety, First Edition. Edited by René R.P. De Vries and Jean-Claude Faber.
© 2012 John Wiley & Sons, Ltd. Published 2012 by John Wiley & Sons, Ltd.

of Belgium, Luxembourg, and the Netherlands. In 1957, the Treaty of Rome created the European Economic Community (EEC), or the "Common Market."

In January 1973, the common construction was enlarged to nine countries, adding to the founding members Denmark, Ireland, and the United Kingdom. The European Parliament increased its influence in EU affairs and in 1979 all their members were elected directly for the first time.

In 1981, Greece became the tenth member of the EU and Spain and Portugal followed five years later (called the Mediterranean enlargement). In 1987, the Single European Act was signed to sort out problems with the free-flow of trade across EU borders and to create the Single Market, which was achieved in 1993.

The 1990s was the decade of two treaties: the Maastricht Treaty in 1993 (establishing the European Union) and the Treaty of Amsterdam in 1999. The "Schengen" agreements gradually allowed people to travel without having their passports checked at the borders (the name comes from a small village in Luxembourg where the agreements were signed on a boat on the Mosel river).

In 1995, the EU gained three more new members: Austria, Finland, and Sweden.

On January 1, 2002, the Euro became the common currency for many Europeans. In 2004, another ten countries joined the EU. This enlargement raised the number of Member States to 25 and Romania and Bulgaria were integrated later. In 2011, negotiations are underway to grant Croatia EU membership.

From the very beginning, the European construction was essentially oriented towards commerce and to the creation of a Common Market. Later on, political aspects gained more and more in importance. Concerning health issues, the situation is somewhat complex and needs some explanation.

Two important principles in the EU need to be mentioned and described at this point: subsidiarity and proportionality.

The EU's decisions must be taken as closely to the citizens as possible. Apart from those areas falling under the exclusive competence of the Community, it does not take action unless this would be more effective than action taken at national, regional, or local level. This principle is known as *subsidiarity* and was reaffirmed in the Lisbon Treaty. Member States have primary responsibility in fields such as health, education, and industry. The EU is to refrain from any action that would detract from the Member States' role in providing services of general interest (and that is health, social services, schools, and so on).

This subsidiarity principle is complemented by the *proportionality* principle whereby the EU must limit its action to what is necessary in order to achieve the objectives set out in the Lisbon Treaty. It is important to mention here that Member States have the right to introduce more stringent protective measures, but they must comply with the provisions of the Treaty.

In the light of the subsidiarity principle, the exclusive responsibility for health issues lies with the Member States: The European Treaty specifies that Community action in the field of public health shall respect the responsibilities of Member States for the organization and delivery of health services and medical care. In particular, measures adopted to set high standards of quality and safety for organs and substances of human origin, blood and blood derivatives, shall not affect national provisions on the donation or medical use of organs and blood. With this a delicate balance is created between the competencies of the EU and those of Member States.

For blood transfusion in the European Community, Directive 89/381/EEC "relating to proprietary medicinal products and laying down special provisions for medicinal products derived from human blood or human plasma" was a milestone in the sense that it established legal provisions for plasma derivatives. It rules that they are to be considered as medicinal products and as such come under Community legislation on medicines; this is true also for the vigilance aspects and in that regard they are covered by pharmacovigilance (as required by Directive 75/319/EEC under article 29a). Blood products are excluded *expressis verbis* from these provisions and therefore do not fall under pharmacovigilance.

In order to understand the evolution of hemovigilance in the EU, one has to go back to the beginning of the 1990s and understand that after "blood scandals" in several Member States, the European Commission (EC) recognized the need to come up with Community legislation on blood matters. The Commission's Communication of December 21, 1994, on Blood Safety and Self-sufficiency in the European Community identified the need for a blood strategy in order to reinforce confidence in the safety of the blood transfusion chain and promote Community self-sufficiency.

The European Council in its Resolution of June 2, 1995, on blood safety and self-sufficiency in the Community, invited the EC to submit appropriate proposals in the framework of the development of a blood strategy. It was proposed to establish a hemovigilance system based on existing networks for the collection of epidemiological data in relation to the blood transfusion chain.

A Colloquium was organized in Adare (Ireland) in September 1996 on "Blood Safety and Self-Sufficiency: an Agenda for the European Community". In its Resolution of November 12, 1996, on a strategy towards blood safety and self-sufficiency in the European Community, the Council invited the Commission to submit proposals as a matter of urgency with a view to encouraging the development of a coordinated approach to the safety of blood and blood products.

Six areas of action were identified for the European Community: one of them was hemovigilance. It was intended to address the subject at Community level, upon a proposal by the EC and referring to a feasibility study for a hemovigilance network within the European Community. The HAEMAN Consortium was constituted in 1997, the Member States met in 1998, and a report on the feasibility was published in 1999 by the EC (at the time DG V/F/4 was in charge of blood issues within Employment, Industrial Relations, and Social Affairs-Public Health and Safety at Work: Communicable, rare and emerging diseases). No further action was taken at that time.

The Treaty laid down in Article 152, 4(a) and (5) "that measures should be adopted setting high standards of quality and safety of organs and substances of human origin, blood and blood derivatives." Mandated by this article, the EC submitted a proposal for a "European Blood Directive," which entered the long and complicated process for adoption by the European Parliament and the European Council (not to be confused with the Council of Europe).

Legal framework set by Community legislation

Between 2003 and 2005, the EU adopted four major pieces of Community legislation:
- Directive 2002/98/EC;[4]
- Directive 2004/33/EC;[5]
- Directive 2005/61/EC;[6]
- Directive 2005/62/EC.[7]

Major efforts and much good will were necessary to coordinate and synchronize the works of the CoE and the EC. The guidance and legislation of these two separate organizations were brought into line in order to avoid two different sets of standards for blood transfusion existing throughout Europe.

Hereafter, the different Directives will be reviewed one by one and legal requirements relevant to hemovigilance highlighted.

Directive 2002/98/EC[4]

This Directive of the European Parliament and of the Council, setting standards for the quality and safety of the collection, testing, processing, storage, and distribution of human blood and blood components, was published on January 27, 2003. This directive is called the "Mother Directive" and has laid down the principles governing blood matters in the EU.

In the legal provisions of this directive, there are two operating articles addressing directly hemovigilance.

Article 14 deals with Traceability and requires that all Member States take all necessary measures in order to ensure that blood and blood components collected, tested, processed, stored, released, and/or distributed on their territory can be traced from donor to recipient and vice versa.

It requires that Member States ensure that blood establishments implement a system for the identification of each single blood donation, and each single blood unit and component thereof, enabling full traceability to the donor as well as to the transfusion and the recipient. The system must unmistakably identify each unique donation and type of blood component and be established in accordance with requirements set out in the directives.

Furthermore, it is required that Member States take all necessary measures in order to ensure that the system used for the labeling of blood and blood components collected, tested, processed, stored, released, and/or distributed on their territory complies with the identification system and the labeling requirements, both defined in the Directive.

Finally, data needed for full traceability need to be kept for at least 30 years.

Article 15 deals with the Notification of serious adverse events and reactions (SAEs and SARs). It requires from Member States that any SAEs (accidents and errors) related to the collection, testing, processing, storage, and distribution of blood and blood components that may have an influence on their quality and safety, as well as any SARs observed during or after transfusion that may be attributed to the quality and the safety of blood and blood components, are notified to the competent authority. Blood establishments must have in place a procedure accurately, efficiently, and verifiably to withdraw from distribution blood or blood components associated with such a notification.

It is required that these SAEs and SARs are notified in accordance with a defined procedure and notification format set out in secondary Community legislation.

In summary, Directive 2002/98 requires in the context of hemovigilance that traceability of blood and blood components from donor to the recipient is guaranteed and that any SAEs and SARs are notified by the blood establishments to the competent national authority.

Although the Mother Directive renders hemovigilance mandatory in the Member States of the EU and regulates to some extent traceability and notification, it should be pointed out that the legal provisions are limitative (see Figure 21.1) and restrict the obligations to

- activities (transfusion or donation) in relation to blood and blood components intended for transfusion and not for manufacturing;
- serious ARs and serious AEs;
- those related to quality and safety of blood and blood components;
- mainly the recipients (this is still under debate).

Figure 21.1 gives a schematic representation of the scope of the Blood Directive. Out of all incidents that (can) happen *only* confirmed SARs and SAEs in relation to quality and safety of blood for transfusion are reportable by Member States to the EC. This is also applicable to donor reactions, and therefore most SARs affecting donors are excluded from reporting as are those incidents in the clinical field, because clinical activities are of the competency of Member States according to the principle of subsidiarity.

The Blood Directive provides that reportable information only concerns "any SAR observed in recipients during or after transfusion which may be attributable to the quality and safety of blood and blood components" and "any SAE which may affect the quality or safety of blood and blood components" (see Figure 21.2).

This is important to understand because in some way it "amputates" hemovigilance at the Community level and "softens" its impact. As already mentioned, these restrictions are to be seen in the light of Article 152 of the European Treaty.

Figure 21.2 illustrates that Member States have to report only a fraction of all reactions (and events) to the EC: Only *serious* adverse reactions (severity grades 2 to 4), which are considered as confirmed (imputability levels 2 and 3) and are linked to a quality and safety problem of the blood products, need to notified through a defined procedure on a defined form. These data also constitute the core information for the annual report of the EC according to the terms of the Blood Directive.

In order to facilitate normative application in the field, three "Daughter Directives" were later

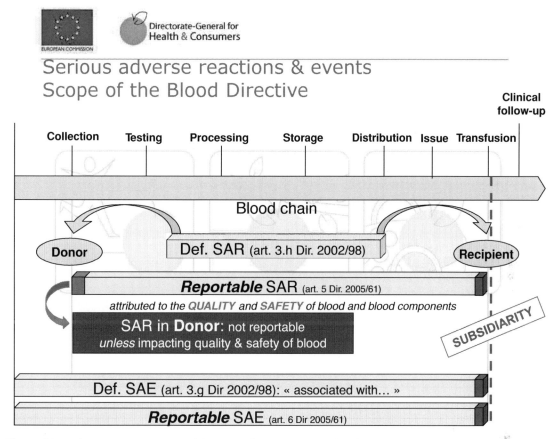

Figure 21.1 Schematic representation of the scope of reporting set by the Blood Directive. ARs and AEs are defined in the Directives as are severity and imputability.

adopted by the EU, as described in the next three sections.

Directive 2004/33/EC[5]

This is the Commission Directive of March 22, 2004, the first so-called Daughter Directive, implementing the Mother Directive as regards certain technical requirements for blood and blood components and determining common definitions and understanding for the technical terminology in order to ensure the consistent implementation of the Directives.

This Directive lays down those technical requirements, which take account of Council Recommendation 98/463/EC of June 29, 1998, on the suitability of blood and plasma donors and the screening of donated blood in the European Community, certain recommendations of the CoE, the opinion of the Scientific Committee for Medicinal Products and Medical Devices, the monographs of the European Pharmacopoeia, particularly in respect of blood or blood components as a starting material for the manufacture of proprietary medicinal products, recommendations of WHO, and international experience in the field.

With regards to hemovigilance, the following issues are covered in this Directive:
• Information to be provided to prospective donors of blood or blood components (so that the donor can understand the educational materials provided,

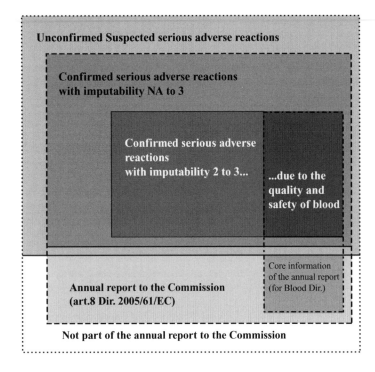

Figure 21.2 Only a fraction of all reactions (and events) happening in the context of blood transfusion are reportable to the EC by EU Member States.

ask questions, get satisfactory responses to any questions asked, and give informed consent to proceed with the donation process).

• Information to be obtained from donors by blood establishments at every donation (including identification of the donor—through unique personal data, and without any risk of mistaken identity, distinguishing the donor—as well as contact details).

• Health and medical history of the donor:
  ○ Health and medical history are to be provided on a questionnaire and through a personal interview performed by a qualified healthcare professional that includes relevant factors that may assist in identifying and screening out persons whose donation could present a health risk to others, such as the possibility of transmitting diseases, or health risks to themselves.
  ○ Validation of the donor interview is done by placing the signature of the donor on the donor questionnaire and countersigning it by the healthcare staff member responsible for obtaining the health history.

• Eligibility criteria for donors of whole blood and blood components:
  ○ Acceptance criteria for donors of whole blood and blood components.
  ○ Deferral criteria for donors of whole blood and blood components (permanent and temporary suspensions).

• Storage, transport, and distribution conditions for blood and blood components.

• Quality and safety requirements for blood and blood components.

In other words, Directive 2003/44/EC is setting a normative frame as well as standards for the donor and donated blood and blood components.

Directive 2005/61/EC[6]

This is the Commission Directive of September 30, 2005, called the second Daughter Directive, implementing the Mother Directive as regards specific technical requirements dealing with traceability and the notification of SARs and SAEs (suspected SARs or SAEs have to be submitted to the competent authority as soon as they become known). It also determines common definitions and understanding for the technical terminology in order to ensure the consistent implementation of the Directives.

The Directive also establishes the notification format defining the minimum data needed, without prejudice to the faculty of Member States to maintain or introduce in their territory more stringent protective measures that comply with the provisions of the Treaty.

In relation to traceability, the following is required: that blood and blood components can be traced through accurate identification procedures, record maintenance, and an appropriate labeling system; that in the blood establishment the tracing of blood components to their location and processing stage is enabled; that each donor is uniquely identified as is each blood unit collected and each blood component prepared; that the facilities can be identified to which a given blood component has been delivered. It is also mandatory to have a system in place to record each blood unit or blood component received, whether or not locally processed, and the final destination of that received unit, whether transfused, discarded, or returned to the distributing blood establishment. Blood establishments need to have a unique identifier that enables it to be precisely linked to each unit of blood that it has collected and to each blood component that it has prepared.

For issuing blood or blood components, blood establishments and hospital blood banks are required to have in place a procedure to verify that each unit issued has been transfused to the intended recipient or if not transfused to verify its subsequent disposition.

In the context of record keeping, blood establishments have to retain data on blood establishment identification, blood donor identification, blood unit identification, individual blood component identification, date of collection, facilities to which blood units or blood components are distributed, or subsequent disposition. Hospital blood banks have to archive data on blood component supplier identification, issued blood component identification, transfused recipient identification, for blood units not transfused, confirmation of subsequent disposition, date of transfusion or disposition, and lot number of the component (if relevant). Archives of these data need to be kept for at least 30 years in an appropriate and readable storage medium in order to ensure traceability.

Notification of SARs needs to be done according to a defined procedure, which is described to some extent in the Directive.

Those facilities where transfusion occurs must have procedures in place to retain the record of transfusions and to notify blood establishments without delay of any SARs observed in recipients during or after transfusion, which may be attributable to the quality or safety of blood and blood components.

These facilities communicate to the competent authority as soon as known all relevant information about suspected SARs. Specially designed SAR notification formats are to be used. One form is for immediate rapid notification, a second one is for confirmation upon adequate investigation, and a third is for annual reporting.

When facilities where transfusions are undertaken encounter a SAR, they are obliged to

• notify to the competent authority all relevant information about SARs of imputability level 2 or 3 (as defined in the Directive), attributable to the quality and safety of blood and blood components;
• notify the competent authority of any case of transmission of infectious agents by blood and blood components as soon as known;
• describe the actions taken with respect to other implicated blood components that have been distributed for transfusion or for use as plasma for fractionation;
• evaluate suspected SARs according to defined imputability levels;
• complete the SAR notification, upon conclusion of the investigation, using the appropriate format;
• submit a complete synoptic report on SARs to the competent authority on an annual basis using the annual reporting form.

Notification of SAEs needs to be in accordance with a defined procedure described in detail in the Directive. It should be noted that the term "event" in the Directive (and therefore in the EU) somewhat differs from the definition used in other parts of the world.

For the purpose of notification, blood establishments and hospital blood banks are required to have procedures in place to retain the record of any SAEs that may affect the quality or safety of blood and blood components.

Those facilities where transfusions are undertaken need to have procedures in place to communicate to the competent authority as soon as known, using the appropriate notification format, all relevant information about SAEs that may put in danger donors or recipients other than those directly involved in the event concerned. Specially designed SAE notification formats are to be used as with the SARs described above for immediate rapid notification, confirmation upon adequate investigation, and annual reporting.

When facilities encounter a SAE, they are required to

- evaluate the SAE to identify preventable causes with a given process;
- complete the SAE notification, upon conclusion of the investigation, using the defined format;
- submit a complete report on SAEs to the competent authority on an annual basis using the form for annual synoptic reporting.

Annual reporting is considered to be of the high importance and priority. Member States have to submit to the EC an annual report (by June 30 of the year following the index year) on the notification of SARs and SAEs received by the competent authority using the defined formats.

In the same spirit, communication of information between competent authorities is regulated in the sense that Member States have to make sure that their competent authorities communicate to each other such information as is appropriate with regard to SARs and SAEs in order to guarantee that blood or blood components known or suspected to be defective are withdrawn from use and discarded.

Member States needed to transpose these legal requirements within a given timeframe: They had to bring into force the laws, regulations, and administrative provisions necessary to comply with this Directive by August 31, 2006, at the latest. They had to communicate to the EC the text of those provisions and a correlation table between those provisions and this Directive.

In summary, Directive 2005/61 requires

- facilities to record the final destination of each received unit, whether transfused, discarded, or returned to the distributing blood establishment;
- facilities where transfusion occurs to retain the record of transfusions and to notify blood establishments of any SAR attributable to the quality/safety of blood;
- blood establishments and hospital blood banks to retain records of any SAE that may affect quality/safety of blood traceability of blood and blood components from donor to the recipient.

Directive 2005/62/EC[7]

This is the Commission Directive of September 30, 2005, the third Daughter Directive, implementing the Mother Directive as regards Community standards and specifications relating to a quality system for blood establishments.

It imposes that a quality system for blood establishments has to embrace the principles of quality management, quality assurance, and continuous quality improvement, and should cover personnel, premises and equipment, documentation, collection, testing and processing, storage and distribution, contract management, nonconformance and self-inspection, quality control, blood component recall, and external and internal auditing.

It must take into account Commission Directive 2003/94/EC of October 8, 2003, laying down the principles and guidelines of good manufacturing practice in respect of medicinal products and investigational medicinal products for human use.

In order to ensure the highest quality and safety for blood and blood components, guidance on good practice had to be developed to support the quality system requirements for blood establishments, taking fully into account the detailed guidelines referred to in Article 47 of Directive 2001/83/EC, so as to ensure that the standards required for medicinal products are maintained.

Good practice is defined as all elements in established practice that collectively will lead to final blood or blood components consistently meeting predefined specifications and compliance with defined regulations.

All blood establishments must have in place a quality system that complies with the Community standards and specifications developed in this Directive:

- quality management and change control;
- personnel and organization;
- premises, including mobile sites;
- equipment and materials;
- documentation;
- donor session;
- processing;
- storage and dispatch;
- quality monitoring;
- quality control and laboratory testing;
- contract management;
- deviations, complaints, adverse events or reactions, recall, corrective and preventive actions;
- self-inspection, audits, and improvement.

It is pertinent to remind that HV is a quality tool in itself. Therefore all the standards and specifications listed in this Directive on quality are relevant for HV. But clearly the requirements in the context of deviations, complaints, adverse events or reactions, recall, and corrective and preventive actions (CAPA) are of particular importance in the light of HV. It is simple logic to anchor the observation, documentation, investigation, and notification of SARs, SAEs, and CAPA in a robust pact for the improvement of quality and safety of blood and blood components.

Member States had to bring into force the laws, regulations, and administrative provisions necessary to comply with this Directive by August 31, 2006, at the latest. They had to communicate to the Commission the text of those provisions and a correlation table between those provisions and this Directive.

Transposition by Member States

In general, EC directives have to be transposed by Member States into national legislation within two years; sometimes a shorter period is set for the transposition. For blood matters, this had to be accomplished for August 31, 2006; in other words all Member States had to integrate all legal dis-

positions into their national laws, including those relevant to hemovigilance. Community procedure requires Member States to inform the EC (as the "guardian" of the European Treaties) each time a directive has been transposed, enabling the Commission to follow the state of advancement.

Difficulties encountered

Community HV is built on existing and developing national systems in Member States of the EU. The national systems must fulfill the minimum requirements set out in Community legislation and they need to be synchronized and coordinated, so that they can fit together at the top, when they are "bundled" at Community level. The relevant data collected by the national HV systems may be "injected" into a single centralized site, an overarching Community structure.

If the European Community succeeds in anchoring quality cycles within a standing and functioning construct, quality and safety of blood transfusion in the Community can improve continuously as expected from a comprehensive quality approach: what is required from the Member States, for example, ensuring quality management at institutional, regional, and national levels, shall not be neglected at Community level.

It should be pointed out that the Community has difficulties in positioning the legal provisions on blood, including, notably, because of the restrictions imposed by the European Treaty, anterior Community legislation, and divergent political views of some Member States:[8–10]

- In drafting the Blood Directives, legislation on medicinal products had to be taken into account and contradictions and inconsistencies had to be avoided. Therefore the Mother Directive's scope states that it shall apply to the collection and testing of human blood and blood components, whatever their intended purpose, and to their processing, storage, and distribution when intended for transfusion. In other words: it regulates processing, storage, and distribution if blood and labile blood components (such as red cells, platelets, plasma) are administered but not if stable plasma derivatives (e.g., albumin, clotting factors, and immunoglobulins) are therapeutically used (here pharmaco-legislation applies). On the other hand, it regulates collection and testing of human blood and blood components, whatever their intended purpose, which means for both lines of products, labile blood components, and stable plasma derivatives.

• A major drawback of the Blood Directives is related to the fact that they ensure only a partial coverage of the blood chain (vein-to-vein). In fact, in order to ensure high quality and safety for the transfused patient, each and every activity along the entire blood transfusion chain needs to be regulated to the same high level. Only in doing so, can this goal be reached in the best interest of the patient who needs a blood transfusion. Unfortunately the Blood Directives mainly regulate the activities of the production segment and, to some lesser degree, the links between the blood establishments and the hospitals. The usage segment of the blood chain (clinical activities in the hospitals) is not covered.

It is well known (from Hemovigilance National Office, Ireland, and Serious Hazards of Transfusion, UK) that hemovigilance data from different Member States of the EU undisputedly show that most of the problems encountered and the majority of the risks inherent in blood transfusion are identified in the usage segment of the blood transfusion chain rather than in the production segment . These are facts, and nobody who is willing to increase quality and safety of blood transfusion in the best interest of the patient is entitled to ignore them.

It is true that some limitations are imposed by Article 152 (5) of the Treaty, but nonetheless many actors in the field are convinced that the least that could be done is to invite the Member States to take national measures ensuring a comparable level of quality and safety for the usage segment (e.g., requiring optimal and safe use of blood components in each and every hospital where transfusions are undertaken, establishing and maintaining transfusion committees in the hospitals in a mandatory way, rendering obligatory proven quality and safety measures in the processes related to the transfusion act, and so on).

Hiding behind Article 152 (5), little has been done to strengthen the clinical part of the transfu-

sion process, which is well known to be the weakest part of the blood transfusion chain. In the light of future experience, time may come to override the restrictions imposed by Article 152 (5) of the Treaty. Otherwise the legal framework for HV will remain fragmented and appear as a patchwork:

• blood for transfusion versus blood for manufacturing;

• blood establishment and hospital blood banks but excluding other units/entities in the hospitals;

• SARs/SAEs as opposed to all ARs/AEs plus nearmisses;

• SARs/SAEs limited to those attributable to quality defects of blood and blood components.

Reporting experiences[11–13]

The annual reporting of SARs and SAEs (called "SAR/E Annual Reporting") is an obligation under the Blood and Tissues Directives, monitors the implementation of the Directives' vigilance provisions at Member States level, and helps the move toward homogeneous understanding and use of vigilance.

The legal tool is in Article 8 of Directive 2005/61/EC, which requires Member States to submit to the EC an annual report, by June 30 of the following year, on the notification of SARs and SAEs received by the competent authority.

The following objectives are pursued at Community level:

• contribute to the improvement of HV across the EU;

• monitor effects of the Blood Directive (trends);

• monitor the implementation of the Blood Directive.

The first reporting to the EC was due on June 30, 2008, concerning information collected during the complete year 2007 (from January 1 to December 31). The notification of SARs and SAEs received by the competent authority is to be done according to procedures and using formats defined in Directive 2005/61/EC.

The form for the annual report of SARs collects basic information (including those on denominators), types of SAR, respective imputability (levels 0–3), and number (total of occurrences and fatalities).

The form for annual report of SAEs reaches out for basic information (including those on denominators), types of SAE (according to activity), total number, and cause at origin of SAE.

What appeared so simple turned to out to be quite complicated, as could be concluded from stakeholders' and competent authorities' feedback: there was a lack of clarity on scope and definitions, a risk of mistake or misreporting, long internal discussions causing delays in response, and so on.

It became apparent that the annual reporting had to be seen as a learning-by-experience exercise. At that point in time it did not yet give a clear view of the reality of SAR/SAE annual occurrences in the EU. It was still considered a snapshot of the Member States' capacity to report accurate data taking due account of the remaining lack of clarity in the reporting requirements as well as the actual ability of the Member States to collect and generate the data.

Thorny discussions turned around denominator data on blood and blood components in the annual activity report and the question remained of which data would best serve the purpose: number of units issued (by country); number of units issued by product (EU); number of recipients transfused (by country); number of recipients transfused by product (EU); number of units transfused (by country); number of units transfused by product (EU).

Another question that was debated intensively concerned the discrimination between SAEs and "background noise" in a given quality system; where to put the delineating line. Some suggested that it would be worthwhile to learn from EUSTITE (European Union Standards and Training in the Inspection of Tissue Establishments) and use an impact matrix.

Clarification was desperately needed on what and how to report. For this purpose a special document was published by the EC: the "Common Approach for Definition of reportable SAR/E as laid down in the Blood Directive 2002/98/EC and Commission Directive 2005/61/EC." This Common Understanding document together with the Standardized Reporting Format was meant to solve the recognized problems.

For the following reporting year, the challenges remained: How to ensure that the reported information is reliable and usable and how to optimize the gathering exercise to avoid unnecessary burden at all stages?

For the second Annual SAR/E Report (launched in June 2009, collecting 2008 data), the experience was similar to the first round. It was decided to publish a second version of the Common Understanding document by the Member States' Expert group, with input from international organizations (e.g., WHO, CoE) and the scientific community (e.g., IHN, ISBT), and to review the online formats to improve user-friendliness.

The third year of annual reporting (launched in June 2010) covered data related to SARs/SAEs that occurred and/or were validated in 2009 (from January 1 to December 31).

In analyzing the data it was interesting to see that only a small fraction of the reported SARs/SAEs were in fact reportable to the EC. 3471 confirmed cases of SARs related to blood or blood components *not* attributable to the quality and safety of the blood/blood component were reported to the Commission by Member States. In this category, the total number of deaths encountered was 73. On the other hand, the EC received 150 confirmed reports of SARs related to blood or blood components that *were* attributable to the quality and safety of the blood/blood component. Among them, five fatal outcomes were reported by Member States to the EC. The data show that there is continuing confusion and uncertainty among Member States on what to report to the EC, even though the Directives are explicit on the reporting requirements of SARs/SAEs: Only those attributable to the quality and safety of blood and blood components are to be reported.

Another interesting conclusion from the analysis of the submitted reports was in relation with the types of SAR reported to the EC by Member States (see Figure 21.3, which shows results from the 3rd Annual Report from the EC for SARs). Except for anaphylactic hypersensitivity, no similarity in classification order between Member States could be found and some types were completely confined in one (or a few) States. The heterogeneity between

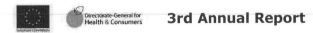 **3rd Annual Report**

SAR – TOP 10

Total sum of all SAR for all blood components for all MS

		Non death	Death
1.	Anaphylactic hypersensitivity	1344	8
2.	Hemolysis - Non-immunological	330	1
3.	Pyrogenic reaction	256	0
4.	TRALI	223	15
5.	Tf transmitted bacterial infection	189	6
6.	TACO	164	7
7.	Febrile non-hemolytic tf reaction	120	0
8.	Hemolysis-Immunological, ABO	119	4
9.	Hemolysis-Immunological, other allo-Ab	108	5
10.	Tf transmitted HBV +HCV	46+60	1+1

Figure 21.3 Results from the 3rd Annual Report (on 2009 data) from the EC for SAR cases.

Member States is evident: the reason for this phenomenon is not clear.

In Figure 21.3, the absolute frequency gives the ranking of the different types of SAR. It shows that there is a marked difference between those SARs that are lethal and those where the patient showing a SAR survives the blood transfusion. For anaphylactic sensitivity manifested as SAR, the fatality rate is 0.59%, whereas for Transfusion Related Acute Lung Injury (TRALI) it is 6.30%, more than 10 times higher lethality.

A similar variability could be observed in the context of reporting SAEs (see Figure 21.4, which shows the results from the 3rd Annual Report). A total of 24,897 cases were reported, with 19,273 from one single Member State (85% being related to product defects, more than half occurring at processing). In this country, most reports included any event that might have endangered the recipient's health even though identified and eliminated according to internal control procedures. Two other Member States showed a similar pattern, although much less pronounced. On the other hand, several States reported not a single SAE in that year.

Despite numerous definitions given in the different directives, important variations exist between Member States and this is particularly true for product defects.

Another lesson learnt from the 3rd exercise was that reporting without differentiation into the "human error" group occurred frequently and was "overfilling" this category. It was felt that this could be improved in the future, to render the data collection and analysis more efficient.

Although not mandatory by the Directives, SARs in donors were reported to the EC. Seven Member States reported 2941 SARs in blood/plasma donors, three reported that they did not record SARs in

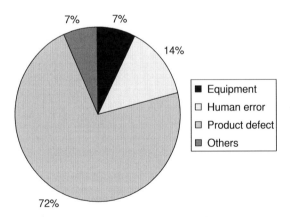

Figure 21.4 Results from the 3rd Annual Report (on 2009 data) from the EC for SAEs. The relative frequencies are derived from the raw data that include the very high numbers of product defects reported from one single country.

donors, and one reported that it was establishing a system for reporting SARs in donors. Because donor vigilance is felt to be important and feasible, it was suggested that in the future annual reporting of SARs in donors continue on a voluntary basis.

There are still numerous unanswered questions around the annual reporting of SARs/SAEs and debates continue around denominators (units issued/transfused, recipients transfused, units produced), numerator data (including/excluding clinical wastage, double-counting or not, reporting SARs associated with multiple blood components transfused), donor incidents (reporting post-donation information and deviations in donor samples) and more.

Some people feel that there are too many categories (a total of 64) and that this is more confusing than helpful to Member States. The distribution pattern supports these views in some way: in 2 out of 64 categories, no SARs/SAEs were reported, in 9 of 64 one SAR/SAE was reported, and in 30 of the 64 categories less than 5 SARs/SAEs were reported.

The question is also asked whether evaluation is possible at all. At this point in time, it may be confirmed that comparing annual evolution is possible, but intra-country comparison is not possible, given the different interpretations and reporting practices.

After three rounds of annual reporting, it is clear that the system is still in a learning phase and that it can be improved stepwise to make it more efficient.

As Step 1, the 2011 round of SAR/SAE reporting (on data collected in 2010) will see a quick quality check after submission of the reports by a team of experts. The common approach document will bring more clarification of the definitions used. In addition, direct contact points will be identified in the national HV systems, alongside the official focal points in competent national authority in Member States.

Step 2 will cover the 2012 SARE report (on data from 2011) and will see a revised template, a revised common approach document (this will be the 3rd edition), and voluntary reporting of SARs in donors: these measures will improve the database. For the analysis of HV data, it is generally felt that expertise and experience in HV and in evaluation are indispensable and should be the route to follow in the future of SAR/SAE reporting and assessing.

In Step 3, a revision of Community legislation may be considered if the need arises.

Basically, the tools used for Member States' Annual Reporting will remain the same:
• common approach document (clarifies the scope of reporting and gives guidance on reportable SARs and SAEs);
• templates (collects the data in a defined format).

The question on who will analyze and evaluate the data collected from Member States in the future remains open at this point.

Figure 21.5 illustrates the EC's tools to collect data in a standardized manner. One of the objectives is progressively to build a comprehensive database on blood activities within the EU.

The annual reports from the Member States will enable the EC to build up a database allowing for comparison and, eventually, for benchmarking in the area of blood (transfusion or donation).

Despite all the problems and difficulties encountered, SAR/SAE reporting has shown its importance to
• providing Member States with reliable and usable data;
• supporting Member States in organizing and developing their systems (e.g., preventive, corrective measures);
• spotting areas where adaptations/improvements of the Blood Directive could be necessary.

Rapid alert

In Europe, rapid alert has two separate arms. One is arranged through the professional/scientific organization dealing with HV, the IHN (formerly the EHN, European Hemovigilance Network) and the other is organized by the responsible Community Authority, the ECDC (European Center for Disease Prevention and Control).

Although rapid alert is not mentioned *expressis verbis* in the operating articles of the Directives, reference to it is made in several "Whereas." Member States are required to ensure that their competent authorities communicate to each other information as is appropriate with regard to SARs and SAEs to guarantee that blood or blood components known

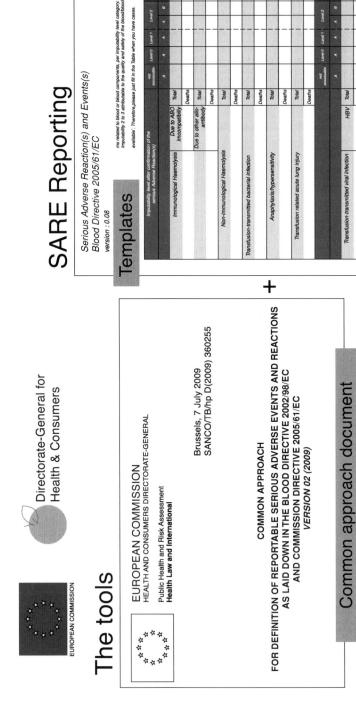

Figure 21.5 Tools that the EC uses to collect data in a standardized way from the Member States.

or suspected to be defective are withdrawn from use and discarded.

The scope of the rapid alerts is on product defects as well as threats to health and blood donations.

Role of ECDC

Established in 2005, the ECDC is an EU agency aimed at strengthening Europe's defenses against infectious diseases. It is based in Stockholm, Sweden.

The ECDC's mission is to identify, assess, and communicate current and emerging threats to human health posed by infectious diseases. In order to achieve this mission, the ECDC works in partnership with national health protection bodies across Europe to strengthen and develop continent-wide disease surveillance and early warning systems. By working with experts throughout Europe, the ECDC pools Europe's health knowledge to develop authoritative scientific opinions about the risks posed by current and emerging infectious diseases.

The ECDC's activities are organized to
• search for, collect, collate, evaluate, and disseminate relevant scientific and technical data;
• provide scientific opinions and scientific and technical assistance including training;
• provide timely information to the EC, the Member States, Community agencies, and international organizations active within the field of public health;
• coordinate the European networking of bodies operating in the fields within the ECDC's mission, including networks arising from public health activities supported by the EC and operating the dedicated surveillance networks;
• exchange information, expertise, and best practices, and facilitate the development and implementation of joint actions.

These tasks are achieved inter alia through rapid alerts.

The ECDC's Epidemic Intelligence encompasses activities related to early warning functions, but also signal assessments and outbreak investigation. It aims to speed up detection of potential health threats and allow timely response. *Epidemic intelligence* is defined as the process to detect, verify, analyze, assess, and investigate public health events that potentially represent a threat to public health. Providing early warning signals is a main objective of public health surveillance systems.

The mandate of the ECDC regarding risk identification and risk assessment is to
• identify and assess emerging threats to human health from communicable diseases;
• establish, in cooperation with the Member States, procedures for systematically searching for, collecting, collating, and analyzing information and data with a view to the identification of emerging health threats that may have mental as well as physical health consequences and could affect the Community.

In the context of HV ECDC has its role in "hot" HV, when threats are emerging in relation to human substances; in 2008 and 2009, rapid alerts were related to Chikungunya, West Nile Virus, Hepatitis A, and vCJD, whereas alerts related to SAEs were quite rare (0 in blood, 3 in tissues).

For all situations outside of "emerging threats", and more precisely outside of constellations representing infectious/contaminating risks, the ECDC does not seem to be the primary organization. According to the Mother Directive, the EC has the mandate to collect the data on SARs and SAEs from Member States and to publish an Annual Report. It has not been stated so far which entity is going to take up the numerous tasks and ensure continuity in analyzing and compiling HV data, producing adequate conclusions, and making necessary recommendations or proposing mandatory measures for the EU.

Figure 21.6 gives a possible scenario that could work at a supra-national level in the EU. It puts together the different elements that currently exist in the EU in the context of HV. The Member States' competent authorities report data of relevance to HV (basically on SARs and SAEs) annually to the EC. Under the EC, a central HV unit could work that deals with the daily business around Community HV and also ensures the link with the ECDC. The EC is assisted by a Regulatory Committee and a Scientific Committee and figures as a platform for issues that are relevant for safety and quality of blood in the EU.

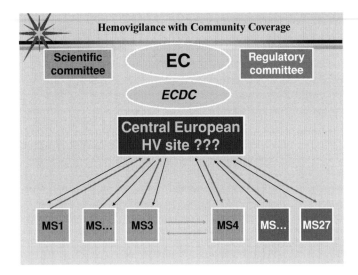

Figure 21.6 Different elements currently existing in the EU as regards hemovigilance. The Community construction is based on national HV systems that vary among Member States.

Future of European hemovigilance

EU legislation is mandatory and the European Communities have issued policies and regulations on different substances of human origin:
- blood and blood components:
  - Blood Directive (2002/98);
  - Commission Directives (2004/33, 2005/61, 2005/62).
- tissues and cells:
  - Tissues and Cells Directive (2004/23);
  - Commission Directives (2006/17, 2006/86).
- Organs:
  - Proposal for an Action Plan and a Directive submitted by the Commission;
  - Co-decision procedure underway in 2011.

It is not surprising that regulatory challenges may arise from the existence of different regulatory frameworks that apply to the different human substances. Efforts are now being undertaken to bring the different pieces of Community legislation into one single legal framework and to avoid problems arising from the legal patchwork (see Figure 21.7).

If the EU succeeds in this endeavor, it will move from hemovigilance to biovigilance, as it exists in other parts of the world.

In the meanwhile, the EC and Member States need to overcome the existing deficiencies and weaknesses in the HV arena in Europe.

Conclusions

At present, HV in the EU has a high priority in most of the Member States and is in place and functioning in nearly all Member States, but it does show significant conceptual differences despite the Blood Directives. Nevertheless, potentially it is a powerful tool to increase safety and quality in blood transfusion.[14] Corrective and preventive actions still need to become an integrated part of it, and there continues to be a need to undergo further standardization and harmonization and also to develop and strengthen further networking.

In the future, HV in the EU may become more integrated into the safety concepts in blood transfusion and develop into a more efficient tool for continuous improvement of quality and safety. In order to achieve this goal, it needs to cover the entire blood transfusion chain, including recipients and donors, processes, blood components, and related services. It also needs be embedded into the quality management systems of all healthcare establishments where blood transfusions are undertaken. In order to gain in value, it needs to be seen as an evolving concept, moving away from reactive to proactive (from corrective to preventive, including more efficient use of data on near-misses). The starting difficulties that have been encountered when collecting and analyzing the

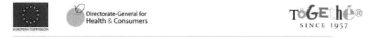

Scope of SAR/E in blood, tissues, cells, organs

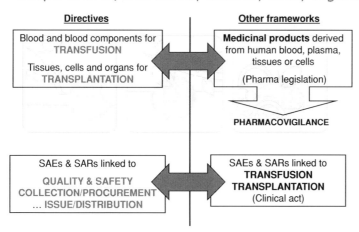

Figure 21.7 Situation in relation to human substances: blood on the one hand; tissues, cells and organs on the other. Each group has its own specific Community legislation and links with other legal frameworks, which sometimes are very voluminous. The cartoon also shows the dichotomy of production (manufacturing activity) and usage (clinical act) for blood and tissues, cells and organs, as well as its impact in the context of SARs and SAEs.

data from Member States will be overcome. Interesting (and hopefully comparable) results will be generated by the different national systems, at the basis for efficient Community-wide hemovigilance.

At the end of the day, Community HV is expected to contribute reliably to the requirement that quality and safety are guaranteed wherever in the EU a patient needs a blood transfusion or a donor proceeds to a blood donation.

References

1 Faber JC, 2000, L'hémovigilance en Europe, *Transfus Clin Biol* **7**: 5–8.
2 Faber JC, 2002, Haemovigilance around the world, *Vox Sang* **83**(Suppl 1): 71–6.
3 Council of Europe, 2002, Guide on the Preparation, Use and Quality Assurance of Blood Components. Recommendation no. R(95)15 (16th edition), Council of Europe Publishing, Strasbourg, France.
4 European Union, 2003, Directive 2002/98/EC of the European Parliament and of the Council of January 2003 setting standards of quality and safety for the collection, testing, processing, storage and distribution of human blood and blood components and amending Directive 2001/83/EC. *Official Journal of the European Union* 8.2.2003: L33/30–L33/40. http://eur-lex.europa .eu/LexUriServ/LexUriServ.do?uri=OJ:L:2003:033:00 30:0040:EN:PDF [accessed February 14, 2012].
5 European Union, 2004, Directive 2004/33/EC of 22 March 2004 implementing Directive 2002/98/EC of the European Parliament and of the Council as regards certain technical requirements for blood and blood components. *Official Journal of the European Union* 30.03.2004: L91/25–L91/39.
6 European Union, 2005, Directive 2005/61/EC of 30 September 2005 implementing Directive 2002/98/EC of the European Parliament and of the Council as regards traceability requirements and notification of serious adverse reactions and events. *Official Journal of the European Union* 1.10.2005: L256/32–L256/40.
7 European Union, 2005, Directive 2005/62/EC of 30 September 2005 implementing Directive 2002/98/EC of the European Parliament and of the Council as regards Community standards and specifications relating to a quality system for blood establishments. *Official Journal of the European Union* 1.10.2005: L256/41–L256/48.
8 Faber JC, 2004, The European Blood Directive: An new era of regulation has begun. *Transfusion Medicine TME* **14**: 257–73.
9 Faber JC, 2005, The European Blood Directive: The impact of Community regulation on EU-Member States. In: *Transfusion in Europe: The White Book 2005*, Rouger P and Hossenlopp C (eds), Elsevier Publications SAS.

10 Faber JC, 2005, Haemovigilance in the European Community. In: *Transfusion in Europe: The White Book 2005*, Rouger P and Hossenlopp C (eds), Elsevier Publications SAS.

11 Brégeon T (European Commission, Directorate General for Public Health and Consumer Protection, Directorate C—Public Health, Unit C6: Health Law and International, Brussels), 2009, personal communication.

12 Siska I (European Commission, Directorate General for Public Health and Consumer Protection, Directorate C—Public Health, Unit C6: Health Law and International, Brussels), 2011, personal communication.

13 Politis C (KEELPNO, Athens), 2011, personal communication.

14 De Vries R, Faber JC, and Strengers P, 2011, Haemovigilance—an effective tool to improve transfusion practice. *Vox Sang* **100**: 60–7.

CHAPTER 22

International Collaboration

Paul F.W. Strengers

Division of Plasma Products, Sanquin Blood Supply Foundation, Amsterdam, The Netherlands

Introduction

The first international meeting on hemovigilance *(1er Séminaire Européen des systèmes d'Hémovigilance)* took place in Bordeaux, France, in 1997, in conjunction with the *2ème Congrès National de Sécurité Transfusionelle et d'Hémovigilance.*[1] Participants were personnel from blood establishments, blood transfusion specialists, clinicians and nurses, lawyers and representatives from insurance companies, and politicians. The necessity of the maximum safety of blood, which forms the basis of the French law of January 4, 1993, was defined in this law in three main elements:

• the objective to satisfy the need of patients regarding blood products;
• the guarantee of the quality of collected blood;
• the start of a system of hemovigilance.

All three were considered as paramount for public health. The word *hemovigilance* had made its entry into blood transfusion medicine.

At the *Séminaire*, the French system was presented of the organization of hemovigilance in cooperation with blood establishments, hospitals, and hemovigilance agencies, and the reporting and analyzing procedures of transfusion incidents. The importance of blood and blood transfusion in medical care made a shift, because from now on blood would be considered not only as lifesaving, but also as the potential cause of (serious) adverse events and reactions. These adverse events and reactions could not only be related to the transmission of blood borne infections, but also

to the nature of blood as a human transplantable substance with potentially immunological reactions in the recipient.

In the scientific program, papers were presented on the prescription and the indications of blood components and medicines derived from blood, including qualitative and quantitative evaluations. The appointments, qualifications, and tasks of the personnel dedicated to blood safety in hospitals were presented, including the procedures that should be followed and the verification and control methods at the bed of the recipient. The safety of blood donors in relation to techniques of blood drawing, the production of blood components, the matching between donor and recipient, and the administration to recipients were also discussed, and methods of improving the exchange of information between blood establishments and hospitals addressed. The authorities announced that all adverse events and reactions after blood transfusion including morbidity and mortality should be presented to the public in official press releases. Transparency about the negative aspects of blood had become the new policy. Finally, the link of hemovigilance with the legal responsibilities of the professionals involved including the consequences for insurance policies were part of a panel discussion that resulted in a heated debate among delegates.

In this way, the concept of hemovigilance was introduced into blood transfusion medicine internationally, which was certainly an innovation in blood safety. The representatives of other blood

Hemovigilance: An Effective Tool for Improving Transfusion Safety, First Edition. Edited by René R.P. De Vries and Jean-Claude Faber.
© 2012 John Wiley & Sons, Ltd. Published 2012 by John Wiley & Sons, Ltd.

transfusion organizations in European countries were made aware of a new way of thinking about blood transfusion.

In the previous years, hemovigilance had been introduced in France by the start of monitoring systems by Blood Transfusion Committees and the founding of the *Centre National d'Hémovigilance*.[2] In Europe, not only blood transfusion specialists but also politicians and civil servants became aware of this initiative and in 1995 the European Council published its Resolution and Communication on "Blood Safety and Self-Sufficiency in the Community,"[3] followed by a report of a feasibility study on the establishment of a hemovigilance network in the European Community.[4] This report included the following:

• items on the identification of objectives, methods, and means related to the establishment of a Community-wide hemovigilance network, which would also serve to improve exchanges of information between the EU Member States;

• promotion of cooperation between the EU Member States on the systematic monitoring of risks and hazards associated with blood collection and transfusion and the provision of guidance in this respect;

• determination of measures that added value to the actions and measures of EU Members States and that needed to be proposed to the European Commission in order to enhance the safety of the blood chain.

The objective of these actions was to improve public confidence in the safety of the blood supply. At the 5th Regional (4th European) Congress of the International Society of Blood Transfusion in the same year, for the first time an international scientific symposium on hemovigilance was organized for professionals working in blood transfusion, and this symposium "Hemovigilance procedures in Transfusion Medicine" concluded that hemovigilance should be considered as part of the quality assurance process in transfusion medicine. Collection of data, the key to quality assurance in medicine, was recognized as being essential, but also that not all data are equally important and that those that are really important should be brought to the surface.[5]

In 1996, at an informal meeting of Ministers of the European Commission in Adare, Ireland, the European Commission organized a Colloquium on Blood, which resulted in the document "Blood Safety and Self-Sufficiency: an Agenda for the European Community" with six areas of action including hemovigilance. These activities could not be without consequences. The European Blood Directive of the European Parliament and of the Council was issued and turned out to be one of the most important documents regarding the quality and safety of blood and blood components both for EU Member States and non-EU Member States,[6] and in a number of countries hemovigilance systems were launched.

International Hemovigilance Network

The first international meeting on hemovigilance in 1997 resulted (in February 1998) in the initiative by five countries of the European Union (Belgium, France, Luxembourg, Portugal, and the Netherlands) of founding a European Hemovigilance Network (EHN), which later changed its name to the International Hemovigilance Network (IHN).[7,8]

The IHN was set up in order to increase blood safety at a European level and to develop and maintain in Europe common structures with regards to safety of blood and blood products. Information on adverse events was pooled, and epidemiological data collected systematically to evaluate differences between countries and to investigate the reasons for the differences. Material-vigilance of blood transfusion devices was developed because it was recognized that specific devices were marketed in several EU countries at the same time and reports were received that locally recalled devices were remarketed elsewhere in Europe. An inventory in all countries showed that legislation and regulation in the field of hemovigilance was either nonexistent or not equal. In some countries, such as Austria, France, Germany, Sweden, and Switzerland, notification of adverse events (AEs) to the authorities is mandatory, whereas in other countries reporting was voluntary, and in Denmark only notification of viral transmission by blood was required. Further, it was recognized that in a mandatory system AEs are not always reported and that underreporting exists.

In order to improve communication, the IHN exchanges valid information between members, increases rapid alert and/or early warning between the members, encourages joint activities between the members, and undertakes educational activities. It assists in the standardization of processes and forms by developing common "mother" matrixes, assists in the compilation and analysis of European data generated by national systems, and helps in the implementation of the European Blood Directive.

The IHN developed forms for a Rapid Alert/Early Warning System (RAS) and for Adverse Reactions to Blood Component Transfusion reporting in order to standardize the information process needed to take appropriate action, while aiming for implementing only one format of adverse events reporting documents in all European hemovigilance systems. The objectives of RAS are enabling corrective actions in the shortest period of time. RAS is being used for signaling the appearance of clusters of clinical signals after transfusion, hidden or apparent defects of disposable materials such as leakage of filter housings, holes in blood bags, defects in apheresis material, and problems with equipment. RAS allows quick and safe transmission of correct and precise data to quality assurance responsible persons in blood transfusion centres and to competent authorities.

The IHN's Adverse Reaction to Blood Component Transfusion report form assists in the investigation of clinical adverse events in order to define the course of action and to try and define the adverse event in the (in most cases complex) treatment of the patient involved.

As a tool for optimal connection and information exchange, the Internet website www.ihn-org.com was developed with two zones of information: a public domain with general information on blood transfusion organizations, data on donors, data on donations, data on blood components; and a protected domain with the Rapid Alert System. The Rapid Alert System, to which only one person per country has access, is used for rapid dissemination of (emerging) threats, clusters of adverse events, and material-vigilance.

After 2000, the number of countries where hemovigilance systems were developed increased and the annual European Seminar on Hemovigilance served in some instances as the starting point of the hemovigilance organization in a specific country. At the Seminars, results were presented on the organization of hemovigilance systems, definitions, the required (type of) data, the data on adverse events related to blood donations, the data on the actual usage of blood components or on specific plasma derivatives such as Anti (D) Immunoglobulin, material-vigilance, and on the security of systems.

After completing the standardization of the definitions, the IHN decided to embark on an ambitious project, that is, the establishment of an international hemovigilance database called ISTARE.

A pilot study on >13,000 adverse reactions with a denominator of >14,000,000 units issued contributed by 12 hemovigilance systems showed that the establishment of such a database is possible and quickly yields relatively valid information. The incidence of ARs varied between countries/systems due to reporting diversities, differences in grading of imputability, and transfusion practices. The compliance with the international definitions was not yet optimal, and the database project will contribute to improving this situation. With these results, it will be possible to do comparisons between data generated by different systems.

Working Party on Hemovigilance of the International Society of Blood Transfusion

The developments of the ISBT Working Party on Hemovigilance that started in 2000 were from the beginning directed to the actual production of blood components and usage of blood products. The activities were presented and discussed from a medical and scientific point of view by the professionals in blood transfusion medicine, and regulatory and control agencies did not participate.

Clinicians, nurses, and other prescribers and users of blood were less represented in this Working Party.

According to the Working Party, hemovigilance covers events surrounding transfusion of donor blood components including all aspects of autologous procedures, including donation. Diagnostic criteria for well recognized types of outcome, along with flowcharts for their investigation and criteria for imputability (i.e., the likelihood that the outcome was caused by the transfusion), were developed (see Appendix B). The Working Party encouraged reporting of new types of adverse outcome associated with transfusion, even though they do not fall within recognized types of transfusion reaction. This is particularly critical at a time when new types of components were emerging, for example, virus-inactivated Fresh Frozen Plasma (FFP), or when procedures such as leucocyte-depletion are being performed on an extremely large scale.

The Working Party encourages "no-fault" reporting so that inherent weaknesses in the transfusion chain can be rectified without fear of disciplinary action. Hazardous events in donors are included in this framework. Recognition that viral epidemiology in donors is an important part of hemovigilance, that studies of "near-miss" events can yield valuable information, and that appropriate blood usage is another element contributing to overall blood safety are among the objectives of the ISBT Working Party on Hemovigilance.

In order to help standardize data elements, the Working Party aims at the development of standard definitions of adverse transfusion events, the creation of new categories of events to be reported as deemed necessary, the identification of denominator data to be used to calculate incidence of adverse events, and the provision of a framework for data reporting at an international level.

In order to exchange information between ISBT members on the operation of different types of hemovigilance systems, and to exchange data on the results, the Working Party examines existing arrangements for "rapid alert" networks in the case of emergence of new infectious or noninfectious transfusion complications, which may have a very low incidence in individual countries. These could be supplemented through this Working Party, if needed. General information exchange would be facilitated by development of a website where non-confidential information could be posted. Finally, the ISBT Working Party on Hemovigilance is a source of information and guidance for countries setting up new hemovigilance systems, including sample documentation and access to expert advice.

Global Steering Committee for Hemovigilance (GloSCH)

In 2005, the WHO issued a guidance document on adverse reporting and learning systems emphasizing that the effectiveness of such systems should be measured not only by data reporting and analysis, but also by the use of such systems to improve patient safety.[9] On June 14, 2007, the launch of World Blood Donor Day took place in Ottawa, Canada, which created the opportunity to organize a WHO Global Consultation on Universal Access to Safe Blood Transfusion. One of the outcomes of that meeting was the agreement to develop a global hemovigilance, surveillance, and alert network, which would provide a platform to countries for sharing key information on blood safety and availability issues, and build a timely response in addressing emerging threats.

In autumn 2007, WHO blood safety officials communicated with officials of the Government of Canada (PHAC and HC) to collaborate on concepts and approaches for the development of such a network. Further meetings followed and in December 2007, at the WHO Global Collaboration for Blood Safety (GCBS) meeting, it was agreed on the importance of hemovigilance as a key element in the management of blood safety globally. WHO GCBS members supported the need to establish a Global Hemovigilance Network to identify existing gaps within the area of hemovigilance, explore opportunities for collaboration with other stakeholders, and avoid potential duplication of efforts. This network needed to consider strategies for local monitoring of complications of donations and transfusions, international benchmarking of rates of donation and transfusion incidents, and the feasibility of a Rapid Alert System.

In February 2008 a meeting took place to discuss various hemovigilance initiatives and to develop collaborative agreements with ISBT, IHN, Canada, USPHS, and WHO concerning the formation of an international collaborative group. Agreement in principle was reached to form a multilateral steering committee with a mandate, to develop a Terms of Reference to support collaborative efforts, and to develop a workplan. Founding members of the new global consortium, the Global Steering Committee for Hemovigilance (GloSCH), are the WHO, Canada, ISBT and IHN, and USPHS.

Since international hemovigilance initiatives were already in place, the goal of GloSCH is to build on global hemovigilance activities and not duplicate them. These goals are to

- provide an ongoing international forum to develop and promote global hemovigilance;
- function as a forum for dialogue, advice, and information gathering;
- promote standardized global hemovigilance reporting tools and determine whether these tools are useful and relevant;
- share information concerning hemovigilance data among member organizations.

The goals could be achieved by recognizing the differences between developing countries and developed countries in the area of hemovigilance, which would be valuable in addressing the improvement of blood safety surveillance in developing countries. In order to achieve this objective, pilot projects were recommended to be established in those countries without existing or emerging hemovigilance systems. The need for the development of additional hemovigilance initiatives in particular directed to low- and medium-index countries was shown by the results of the WHO Survey Results (2004), according to which a national hemovigilance system should be present in 42 (40%) of 105 countries.

Members of GloSCH should work within the mandate of their parent organizations to support developing countries to establish pilot projects for hemovigilance, surveillance, and alert, with a number of steps including the following:

- identify and discuss the need for pilot projects;
- help design and launch the pilots and provide ongoing assistance;
- develop a template for data/information collection and analysis;
- provide an international mechanism for timely information-sharing among pilot participants on matters such as adverse events, emerging blood-borne pathogens, and so on.

In order to achieve these goals it was important to link the pilots with regional and international systems, and to facilitate effective alert, response, and precautionary action to provide capacity-building for blood safety within pilots. Collaboration with other hemovigilance systems could help by providing training for the operators of the pilots in terms of how other systems work, for example, in IHN, ISBT, and so on. GloSCH members agreed unanimously that effort should be placed on development of two documents: (i) on the development of WHO Recommendations on the establishment of National Hemovigilance Systems and (ii) a technical and/or guidance document to support standardization of hemovigilance reporting.

Objectives of international collaboration between organizations

Hemovigilance goes beyond borders. This is not easy to understand because every blood component product, that is, an erythrocytes-concentrate product, a platelet concentrate, or a unit of plasma for transfusion (FFP), is a single product produced from one unit of blood donated by one blood donor. In general, due to the relative short shelf life, blood components are transfused in the country where the production and release take place. Borders are not passed.

In contrast to blood components, plasma-derived blood products are also manufactured from blood or plasma but during the production process many units are pooled together in order to obtain a sufficient yield of a specific protein, which in itself is present in plasma at a very low concentration. For the manufacturing of intravenous immunoglobulin, pooling of more than 1000 plasma units is also essential in order to get a spectrum of antibodies broad enough to give the receiver of the product, the immune deficient patient, sufficient protection against viruses and bacteria. As outcome of this production process a great number of vials of final product, a batch, is obtained from a certain production volume of plasma and a great number of patients receive products from this batch. If a vial of a specific batch is implicated in a serious adverse event, other vials from the same batch might be implicated as well and actions have to start in order to protect the other receivers from vials from that same batch. Vials of the final product may be used in more than one country, and so it is understandable that pharmacovigilance of plasma-derived products implies going beyond borders.

The fact that hemovigilance goes beyond borders is related to international collaboration on other elements that are important for the blood-components producers and users, and this information has to be disseminated in order to protect patients from adverse events inherent to the use of blood components. Collaboration on hemovigilance implies sharing information and experience, and learning from each other. IHN seminars showed other hemovigilance organizations which type of adverse events occur with blood components, that the incidence of these events is higher than reported, and that most of these events can be prevented by appropriate measures.

Transparency and sharing data on adverse events after blood transfusion turned out not to be negative but an important contribution to quality improvement of the blood transfusion process from donor to recipient. By comparing the data on the efficiency of different hemovigilance systems (voluntary or compulsory reporting), the efficacy of the systems turned out not to be relying on imposing regulations by authorities but on creating confidence with the actual prescribers and administrators of blood components in the hospitals. Informing and educating the physicians and nurses on the side effects of blood transfusion contributes significantly to the safety of it.

Having common regulations in one geographical area helped in bringing forward the need for a paradigm shift. In the first phase of hemovigilance, emphasis was laid on Rapid Alerts. In particular regarding adverse events caused by deviations in devices, it was important that these events were reported in an information structure that allowed users of these devices in different countries to take the appropriate measures. Although Rapid Alerts are still considered very important, the alertness on the occurrence of adverse events as the results of the usage of common devices with insufficient quality is not developed sufficiently well. Fear for litigation in the case of an insufficient causality assessment may play a role, but experience shows that it is hardly acceptable that the receiver of the product may be harmed due to negligence.

Collaboration between hemovigilance organizations played a very important role in creating common definitions on hemovigilance. It is quite unique that after an intensive discussion process, the IHN and the ISBT Working Party on Hemovigilance were able to define different (aspects of) adverse events and reactions in component production, patients, and donors in the same manner (see Appendix B). Common definitions are very important for adverse event reporting, data gathering, data analyses, and reporting to authorities and in the scientific literature. This collaborative work resulted in the acceptance of these definitions by the European Commission as the basis for the required report structure on hemovigilance by the EU Member States.

Comparability helps in improving procedures to prevent the occurrence and reoccurrence of adverse events, in particular these adverse events related to immunological reactions. The introduction of only male plasma for transfusion in order to prevent transfusion related acute lung injury (TRALI) may be considered as a successful measure resulting from hemovigilance data analyses. Introduction of improving methods in blood drawing by discarding the first part of the donated blood has decreased the occurrence of bacterial contamination of blood components in particular platelet concentrates. International collaboration has set the basis for quality assessment in hemovigilance. Introduction of common approaches, standard operating procedures, and quality indicators is taking place after seminars and symposia in which the participants are informed on the magnitude of the problem and the potential consequences of the implementation of the proposed actions.

Regarding improving transfusion practices, the medical professionals in the hospitals are very much involved, but unfortunately in a great number of countries blood establishments do not have sufficient access to the wards or operating theaters. Experience with the actual transfusion practices of blood components to recipients and reporting of bedside adverse events became much more important after the introduction of hemovigilance and the data collection on incorrect blood component transfusion. The move in thinking about blood transfusion from basic blood transfusion science and component production to blood transfusion medicine implied a move from blood establishments to blood-using wards and operating theaters.

The effects of international hemovigilance seminars organized by IHN were significant in this respect. The seminars not only served as a scientific forum of information and exchange of data, but also as the start of hemovigilance systems in a number of countries such as Greece, the Netherlands, and Portugal. Introduction of experiences in vigilance activities of cellular products formed the start of the biovigilance initiatives in the US and the worldwide collaboration that formed the basis for the GloSCH initiatives.

References

1 Programme definitive, Livre de résumés, 2ème Congrès National de Sécurité Transfusionelle et d'Hémovigilance/1er Séminaire Européen des systèmes d'Hémovigilance. Bordeaux, France. November 6–8, 1997.

2 Salmi R, 1994, Les supports épidémiologiques de l'hemovigilance. *Transf Clin Biol* **6**: 421–4.

3 European Union, 1995, Council Resolution of 2 June 1995 on blood safety and self-sufficiency in the Community, *Official Journal of the European Communities* **C164**, 30/6/95, p. 1.

4 European Union, 1998, The establishment of a haemovigilance network in the European Community: A feasibility project carried out by Haeman Consortium. December 1998.

5 Strengers PFW, and Heier H-E, 1997, Haemovigilance procedures in Transfusion Medicine. In: Proceedings of the ISBT 5th Regional (4th European) Congress, Rossi U, Massaro AL, and Sciorelli G (eds), p. 953.

6 European Union, 2003, Directive 2002/98/EC of the European Parliament and of the Council of January 2003 setting standards of quality and safety for the collection, testing, processing, storage and distribution of human blood and blood components and amending Directive 2001/83/EC. *Official Journal of the European Union* 8.2.2003: L33/30.

7 Faber J-C, 2001, Haemovigilance in Europe: The European haemovigilance network. *Transf. Clin Biol* **8**: 285–90.

8 de Vries RRP, 2009, Haemovigilance: Recent achievements and developments in the near future. *ISBT Science Series* **4**: 60–2.

9 WHO, 2005, Guidance on Adverse Event Reporting and Learning Systems, http://www.who.int/patientsafety/events/05/Reporting_Guidelines.pdf [accessed February 17, 2012].

CHAPTER 23

Hemovigilance in Developing Countries

Jean-Claude Faber

Blood Transfusion Service of the Luxembourg Red Cross, Luxembourg

Introduction

This chapter focuses on transfusion medicine and blood-safety measures in developing countries, identifying severe deficiencies in the production and usage segments of the blood chain. A model to start hemovigilance (HV) in developing countries is given as a practical first step toward HV being a tool for quality and safety in blood transfusion. The pre-eminent role of the World Health Organization (WHO) is identified as well as the many different activities of its Blood Transfusion Safety Program and their vision to make "universal access to safe blood and blood products for transfusion" a reality. WHO considers HV to be a vital "pillar" in the context of safety, quality, and supply of blood and blood products.

Based on the United Nations' (UN) Human Development Index (HDI), for the present purpose "developing" countries are defined as those with a low HDI, and some with a medium HDI, in contrast to "developed" countries, which have a high HDI.

(Although recently the above-mentioned categorization has been reviewed and only very-high HDI countries are now labeled as "developed", and all the others—from high- to low-HDI—are called "developing" countries, in this chapter, the former approach is used.)

Developing countries have numerous significant and urgent problems particular to them, in addition to the risks and threats to the blood supply identified in the developed countries.

Very generally speaking, developing countries show the following similar and comparable key characteristics:

- lack of funds;
- lack of facilities, equipment, and material;
- lack of staff;
- lack of leadership, guidance, management, governance, and so on;
- hostile environments (in terms of climate, geography, topography, politics, and so on).

Blood system level

At a national level in developing countries, deficiencies may be encountered in different areas. Frequently, a national policy on blood transfusion does not exist, so that political commitment is not documented. Furthermore, comprehensive legislation on blood transfusion is missing; in the best of cases, fragments of legal instruments are in place and noncompliance and violation may be yet another important aspect of it.

In general in developing countries, overall organization is absent, inadequate, or fragmented—in many cases, unified national blood services just do not exist. In addition, governance structures are poorly developed and skilled management is lacking. These weaknesses are aggravated by the fact

Hemovigilance: An Effective Tool for Improving Transfusion Safety, First Edition. Edited by René R.P. De Vries and Jean-Claude Faber.
© 2012 John Wiley & Sons, Ltd. Published 2012 by John Wiley & Sons, Ltd.

that quality culture and behavior are underdeveloped at most levels. Finally, with very few exceptions, available funds in the blood system (to cover investment and running costs) are not sufficient and most of the time not sustainable; costly duplication of efforts, infrastructures, equipment, and so on, and counterproductive competition, render the financial situation even more precarious.

Therefore interventions at a national level are often urgently needed and should be oriented toward the following:

• a National Blood Policy (NBPol) to be adopted;
• a National Blood Program/Plan (NBProgr) to be agreed;
• a National Blood System (NBS) to be created in a uniform, balanced way through vertical integration and horizontal coordination;
• a National Blood Transfusion Service (NBTS) to be organized;
• legal instruments to be adopted and enforced;
• regulatory authority to be set up to ensure compliance with, for example, quality management (QM), Inspection and Accreditation (I&A), HV, and so on;
• funding to be sufficient to ensure sustainability.

Taking these aspects into account, it comes as no surprise that in many developing countries HV is often absent or in its early infancy.

The WHO Global Database on Blood Safety[1] (see Figure 23.1) shows that the HV pattern at national level in developing countries is significantly different from that in developed countries. Although in the latter there is still potential to develop national HV (two thirds have a national system in place), it is indisputable that in developing countries a majority have not (yet) set up national HV (around 80%).

Building up a HV system is only one challenge, however; maintaining it over time is another. Also, rendering it functional, efficacious, and efficient (in the sense that as a final result of HV, actions are triggered and conducted to improve quality and safety in the context of blood transfusion) is certainly a difficult goal to achieve.

The world map in Figure 23.2 shows that a large part of the globe is not covered by HV (or it is not known whether it is covered by HV).

Entire continents are currently deprived of HV (at least at a national level):[2–6] Africa, the Americas (with the exception of Canada and the US), Asia (with the exception of Russia), and Oceania/

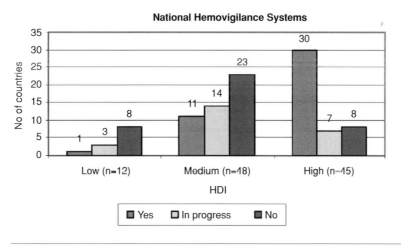

Yes: 42; In Process: 24; No: 39   Data from 105 countries: *WHO Global Database on Blood Safety 2004–05*

Figure 23.1 The situation in relation to the National Hemovigilance System in the countries grouped according to the Development Index and based on data from WHO Global Database on Blood Safety 2004–2005: the differences are striking between LDI, MDI, and HDI countries when it comes to the presence or absence of functioning countrywide surveillance systems for blood. (*Source*: http://www.who.int/bloodsafety/global_database/en/ [accessed April 2012]. Reproduced with permission from WHO.)

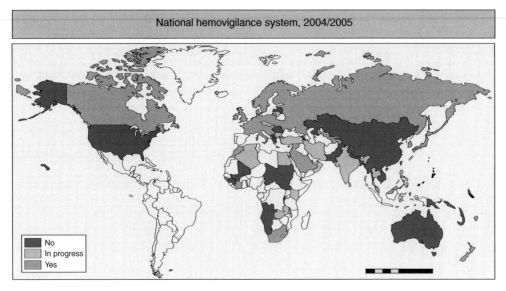

Yes: 42; In Process: 24; No: 39   Data from 105 countries: *WHO Global Database on Blood Safety 2004-05*

Figure 23.2 The geographical distribution of countries with a functioning National Hemovigilance System and those without such a system, based on data from WHO Global Database on Blood Safety 2004–2005: it is notable that for many countries no data are available and for others it is uncertain whether the concept of national surveillance for blood transfusion is correctly understood. (*Source*: http://www.who.int/bloodsafety/global_database/en/ [accessed April 2012]. Reproduced with permission from WHO.)

Pacific. In Europe, HV is spreading throughout the continent and this is mainly due to legislation rendering HV mandatory in the European Union (at least for defined areas of it).

In developing countries, the different segments of the blood chain are overshadowed by typical deficiencies[7,8] and the following section describes them.

Production segment

Blood establishments (BEs) are the sites of the production segment of the blood chain: they convey blood donors, take blood donations, test them, process whole blood into the different blood components, and store and distribute the latter. All these activities are carried out under strict quality and safety precautions and in accordance with good practice.

The above description represents an ideal and desirable situation, but in developing countries the reality is often quite different.

Blood donors

Blood donors represent one of the most important elements of any blood system. Developing countries commonly struggle with more or less severe shortages of blood donors (in absolute numbers) and an uneven geographical distribution of them (urban versus rural).

When it comes to the type of blood donors (and inherently the safety of blood products), the situation in developing countries is habitually characterized by the existence of paid donors, the reliance on family/replacement donors, and a liberal interpretation of voluntary non remunerated blood donors. In addition, low-return rates of blood donors and a concomitant high proportion of first-time donors pose a significant problem as do high-deferral rates of donor candidates (e.g., anemic, HBsAg carrier, and so on) and negative KBA (Knowledge, Behavior, and Attitude) in the general population and even in the active blood donor pool.

Blood donations

Blood donations are encumbered by shortages (in absolute numbers), spotted geographical distributions, and seasonal fluctuations (e.g., school holidays, New Year festivities, rain period with floods and earth-slides, and so on). A major drawback in developing countries is the low-collection volume (200–250 ml or 300–350 ml blood donations): there is practically no scientific data available to demonstrate that in donor populations in developing countries an increase in collection volume to the internationally agreed standard volumes (e.g., of 450–500 ml) is either safe or poses a potential risk for the donor. Therefore, habits and irrational approaches continue and collection amounts remain low, which significantly impedes on the blood supply.

Another important burden on the blood supply is the high-discard rates related to quality problems at the moment of blood drawing. The process of identifying the collected units (as well as blood donors) is also often critical. The success of blood drives is also hampered by uncomfortable donation/collection conditions (in terms of temperature, hygiene, access, and so on).

Testing

Testing of donated blood is obstructed by a lack of uniform national screening policies/practices and the absence of precise, detailed national standards and guidelines (S&G) as well as algorithms. In developing countries, manual screening methods are used in many instances and often show large variations and numerous deviations from good practice. Frequently, testing techniques are obsolete (e.g., blood grouping on tile, crossmatching on glass slide, and so on) and inadequate reagents are used (with low sensitivity and poor specificity, not approved, not validated). Disruptions in the supply of reagents add to the already fragile situation in these important activities. The widespread use of rapid tests in Transfusion Transmissible Infection (TTI)-screening is a particularly difficult subject, which needs balancing of the advantages (in terms of easier practicability) and disadvantages (in terms of lower test performance).

Inappropriate and poor testing facilities as well as ancient and obsolete testing devices constitute yet another hazard in the testing arena. One of the most important problems here is maintenance of laboratory equipment (old or newly acquired): absent or poor care of pieces of equipment directly impacts on technical sustainability or maintainability and therefore constitutes a threat of its own for a properly tested and screened blood supply. Insufficiently qualified and trained laboratory personnel is another jeopardy to safety and quality. In general, quality control (QC), quality assurance (QA), QM (when enshrined in a system, known as QMS) are largely underdeveloped or just absent. But this is not only true for the testing activities; it also applies to most processes, subprocesses, and activities in the production segment of the blood chain.

Processing

Processing of whole blood and preparation of blood components (BCs) in developing countries is often characterized by premises in critical conditions, poor and old equipment, and scarce qualified and trained staff in addition to low good manufacturing practices (GMP) compliance. Substandard and suboptimal processing techniques further hamper the production activities (e.g., platelet rich plasma method for platelet concentrate production, inappropriate freezing techniques for plasma, open system in the preparation of BCs with subsequent sharply shortened expiry date). As already mentioned in the context of testing, inefficient or absent maintenance and repair of equipment is one of the most striking problems in all activities requiring technical devices (machines, instruments, and so on).

Regularly, blood transfusion shows a low proportion of BCs (as compared to whole blood being transfused). It is not always clear what causes this imbalance in therapeutic practice—perhaps inadequate or absent equipment in BEs (in terms of refrigerated production centrifuges, separation devices, and so on) or low demand for and prescription of blood components by the clinicians—but no matter what, the result is that whole blood is transfused as a medical preference.

Storage and transportation

Storage and transportation of blood and blood components as well as logistics are affected by extreme natural surroundings (e.g., in terms of temperature, humidity, dust), very challenging conditions (e.g., road infrastructures, distances, topography), and unreliable power supply (voltage fluctuations, power cuts, uncertain emergency generators, and so on). These activities are particularly dependent on technical means and threatened by technical weaknesses such as lack of adequate blood cold chain equipment (BCC), irregular QM of equipment (in terms of validation, calibration, checks, and so on), inefficient and insufficient maintenance of existing equipment (including lack of awareness, problems in organization, delegation and responsibility, lack of funds for spare parts), and shortages in transport vehicles.

Usage segment

Hospitals are the sites of the usage segment of the blood chain: they care for the patients, diagnose and treat them, order the blood components if a blood transfusion is prescribed, undertake the pretransfusion testing and administration of the transfusion, as well as the surveillance and follow-up of the recipients. In these activities, hospital blood banks play an important part. Strict quality and safety precautions should apply and good practice is the ultimate command.

Again, the above represents the ideal, desirable situation, but in developing countries the reality is often far from optimal.

As already mentioned, national blood systems are frequently fragmented and include a patchy hospital sector. As a result, planning is often inadequate and activities are collection-driven, not demand-driven as in an efficient system. On top of this, obsolete transfusion practices result in routine administration of whole blood instead of specific BCs. Furthermore, the absence of adequate structures in the clinical segment is reflected by the fact that rarely are Hospital Transfusion Committees (HTCs) in place (see Figure 23.3), and so important functions are missing, such as setting

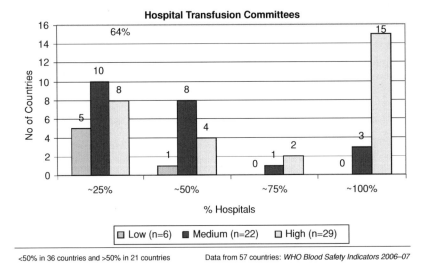

<50% in 36 countries and >50% in 21 countries   Data from 57 countries: *WHO Blood Safety Indicators 2006–07*

Figure 23.3 The situation in relation to Hospital Transfusion Committees in hospitals in the countries grouped according to the Development Index and based on data from WHO Global Database on Blood Safety 2006–2007: the differences are again striking between LDI, MDI, and HDI countries when it comes to the presence or absence of functioning Hospital Transfusion Committees (HTCs) according to the proportion of healthcare institutions having a HTC. It should also be kept in mind that data are available only from 57 countries out of the nearly 200 nations recognized by the UN. (*Source*: http://www.who.int/bloodsafety/global _database/en/ [accessed April 2012]. Reproduced with permission from WHO.)

internal procedures for the blood transfusion process, training of clinical staff, reviewing transfusion practice based on peer review of patient transfusion dossiers, and organizing local hemovigilance (HV). Very often, no S&Gs are in place for appropriate clinical use of blood (ACUB), compromising access to blood transfusions (obstructed by patient's financial difficulties, inadequate logistics, and so on).

The WHO Blood Transfusion Safety (BTS) Database shows that only 41% of hospitals performing transfusion in developing countries and 52% of hospitals in transitional (that is, from developing to developed) countries have systems for reporting adverse transfusion events, including transfusion reactions, as compared to 93% of hospitals in developed countries.

Vigilance of donors, recipients, and products/processes in developing countries

Nowadays, modern HV is conceived as a triple approach in a single concept comprising surveillance of donors, recipients, and products/processes at an equal level with the ultimate goal to improve quality and safety in a broader blood scope (see Figure 23.4).

The basic problems affecting HV in developing countries are the consequences of the fact that QM is missing (in most cases QM is quasi-inexistent; in some cases it is in an embryonic stage), that general organization, management, and communication are sub-standard, and awareness and knowledge of the use of blood transfusion are underdeveloped or absent.

The challenges and barriers to establishing HV systems are similar to those in developing countries:

• no or little tangible advance is seen to minimize preventable transfusion errors while TTIs continue to attract considerable attention;
• transfusion errors remain largely under-reported due to the lack of awareness among hospital staff about transfusion-related adverse events (AEs) and the inadequacy of feedback systems;

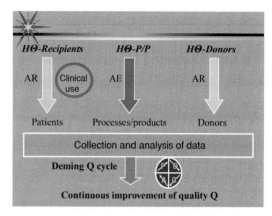

Figure 23.4 A schematic representation of hemovigilance nowadays as a triple approach in a single concept: systematic surveillance approaches of adverse reactions (AR) and adverse events (AE) in donors, recipients, and products/processes (P/P) become emancipated with a final goal to improve quality and safety symbolized by the Deming Quality Cycle of (Plan, Do, Check, Act).

• transfusion data are scarce and unreliable and major gaps exist in monitoring systems for transfusion practices;
• blood usage and clinical transfusion practices are issues that have not yet raised global concern.

Donor vigilance

In developing countries, BEs have often put in place donor vigilance and it is directly proportional to the degree of development and implementation of QM in the given institutions. Some BEs have excellent records in relation to blood donors including complications, but there is also wider demographic data. Nevertheless it must be recognized that in most cases the activity is spontaneous, episodic, and not systematic. Also, improvement in donor management and care is rarely triggered through donor vigilance.

Patient hemovigilance

As in the developed world a decade or two ago, HV has the best chance to take-off with organized surveillance of the transfused patients. Naturally, in the beginning the serious and very serious (fatal) adverse reactions (ARs) in hospitalized recipients

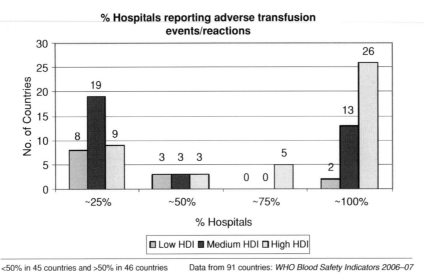

Figure 23.5 Participation of hospitals in the countries grouped according to the Human Development Index and based on data from WHO Global Database on Blood Safety 2006–2007. The pattern reflects the adequate role of the hospitals in the HDI countries (although progress is still possible) and a challenging situation in the hospitals of MDI and LDI countries. (*Source*: http://www.who.int/bloodsafety/global_database/en/ [accessed April 2012]. Reproduced with permission from WHO.)

are scrutinized and recorded locally, and sporadic reporting already exists here and there. It is not uncommon that HV-like activities are started by a motivated competent individual in the hospital as a "one-man-show". Later in the evolution of HV, it becomes routine that wards transmit the information on incidents to the hospital blood banks (hBBs) where it is documented. In the best of cases, the hBB will then contact the concerned BE and communicate about ARs/AEs after transfusion of their product(s).

The roles and responsibilities of hospitals, as healthcare delivery institutions, are obvious in the context of hemovigilance: without the active and reliable input of hospitals where blood transfusion is performed the surveillance system cannot be effective. Figure 23.5 shows that there is a long way to go before the entry into the systems (when they exist) is on solid ground.

In developed countries, the participation of hospitals in reporting ARs/AEs looks satisfactory at first glance (60% of responding high-HDI countries report notification from 100% of the hospitals on their territory)—but this also means that 40% have

not yet achieved total coverage, and 20% are even very low in hospital response (25% or less). In low-HDI countries, the situation is just the opposite, with low and fragmented coverage. The split between participating and nonparticipating hospitals is very pronounced in medium-HDI countries. This may be due to the fact that very often in these countries hospitals in the capital and the large cities are making progress in terms of organization, personnel (including their educational and professional levels), and equipment, but in rural or nonurban areas this is far from being the case. Beside the occurrences most reported in HV systems in developed countries (e.g., NHFTR, allergic/anaphylactic, Transfusion Related Acute Lung Injury (TRALI), Transfusion Associated Circulatory Overload (TACO), Transfusion Associated Graft-Versus-Host Disease (TA-GVHD), post-transfusion purpura (PTP), and so on), in developing countries there are probably numerous ARs/AEs in transfused patients that are directly linked to the deficiencies identified at the beginning of this chapter.

In developing countries there are scarce HV data available in relation to blood-transfusion recipients.

Therefore, one can only presume that additional risks and dangers are incurred by transfused patients based on reasonable assumptions from observations in the field:

- bacterial contamination of blood and blood components (due to inadequate storage and transport conditions);
- viral transmission through blood transfusion (due to omitted, partial, or incorrect TTI screening of donated blood);
- hemolysis (provoked by allo-antibodies missed by the use of pre-transfusion testing techniques with low sensitivity, caused by ABO-incompatibilities due to wrong blood grouping or errors, or induced by defective blood and blood components due to inadequate storage and transportation);
- others risks of different types.

In general, the clinical use of blood is documented although it is restricted to the most basic data such as patient ID and blood unit number (and blood group). This is often through the billing system of the blood transfusion to the recipient (or to family or health insurance, where it exists). Commonly, little is known about the clinical aspects of the patient, the rationale (or the *irrationale*) of the medical prescription, and the follow-up of the blood transfusion.

Reliable data on patient blood management are available only in those hospitals where HTCs are functioning (meaning productive work according to the predefined responsibilities) and these are rather rare in developing countries.

Product and process vigilance

It has already been mentioned that QM and GMPs are largely underdeveloped in establishments concerned with blood transfusion (BEs and hBBs) of developing countries. Therefore it is not surprising that key functions in quality (according to the Deming Quality Cycle: plan, do, check, act) are missing and vigilance of products (whole blood and labile blood components) and processes (for realization—collection, testing, processing, storage, and distribution—for support, and for management) is also absent. It should be mentioned that here and there institutions may mark an exception

to this general rule because they have developed, set up, and maintained a robust QMS, often under the leadership of a highly motivated individual in a position allowing that person to take decisions fostering growth of quality in products, processes, and services.

In most developing countries it appears that the development of product/process vigilance in the establishments concerned is directly linked to the maturity of the QMS in these institutions.

Key factors in this context are as follows:

- A national hemovigilance system can be set up and maintained only when effective mechanisms exist for data collection in hospitals and when there is adequate coordination at the national level.
- Data need to be collected from:
  - blood centers (BEs);
  - hospital blood banks (hBBs);
  - hospitals practicing transfusion at provincial/regional and district levels.
- Standardized tools have to be used to improve national coverage, data quality, and monitoring procedures.
- Corrective and preventive actions (CAPAs) are to be identified and implemented in an appropriate and timely manner.
- A stepwise and locally suitable implementation is essential.

Proceeding with HV in developing countries

In many developing countries there is nowadays a great deal of interest in HV because it is widely recognized that it is one of the most effective and efficient tools to improve quality and safety in blood transfusion. Therefore, the question arises again and again of how to proceed in setting up, running, and maintaining HV (built into a national system).

Right from the beginning it should be made clear that there is no universal solution that would work in a general way in developing countries.

Once the decision is taken in principle to introduce HV at the different levels, it is clear that political commitment and the support of key political figures are desperately needed.

Hemovigilance: From basic to comprehensive

A sequential and stepwise approach in the context of HV is highly recommended. The most basic prerequisite in HV is bi-directional traceability (link from donor to recipient and vice versa). At the beginning, stands the simple collection of key data (core information). If this becomes an ongoing activity, a database can be established. Analysis and evaluation of data and datasets can lead to improvement of quality and safety through corrective and preventive action triggered by recommendations and instructions, investigation and research, reports and feedback. Finally, the ultimate step is to produce proof of outcome and improvement, closing the Deming Quality Cycle.

The following questions require answers before proceeding with HV:
• Should it be a national system with central, regional, local, institutional activities?
• Should participation be voluntary or mandatory?
• What is to be reported and notified: adverse reactions, adverse events, incidents, untoward occurrences; all or only serious ones?
• What is included: transfusion recipients, blood donors, blood products or processes in this context? What about documenting and reporting deviations, errors, near-misses?
• Is notification anonymous or not?
• Is this going to happen in a punitive or nonpunitive environment?
• What are the links of the actors and institutions involved with regulation and governance?
• What about issues such as costs, funds, and so on?

Taking all this into account it becomes obvious that a logical and realistic long-term strategy is needed based on separate modules that are timely aligned. In order to develop such a strategic plan, it is necessary to undertake a detailed assessment of the existing situation and to elaborate assumptions for the future development of the blood sector in the country.

Such an assessment should
• have a national coverage;
• look into the existing blood system with a national scope;
• include all segments of the blood chain (vein-to-vein);
• identify existing elements useful for HV;
• detect the gaps and obstacles for HV construction.

Prerequisites for setting up HV

First and most important, there should be a strong political will to practice HV and this *political commitment* should be documented in the National Blood Policy.

An adequate *legal framework* needs to be in place defining principles, general aim, specific objectives, actors, tools, charges, and practicalities in the context of HV.

Specific *regulations* on HV are needed to
• define the scheme (with different levels: national-central/regional/local-institutional);
• ordain the respective mandates and responsibilities;
• organize rapid alert and early warning;
• institute a centralized evaluation and analysis site;
• delineate modalities (voluntary or mandatory participation; notification of all or only serious occurrences; notification anonymous or not);
• lay out definitions;
• standardize reporting procedures and report formats;
• coordinate the different actions, especially corrective and preventive ones;
• establish communication channels and feed-back to those concerned;
• train staff involved (prescribing doctors, transfusion nurses, laboratory technicians, transfusion safety officers, hemovigilance officers, and so on);
• set up HTCs;
• ensure appropriate funding of the different components of the system;
• facilitate international cooperation.

A *master plan* needs to be elaborated: it should reflect a sequential and stepwise approach and may include pilot, first, second, and final phases. A situation assessment in the country is necessary to determine the assets. Based on the existing resources and potential in the country, a master plan can be drafted and agreed on consensus.

As an example, the outline of a master plan with a possible roadmap and timeline is given below:

- *Pilot (for 6 months):*
  - including the best performing elements in the blood system (generally some BEs—the National Blood Transfusion Center (NBTC) and one of several Regional Blood Transfusion Centers (RBTCs) with their associated hospitals);
  - requiring mandatory notification of serious ARs in donors by these BEs;
  - calling for voluntary notification of serious ARs in recipients by selected hospitals.
- *First phase (for 6 months):*
  - making voluntary notification of serious ARs in recipients mandatory for the participants in the pilot;
  - adding mandatory notification of serious AEs (in BEs as well as in hospitals).
- *Second phase (for 12 months):*
  - expanding the coverage and adding more RBTCs and their associated hospitals with mandatory notification of serious ARs in recipients and donors as well as serious AEs (in BEs and in hospitals).
- *Final phase:*
  - based on the experience from the above phases, including the remaining BTCs and hospitals where blood transfusions are undertaken.

The above timeline is quite ambitious: If the situation in a given country requires, it may be stretched to establish HV in a proper and robust way.

Experience in the field shows that implementation is often hampered by missing elements. Therefore, setting up right from the beginning the basic components of HV (from hospital up to national level) is crucial. Coordination of the functional elements in the network is vital, bringing together hospitals (wards, hBBs, HTC), blood establishments (QA department), competent authority (I&A), and National Hemovigilance Office (NHO).

National *Standards and Guidelines* (S&G) for the activities in blood transfusion are needed as a reference for different purposes; this is particularly true for HV. Such S&Gs should be drafted, taking into account existing references that have proved effective, for example, those developed in the EU, by the Council of Europe, International Hemovigilance Network (IHN)/International Society of Blood Transfusion (ISBT), or national ones such as in the UK, Ireland, France, Canada, and so on. These S&Gs in the context of HV should be elaborated with a consensus of the national stakeholders in blood safety, adopted by the competent authority (in most instances the MoH), circulated through existing channels, applied in the field, and assessed by the regulatory authority. They need to be updated periodically and whenever there is a need to do so, according to predefined procedures.

Training of all the actors involved in HV is essential (doctors, nurses, midwifes, lab technicians, and so on). Educational activities should not only confer the necessary knowledge, but also generate the necessary amount of motivation needed for a well-functioning HV system. Training is needed at all levels of the system: at institutional level (in the hospitals, organized under the responsibility of their HTC; in the BEs, administered through their QA dept.); at regional level (through periodic workshops); and at national or central level (through annual conferences and participation in international events on HV). Each echelon should benefit from specific educational activities tailored to their actors and their interests as well as their responsibilities.

As for most key activities, *funding* is vital. Resources must be made available to cover the costs of running a HV system (e.g., material, personnel, IT, training, publications). Decision-makers must be aware that HV costs money and is not free. The primary investment may appear important, but it will pay off later (when the system works and improvements are being achieved).

Caveats must be taken into account and *threats* to HV initiatives may be poor participation, lack of confidence, fear of punishment, additional work, and reluctance to change.

For HV, very different approaches exist worldwide. The systems in place are under the responsibility of the national regulator, the producer of BCs, or the clinical professionals. Hybrid systems exist too. The past has shown that whatever system is chosen, it can work in a given setting and fulfill the objectives set out. At the end of the day, all depends on how those involved in blood transfusion give input and show active participation and how the HV results obtained are used to improve quality and safety for patients and donors in terms of products and processes.

Experience has also led to the formulation of generic advice when it comes to HV, which is also valid in developing countries: HV should be started in a carefully planned way and show a gradual pattern, but there is no way around the fact that it has to be started at some point, and the sooner the better.

In developing countries, the future of blood transfusion will see
- blood systems developing further;
- hemovigilance becoming part of the progress;
- hemovigilance being feasible but needing the unconditional will of the different actors involved in blood transfusion;
- hemovigilance being implemented stepwise and primarily bottom-up (with some top-down aspects);
- quality and safety of blood transfusion increasing;
- hemovigilance playing a crucial role in the improvement of blood transfusion and needing to be integrated into QM.[9]

A final consideration

In developing countries, the blood system is very often fragmented and displays many weaknesses and deficiencies that can result in all kinds of risks and dangers not only for the patients, but also for the donors. In most instances, HV is absent or in an embryonic stage. This is particularly regrettable because in developing countries it is vital to define priorities when it comes to investment in the blood system to eliminate the most important dangers in relation to blood transfusion. As HV often does not exist, there are very little data and objective information available to make the right decisions of where to put the scarce financial resources with the highest probability of getting the best added value. Therefore it is extremely important to set up HV as soon as possible in developing countries.

WHO and hemovigilance

The World Health Organization is a specialized agency of the UN that acts as a coordinating authority on international public health. It was established on April 7, 1948, with headquarters in Geneva, Switzerland.

Framework

WHO has two sets of legal entities: the Governments of 193 member countries (as of the beginning of 2011) and the Secretariat. The Governments meet annually at the World Health Assembly (WHA) and decide on resolutions, which set the agenda for what the Governments want the Secretariat to do.

As a global player, WHO has a worldwide representation starting with the Regional Offices (RO):
- AFRO: The Regional Office for Africa, with headquarters in Brazzaville, Republic of Congo, includes most of Africa, with a few exceptions;
- EURO: The Regional Office for Europe, with headquarters in Copenhagen, Denmark;
- SEARO: The Regional Office for South East Asia, with headquarters in New Delhi, India;
- EMRO: The Regional Office for the Eastern Mediterranean, with headquarters in Cairo, Egypt. It includes the countries in the Maghreb and those in Africa that are not included in AFRO, as well as the countries of the Middle East;
- WPRO: The Regional Office for the Western Pacific, with headquarters in Manila, Philippines. It covers the countries in Oceania and all the Asian countries not served by SEARO and EMRO;
- AMRO: The Regional Office for the Americas, with headquarters in Washington, DC, USA. It is better known as PAHO, the Pan American Health Organization.

WHO also has Country Offices in Member States, which develop the many different activities in the field, particularly in developing countries.

Altogether, WHO-HQ, WHO-RO, and the Country Offices ensure a global coverage: In developing countries, the presence and the activities of WHO are of outstanding importance.

Concerning blood transfusion, WHO has a long tradition when it comes to the safety, quality, and supply of blood.[1,10–14]

At HQ level in Geneva, WHO has a Blood Safety Unit (with a dedicated team), which is part of the Essential Health Technologies. At RO level, there are specific programs for blood transfusion that are integrated into other sectorial programs.

Aims and responsibilites

Since 1975 the WHA has adopted several resolutions on blood safety; the most important ones are listed in Figure 23.6.

In the context of fighting AIDS/HIV through blood transfusion, the WHA approved the following resolutions on blood safety:
- global strategy for the prevention and control of AIDS WHA 40.26;
- global strategy for the prevention and control of AIDS WHA 45.35;
- Paris AIDS Summit WHA 48.27.

For blood matters, WHO runs a special Blood Transfusion Safety (BTS) program with the vision to make "universal access to safe blood and blood products for transfusion" a reality.

The mission of WHO BTS is twofold and is of particular importance for developing countries:
- to facilitate equitable access and appropriate use of safe and quality blood and blood products worldwide;

- to ensure donor and patient safety, and the contribution of blood transfusion to patients' health and survival.

The strategic directions of WHO may be summarized as follows:
- take forward the WHA-defined agenda on global blood safety with the objective of universal access to safe blood and blood products for transfusion and safe transfusion practices, aligned with WHO's strategic objectives and operational planning with clear objectives, milestones, and targets;
- foster dialogue, collaborations, networking, and information-sharing between WHO Collaborating Centers, Expert Panel members, and international organizations;
- strengthen mechanisms for the engagement and involvement of WHO Collaborating Centers, Expert Panel members, and international organizations in developing and implementing work plans to achieve WHO's strategic objectives;
- strengthen its communication with international organizations to advocate WHO's policies, strategies, guidelines, and strategic objectives;
- convene global consultations and forums and provide consultative platforms to engage key international partners in addressing issues of global concern requiring strategic and/or urgent attention for global blood safety and universal access to safe blood and blood products such as the biennial Global Forum (the GFBS) and Global Blood Safety

1975	WHA28.72	Development of National Blood Transfusion Service based on voluntary non-remunerated blood donors
1987	EB79.1	National blood policies (Executive Board)
1995	WHA48.27	International collaboration
2000	WHA53.14	Blood Safety as a priority & World Health Day 7 April, Global strategy for blood safety
2002	WHA55.13	Quality of care: patient safety
2005	WHA58.13	World Blood Donor Day, 14 June
2007	WHA60.24	Health promotion in globalized world
2007	WHA60.29	Health technologies
2010	WHA63.12	Availability, safety and quality of blood products

Figure 23.6 WHA resolutions on blood safety.

Network (the GBSN, formerly GCBS), both feeding into the biennial planning process of the work of the WHO secretariat.

The following recent achievements should be mentioned: WHO Global Consultation on Universal Access to Safe Blood (in Ottawa 2009), WHO Global Forum for Blood Safety on Patient Blood Management, and WHO Global Blood Safety Network (in Dubai 2011).

A milestone for the work of WHO in the field of blood safety is without doubt the recent WHA Resolution, WHA 63.12. In May 2009 and January 2010, the WHO-Executive Board (EB) discussed the agenda on "Availability, quality and safety of blood products." In January 2010, the EB adopted a resolution (EB126.14) addressing the issues of availability, quality, and safety of blood products. In May 2010, this EB resolution was presented to the 63rd World Health Assembly (WHA) for further deliberation and was adopted as a WHA resolution.

This resolution requests among other things the following:
• to establish, implement, and support nationally coordinated, efficiently managed, and sustainable blood and plasma programs, with the aim of achieving self-sufficiency;
• to update national legislation on donor assessment and deferral, the collection, testing, processing, storage, transportation, and use of blood products and operation of regulatory authorities;
• to establish quality systems, for the processing of whole blood and BCs and GMPs for the production of plasma-derived medicinal products and appropriate regulatory control;
• to build human resource capacity through the provision of initial and continuing training of staff to ensure quality of blood services and blood products;
• to establish or strengthen systems for the safe and rational use of blood products;
• to provide training for all staff involved in clinical transfusion;
• to implement potential solutions to minimize transfusion errors and promote patient safety;
• to promote the availability of transfusion alternatives including, where appropriate, autologous transfusion and patient blood management;

• to ensure the reliability of *mechanisms for reporting serious or unexpected adverse reactions* to blood and plasma donation and to the receipt of blood components and plasma-derived medicinal products, including transmissions of pathogens.

Although HV has been addressed several times in the past by WHO, it is now enshrined in WHO's overall strategy for safe blood transfusion (see Figure 23.7).

WHO is the leading promoter of voluntary, non remunerated blood donors and donations, not only for ethical but also for safety reasons. It is evident that WHO is a strong advocate for testing all donated blood and for the safe and rational use of blood (transfusions): the "pillars" in Figure 23.7 do not need further explanation. It is also easy to understand that all the activities along the blood chain (vein-to-vein, from donor to recipient) need to be undertaken according to minimum quality standards: these need to be turned into quality products and services in the context of blood through adequate quality systems, both in the BEs (the producers) and in the hospitals (the users). Hemovigilance, another main WHO pillar for blood safety, plays a crucial role in quality improvement and safety enhancement because it fuels the quality cycle, resulting in better products and activities in the context of donation and transfusion.

WHO BTS

The priorities are set for the WHO BTS Program and focus on Safe Blood Policy, Blood Safety Standards, and Safe Transfusion Practice.

Safe Blood Policy

The Safe Blood Policy addresses the strengthening of the capacity of countries to develop national policies/plans for the national blood program including the following:
• Universal Access to Safe Blood Transfusion & Safe Blood for Safe Motherhood;
• resolutions on blood safety;
• Global Database on Blood Safety;
• collaborations, networks and partnerships;
• World Blood Donor Day.

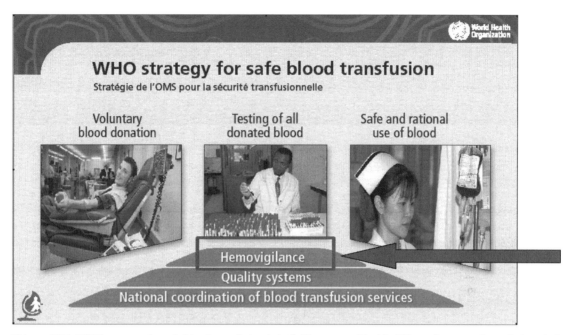

Figure 23.7 WHO's strategy for safe blood transfusion is built like a pyramid with different layers, each one being vital for the stability of this safety construction. (*Source*: http://www.who.int/bloodsafety/global_database/en/ [accessed April 2012]. Reproduced with permission from WHO.)

Blood Safety Standards

The Blood Safety Standards help to ensure the quality and safety of blood and blood products through

- organization and management;
- quality management (QM);
- voluntary non remunerated blood donation (VNRBD);
- blood donor selection and donor counseling;
- screening blood for TTIs;
- Blood Collection and Component Program.

Safe Transfusion Practice

Safe Transfusion Practice assists promoting and supporting best practices for the safe and rational use of blood and blood products, mainly through

- patient safety in blood transfusion;
- safe clinical transfusion and patient blood management;
- hemovigilance and surveillance;
- blood cold chain strengthening.

Since 1975, WHO has been at the forefront of the movement to improve global blood safety as mandated by successive WHA resolutions. In developing countries, the role of WHO in blood transfusion has been particularly prominent and had a significant impact.

BTS focus

The BTS program within WHO focuses on several key areas of work:

- blood system strengthening, including national blood policy, plans, quality, education and training, and universal access to safe blood transfusion;
- quality systems;
- VNRBD;
- donation testing;
- donation processing;
- safe and appropriate blood use;
- hemovigilance;
- collaboration and partnerships;
- Global Database for Blood Safety.

WHO publications

Many publications have been extremely helpful for developing countries serving advocacy and guidance. Among the best known are the following documents on

- Blood Safety (for National Blood Programs);
- Good Policy Process for Blood Safety and Availability;
- Developing a National Blood System;
- Quality Systems for Blood Safety;
- Clinical Use of Blood;
- Safe Clinical Transfusion Process and Patient Safety.

WHO has also issued many recommendations on all possible topics in relation to blood matters, some more general, some quite specific and detailed. In this context should be recommendations on "Developing a National Policy and Guidelines on the Clinical Use of Blood."

WHO has also published recommendations on hemovigilance and its basic requirements:

- use patient wristbands to reduce incorrect patient identification;
- establish traceability (document trail) from the blood donor and blood unit to recipient and vice versa, so that adverse events can be investigated and corrective action taken;
- organize an efficient national system, involving all relevant stakeholders;
- include as an integral part a quality system of the healthcare establishment, covering the entire transfusion chain;
- define adverse events, near-misses, and reactions;
- establish a voluntary and nonpunitive system;
- maintain a system to minimize recurrence
- analyze reported events in a timely way;
- act through recommendations for corrective and preventive actions in a timely manner;
- have written procedures to initiate and coordinate retrieval and recall of blood and BCs involved in untoward occurrences;
- maintain confidentiality;
- have a standardized report format.

Also, WHO has developed a wide range of educational initiatives in form of workshops, training materials, and open learning materials.

Well known is the Global Database on Blood Safety (GDBS), which WHO established in 1998 to address global concerns about the availability, safety, and accessibility of blood for transfusion. The objective of this activity is to collect and analyze data from all countries on blood and blood product safety as the basis for effective action to improve blood transfusion services globally.

In the future, the WHO BTS Program plans to intensify its efforts mainly in the following areas:

- high-level advocacy on developing national blood systems inclusive of clinical transfusion in patient blood management;
- provision of assessment, audit, and monitoring and evaluation (M&E) tools for rational blood use;
- result-based collaborative and structured efforts;
- guidance, capacity building, and country support for
  - implementing effective blood use and patient blood management systems;
  - establishing HV systems.
- strategic information and evidence on
  - blood utilization patterns in different regions and countries;
  - key indicators for its monitoring.

WHO and hemovigilance with special emphasis on developing countries

Right from the beginning, WHO advocated that "hemovigilance is required to identify and prevent occurrence or recurrence of transfusion related unwanted events, to increase the safety, efficacy and efficiency of blood transfusion, covering all activities of the transfusion chain from donor to recipient."

The WHO draft guidelines on "Adverse event reporting and learning systems: From information to action" emphasize the fundamental role of reporting systems in enhancing patient safety by learning from failures of healthcare systems. Effectiveness of such systems should be measured not only by data reporting and analysis, but also by the use of such systems to improve patient safety.

WHO has always supported the view that a hemovigilance system must be an integral part of QM in a blood system, developed for continual improvement of quality and safety of the transfusion process, and that it should cover processes throughout the entire transfusion chain, from blood donation, processing and transfusion to patients for the monitoring, reporting and investigation of adverse events and reactions and near-misses related to blood transfusion. WHO has claimed that clear definitions of adverse events, near-misses, and reactions need to be established.

In accordance with other organizations dealing with HV, WHO has recognized that a HV system is dependent on the traceability of blood and blood products from donors to recipients, spontaneous reports of transfusion adverse events/reactions and rigorous management of information related to the transfusion process. Information generated through this system is key to introducing the required changes in the transfusion policies, improving transfusion standards, assisting in the formulation of transfusion guidelines, and increasing the safety and quality of the entire transfusion process.

WHO has asserted that a HV system should involve all relevant stakeholders, and should be coordinated between the blood transfusion service, hospital clinical staff and transfusion laboratories, hospital transfusion committees, regulatory agency and national health authorities. It should include identification, reporting, investigation, and analysis of adverse events, near-misses, and reactions related to transfusion and manufacturing.

As already mentioned, WHO emphasizes the role of traceability (document trail) from the blood donor and blood unit to the recipient of the transfused blood or blood product, and vice versa, to enable adverse events and reactions to be investigated and corrective action taken to minimize the potential risks associated with safety and quality in blood processing and transfusion. It should be voluntary and nonpunitive. Staff and organizations should be encouraged to report adverse events and near-misses that may affect blood product quality and safety and other safety concerns related to blood transfusion.

WHO response to make HV a reality in its member states

The WHO BTS program organized a Global Consultation on Universal Access to Safe Blood Transfusion, which coincided with the global launch of World Blood Donor Day in June 2007 in Ottawa, working in collaboration with the Public Health Agency of Canada, Health Canada, Canadian Blood Services, and Héma-Québec.

One of the key recommendations made by the participating experts was for WHO "to develop a global hemovigilance, surveillance and alert network, which would provide a platform to countries for sharing key information on blood safety and availability issues and build a timely response in addressing emerging threats."

Following this consultation, WHO BTS has been working with key programs in the Public Health Agency of Canada and Health Canada to elaborate concepts and approaches for the development of such a network. This stands at the beginning of a new global consortium in which the founding members are WHO, ISBT, EHN/IHN, Government of Canada, and USPHS (Public Health Services of the United States of America).

At the 8th Global Collaboration for Blood Safety (GCBS) meeting in December 2007 in Geneva, this topic was discussed with key international organizations concerned with global blood safety. The GCBS participants agreed on the importance of HV as a key element in the management of blood safety globally and on the need to establish a global HV, surveillance, and alert network.

The GCBS tasked interested participants and members to convene and participate in a meeting to identify existing gaps, explore opportunities for collaboration, and avoid potential duplication of initiatives for a global HV network. In this context, it was requested to consider strategies for

• local monitoring of complications of donations and transfusions;
• international benchmarking of rates of donation and transfusion incidents;
• rapid alert systems.

GloSCH: A worldwide HV initiative

In the beginning of 2008, collaborative arrangements were discussed with the International Society of Blood Transfusion and the International (formerly, the European) Hemovigilance Network to establish an informal collaborative mechanism, as a global committee in the area of hemovigilance.

It was agreed that the WHO BTS program, the Public Health Agency of Canada and Health Canada (Federal Government of Canada), and the ISBT and IHN would participate as core agencies of this committee.

This multilateral consortium is now known as GloSCH (Global Steering Committee for Hemovigilance) and has the mandate to support collaborative efforts and to develop a global workplan in the context of HV.

Based on the agreed principle to build on global HV activities (and not duplicate them), the goals of this collaborative initiative are to

• provide an ongoing, international forum to develop and promote global HV;
• share information concerning HV data;
• function as a forum for dialogue, advice, and information-gathering;
• develop and promote standardized global HV-reporting tools and determine whether these tools are useful and relevant.

The main objectives for this international consortium are

• to work toward improving international and national systems for the identification and assessment of adverse events, risk of infections transmission, existing and emerging threats to blood safety;
• to work toward improving global collection, analysis, and sharing of blood surveillance data/information, drawing on data/information from individual nations and organizations in a bottom-up approach;
• to assist blood safety authorities internationally and within nations to deal with the alert/response function for threats to blood safety;
• to identify, assess, and share information on best practices in the field of HV;
• to promote new science, research, and knowledge generation in key areas of HV;
• to encourage knowledge transfer respecting HV to developing countries;

• to assist in the provision of technical assistance concerning HV to developing countries;
• to explore the development and distribution of related communication and educational materials.

GloSCH members agreed that efforts should be placed first on development of a Hemovigilance Guidance Document identifying the need for HV, requirements of HV, models for implementing HV, and technical aspects of reporting, validating, and analyzing HV data.

In conclusion, WHO has played and will continue to play a leading role when it comes to blood safety and HV, with special emphasis on developing countries because the need there is the most urgent and the expected benefit the most significant.

References

1 WHO, 2008, Global Database on Blood Safety (2004–2005), World Health Organization, Geneva, Switzerland. http://www.who.int/bloodsafety/global_database/GDBSReport2004-2005.pdf [accessed February 21, 2012].

2 Faber JC, 2003, Haemovigilance: Definition and Overview of Current Haemovigilance Systems. *Transfusion Alternatives in Transfusion Medicine* **5**(1): 237–45.

3 Faber JC, 2004, Worldwide overview of existing haemovigilance systems. *Transfus Apher Sci.* **31**(2): 99–110.

4 Arslan O, 2005, Haemovigilance in developing countries. *Hematology* **10**(Suppl 1): 79–81.

5 Faber JC, 2002, Haemovigilance around the world. *Vox Sang* **83**: 71–6.

6 International Forum, 2006, Haemovigilance. *Vox Sang* **90**: 207–41.

7 Sharma RR, Kumar S and Agnihotri SK, 2001, Sources of preventable errors related to transfusion. *Vox Sang* **81**: 37–41.

8 Tayou Tagny C, Mbanya D, Tapko J-B, and Lefrère J-J, 2008, Blood safety in Sub-Saharan Africa: a multifactorial problem. *Transfusion* **48**: 1256–61.

9 Nel TJ, 2008, Clinical guidelines, audits and haemovigilance in managing blood transfusion needs. *Transfusion Alternatives in Transfusion Medicine* **10**: 61–9.

10 World Health Organization, 2005, WHO Guidelines for Adverse Event Reporting and Learning Systems. http://www.who.int/patientsafety/events/05/Reporting_Guidelines.pdf [accessed February 21, 2012].

11 World Health Organization, 2008, Report Blood Safety Indicators 2006. http://www.who.int/bloodsafety/global_database/FactSheet279-2008BSDonation.pdf [accessed February 21, 2012].

12 World Health Organization, 2008, Universal Access to Safe Blood Transfusion. http://www.who.int/bloodsafety/publications/UniversalAccesstoSafeBT.pdf [accessed February 21, 2012].

13 World Health Organization, 2008, Recommendations: Basic Requirements for Blood Transfusion Services.

14 Dhingra N, WHO Blood Programme (personal communication).

PART 5
Achievements

CHAPTER 24

Achievements Through Hemovigilance

Jean-Claude Faber[1] and Fátima Nascimento[2]
[1]Blood Transfusion Service of the Luxembourg Red Cross, Luxembourg
[2]Transfusion Medicine, General Directorate of Health, Lisbon, Portugal

Introduction

Hemovigilance (HV) has existed in a primitive form since the beginning of blood transfusion as a treatment for the ill. When Jean-Baptiste Denis undertook transfusions in 1667–1668 and the King of France reacted and prohibited transfusions owing to numerous fatal outcomes, it was nothing less than the beginning of HV. When Karl Landsteiner in 1900 undertook his revolutionary studies and created the basic rules for blood transfusion, it was the first preventive action based on data and its analysis. In 1939, Landsteiner/ Wiener and Levine/Stetson observed a similar phenomenon linked to the Rhesus system and came up with rules to avoid hemolytic disease of the newborn (HDN), another example of early HV. During the 1950s, transmission of syphilis through blood transfusion was observed and testing was introduced to eliminate what was identified as the first transfusion-transmitted infection (TTI)...again this was applied HV. And so it continued in the 1960s with HBV, through the mid-1980s with HIV and a few years later with HCV. Look-back studies and systematic screening of patients after transfusion are nothing else than the modern instruments of surveillance.

HV was created as a reaction to the numerous infections through transfusion of contaminated blood products and to blood scandals in several countries. It targeted in a first instance patients (or recipients) and focused on the protection of their health. In order to uncover risks, problems, and harm for the transfused patient, it was realized that sufficient hard data were needed for assessment and decision-making.

HV was and is intended to improve quality and to increase safety in the context of transfusion. Soon, it became obvious that HV could significantly contribute to these objectives and therefore offer substantial "added value."

The general feeling is that HV has contributed substantially to increased transfusion safety and improved quality of products for administration. Nevertheless, if "system thinking" is strictly applied (Figure 24.1), the conclusion may appear to be less clear and less obvious. In the present context, "inputs" in the figure comprises all kinds of observations, reports, data collections, information gathering, studies, inquiries, and so on.

When it comes to "process" (and subprocesses) and the initiated change, the situation becomes more mitigated due to the technical, organizational, and legal complexity. Therefore, in most cases "change" means "changes" with the intended modification being the most apparent one. But concomitant alterations happen, and they are often less obvious, less visible, and consecutive with a defined action.

Consequently, "outcome" also should come in the plural. As seen before, each and every single change (intended or not, major or apparently minor) may result in an outcome or several ones.

Hemovigilance: An Effective Tool for Improving Transfusion Safety, First Edition. Edited by René R.P. De Vries and Jean-Claude Faber.
© 2012 John Wiley & Sons, Ltd. Published 2012 by John Wiley & Sons, Ltd.

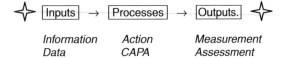

Information   Action   Measurement
Data   CAPA   Assessment

Figure 24.1 How the system model is applied to hemovigilance (CAPA = corrective and/or preventive action).

From the beginning hemovigilance systems are known to cause expense, therefore the questions of efficacy and efficiency are inescapably posed. Hemovigilance systems do not come at zero cost.

In a very simplified costing model, the expenses that a hemovigilance system cause can be classified according to their nature:

• *Direct versus indirect costs:* Direct costs are those visibly related to personnel employed, to infrastructures, to material, and so on, all for the sole or predominant purpose of HV. Indirect costs are less apparent but can nevertheless be substantial, for example, the voluntary unpaid contribution of many different actors and contributors to HV.

• *Intrinsic versus subsequent costs:* Intrinsic costs are those generated by the setting up and running of a hemovigilance system at different levels. Subsequent costs are those encountered primarily to put into action the conclusions and recommendations of HV (in blood establishments (BEs), hospitals, or more generally, in the healthcare sector).

There are striking differences between the national HV systems: some have a low absolute and relative cost (e.g., Luxembourg) and some cause high absolute and relative costs (e.g., France). These differences do not relate only to the size of the system.

In Luxembourg, for example, the direct costs of the HV system itself are quite low because the system is managed by the sole existing BE for the national level, assuming cooperation of the users, mainly the hospitals, for the recipient segment and also integrating logically the donor segment. It is patronized by the Ministry of Health, the competent authority for blood matters (donation and transfusion activities) and blood products (labile components and stable derivatives).

In France, on the other hand, the HV system is characterized by its high complexity, existing parallel routes, different levels and layers in the structure, and a significant number of employees working full time and exclusively in HV and many others working there part time. The authors are not aware of any published detailed analysis of the costs of the French system, but in our view its overall annual cost must be substantial.

At times of budget constraints for healthcare all over the world, efficacy and efficiency have increased in priority and have significantly influenced the discussions, decisions, and actions in this context. So, questions concerning results and outcomes are now of high interest.

According to the Deming Quality Cycle (summarized as "Plan, Do, Check, Act") and following its transposition on the blood chain, the graph in Figure 24.2 illustrates the rationale along the chain.

Starting from this flowchart, it becomes obvious that certain caveats, difficulties, and problems may arise in the analysis of pertaining data and the discussions around "Change" and "Outcome."

In the EU (and its 27 Member States), there are tremendous variations when it comes to routines (in BEs, in healthcare institutions, and so on) in relation to donors, recipients, and products/processes, despite the fact that there is a body of mandatory Community legislation in the form of

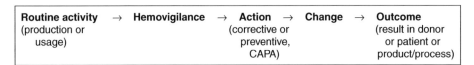

Figure 24.2 How the improvement of safety and quality in blood-related activities is achieved through application of the basic principles of the Deming Quality Cycle: corrective and preventive actions (CAPA) are the promoters to increase safety and quality levels in relation to blood donation and blood transfusion.

four "Blood Directives"[1] ruling on blood matters.[2] From a worldwide view this range is even wider:[3]

• "Routine": Comparison of routines is tricky and has many caveats. The variation in techniques, materials, experience, and skills of personnel is astonishing, from one country to another, and between BEs within the same country.

• "Hemovigilance": The diversity here is also striking.

• "Action": Approaches in terms of CAPA appear more similar or standardized, but may not be identical, from one country to another, from one BE to the next, from one hospital to the next clinic. As an example, one might cite leuco-depletion of blood components where the performance in terms of residual leucocytes in the final product is significantly influenced by the filter device manufactured by one company to the next, the production procedures applied in one BE to another, the counting methods in different quality control (QC) laboratories, and so on.

• "Change": Also not easy to assess and to compare for different reasons (technological complexity, multifactorial nature, and so on). For example, the switch in production method of platelet concentrates from "platelet rich plasma" to "buffy coat" influences many different parameters at the same time.

• Results/"Outcomes": These may be measurable, objectively assessable, or not at all...or not in substantial numbers. As a positive example in the context of outcome, one might come up with the introduction of "male-only" plasma for transfusion: it has led to a striking reduction of TRALI incidence in patients receiving Fresh Frozen Plasma (FFP). As a negative example, one might cite the change in donor selection to prevent transmission of prions to transfused patients: in EU Member States vCJD is quasi-absent,[4] making it impossible to assess the situation before and after the introduction of permanent deferral for donors who have spent a certain period of time in the UK and to express the impact in terms of outcome of this preventive action triggered by HV.

All these limitations have to be kept in mind because they may constitute a real hindrance in the debate on efficacy and efficiency.

One additional fact complicates the debate on outcome, at least at the moment of writing: in many countries around the globe hemovigilance systems are just building up or have been set up only recently, which makes it impossible to form conclusions because of insufficient follow-up (reference points are needed to make objective comparisons and assessments).

Taking all this into account, it is evident that achievements through hemovigilance are not so apparent of where change induced by hemovigilance has resulted in hard-evidence outcomes with a direct mono-causal link.

Methods

Two different ways were used to collect information on subjects from different countries and their national hemovigilance systems:

• *A questionnaire* was developed especially for this purpose. Essentially three questions were asked:
  ○ In your country, which risks/problems have been detected through hemovigilance?
  ○ In your country, have there been (corrective) actions or (preventive) measures put in place following recognition of risks/problems?
  ○ Have they generated specific outcomes and resulted in measurable improvements of the blood chain?

The questionnaire was sent to all official contact persons (OCPs) of the International Hemovigilance Network (IHN) members ($n = 28$). Responses were received from 23 national HV systems (82%), some rather concise and others very elaborate as we illustrate later in this chapter. When questions arose during the evaluation of the data reported in the questionnaire, clarification was asked from the respective OCP.

• *Published annual reports* of different national HV systems are a great source of information. Apart from their use in connection with the present subject, it is highly recommended to read carefully through these reports because they contain valuable descriptions on the respective structure, modus operandi, results, conclusions, recommendations, actions, and impacts. The addresses of the websites where the Annual Reports can be found are available from the IHN website (www.ihn-org.com).

Longitudinal analysis using UK data

The UK's SHOT is one of the oldest HV systems in place, starting as a voluntary reporting system for Serious Hazards of Transfusion (see Chapter 14). Using the example of the UK, we try in this chapter to come up with a longitudinal cut-through of a HV system/scheme.

We chose to do this exercise using the SHOT information[5] for several reasons:
• its long run (nearly 15 years), thus allowing continuity and continuous improvement;
• its regular detailed Annual Reports from the beginning;
• it broad scope;
• its trigger of multiple actions for correction and prevention.

Figure 24.3 shows the evolution of the reports (in number and category) since 1996:

Incorrect blood component transfused (IBCT) is the most common event reported (39.6% of all

reports). Some events—inappropriate and unnecessary transfusion (I&U), handling and storage errors (HSE), and anti-D-related events—have been withdrawn from IBCT over the years, due to their importance and/or frequency.

Adverse reactions, such as acute transfusion reactions (ATR), hemolytic transfusion reactions (HTR), and Transfusion Related Acute Lung Injury (TRALI), are also reported as clinical situations after transfusion. Less frequent are post-transfusion purpura (PTP), Transfusion Associated Graft-Versus-Host Disease (TA-GVHD), and transfusion-transmitted infections (TTIs). Transfusion Associated Circulatory Overload (TACO) and Transfusion Associated Dyspnea (TAD) were reported for the first time, as an independent entity, in 2008 and the number of reports is increasing.

Regarding the seriousness of these adverse reactions/events, TA-GVHD has been fatal in all cases and TRALI has had a high incidence of death during the last 15 years.

To prevent/decrease the potential injuries related to blood transfusion, SHOT has recommended numerous actions. We analyzed the impact of these measures and highlight the outcomes reflecting improvements of the blood transfusion chain below.

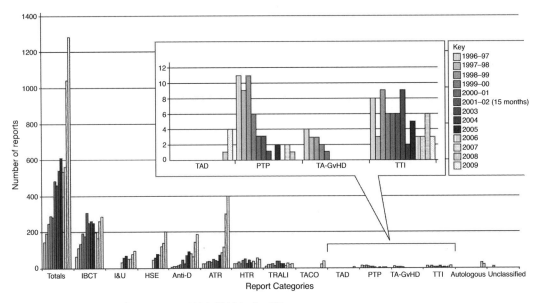

Figure 24.3 Comparison of report types 1996–2009 in the UK.

General recommendations

General recommendations to enable an increase in the number of reports and to diagnose accurately the adverse reactions/events were issued by SHOT from the beginning and on an ongoing basis:

- Each hospital shall have a Hospital Transfusion Committee (HTC; a recommendation issued 1996/97).
- Clinicians are encouraged to report ALL types of serious unexpected reactions associated with transfusion (1997/98).
- Local initiatives to disseminate the main messages of the SHOT report are essential in order to derive full benefit for patients and staff from the SHOT scheme (2001/02).
- Clear policies must be developed for communicating special transfusion needs of patients to other hospitals or units that may share their care (2001/02).
- Hospital blood bank laboratory staffing must be sufficient for safe transfusion practice (2003).
- Pediatric units undertaking transfusion must ensure that staff members are educated in special transfusion requirements of children (2003).
- Laboratory IT systems should be regularly updated to support implementation of new guidelines (2003).

As a consequence, participation in HV has increased gradually (quantitatively and qualitatively), demonstrating the acceptance of HV as a quality tool and its integration into quality management systems (QMS).

Specific recommendations

SHOT has also issued specific recommendations, according to the main adverse reactions/events detected, and these have accumulated over the years.

To avoid/decrease TA-GVHD:

- 1996/97:
  ○ a single national laboratory for investigation of suspected cases should be designated;
  ○ guidelines should be reviewed considering whether B-cell lymphoid malignancies should be added to the indications for irradiated blood components.
- 1997/98:
  ○ investigation of the donor in cases of suspected TA-GVHD should be performed;

○ a standard protocol for investigation of TA-GVHD should be developed;
  ○ BCSH Guidelines for Irradiation of Blood Components should be reviewed for consideration of inclusion of patients with B-cell lymphoid malignancy;
  ○ the additional risks of fresh blood should be borne in mind if such blood components are ordered for cardiac surgery.
- 1999/2000:
  ○ patients at risk should carry a card to indicate their need for irradiated components.
- 2001/2002:
  ○ all blood components from family members should always be irradiated;
  ○ new chemo-immunotherapies should be assessed for their potential to cause TA-GvHD.
- 2003:
  ○ gamma- or X-ray irradiation with 25 Gy of blood components for those at risk of TA-GvHD remains essential.
- 2007:
  ○ the importance of irradiation and the rationale behind TA-GVHD should be focused on during teaching of junior hematology and oncology doctors.

The implementation of the recommendations to eradicate TA-GVHD can be considered a full success: Since 2000/01, cases of TA-GVHD have been "knocked out" and no longer reported.

To avoid/decrease TRALI:

- 1996/97:
  ○ donors implicated in cases of TRALI should be withdrawn from donor panels.
- 1997/98:
  ○ blood services should develop systems for ensuring appropriate donor investigation of cases of suspected TRALI;
  ○ a standard protocol for investigation of TRALI should be developed.
- 1999/2000:
  ○ unnecessary transfusion of plasma-rich blood components should be avoided.
- 2000/01:
  ○ in a more general context, better epidemiological data are required to understand patterns of usage of blood components.

- 2001/02:
  - FFP should be sourced from untransfused male donors and platelets should be suspended in a plasma-free medium.
- 2003:
  - whole blood transfusions are discouraged.
- 2004:
  - blood services should continue to consider strategies to minimize the risk of TRALI from apheresis platelets.
- 2008:
  - blood services that have not yet achieved 100% male FFP and a plasma-free medium in platelet pools must make this a priority.

After stepwise introduction of untransfused male plasma in 2003, the number of fatalities due to TRALI started to decrease. In the few residual cases reported after 2003, most of them are related to female-plasma transfusion. The action taken has achieved a clear-cut improvement for the patients in need of a FFP transfusion and therefore is considered a successful initiative.

To avoid/decrease IBCT:

- 1996/97:
  - pre-labeled sampling tube should not be used;
  - previous transfusion records of each patient should be accessible;
  - hospitals should have a procedure to identify the patient at the time of blood sampling and before the transfusion.
- 1997/98:
  - hospitals should review their current system to ensure that errors in this area can be prevented;
  - appropriate staff training is essential;
  - standards should be set for a minimum identification requirement to be used when a blood component is collected.
- 1998/99:
  - hospitals must ensure that staff working with blood transfusion receive correct education and training;
  - hospital systems must ensure that there are no exceptions with regard to the provision of patient identity wristbands or their equivalent;
  - IT as an aid to transfusion safety should be assessed and developed at the national level.

- 1999/2000:
  - every patient should be uniquely and positively identified using a wristband or equivalent and there should be no exceptions;
  - hospital transfusion laboratories must have protocols for the timely removal of expired blood components from blood banks.
- 2004:
  - training and competency testing of all staff involved in the transfusion process must emphasize the importance of positive patient identification, with particular attention paid to critical-care situations.
- 2005:
  - blood transfusions outside of core hours should be avoided.
- 2007:
  - staff involved in blood component transfusion must be aware of their professional accountability and responsibility;
  - transfusion medicine needs to be a core part of the curriculum.
- 2008:
  - the UK Transfusion Laboratory Collaborative has recommended minimum standards for hospital transfusion laboratories in terms of staffing, technology, training, and competence;
  - all staff must be trained (and competency-assessed) in recognizing the different blood components and their labels.
- 2009:
  - a transfusion checklist should be developed, ideally with an accompanying transfusion record section;
  - the existence, and the importance, of special transfusion requirements must be taught to junior doctors in all hospital specialties;
  - the IT system should be configured to flag a blood component discrepancy between that ordered and that issued, and the system should be fully validated;
  - guidance should be provided regarding the removal (and return, should it not be required) of every blood component from validated storage areas;
  - as part of the competency-assessment process, the importance of checking the expiry

date during the collection/final patient identity checks must be emphasized to all practitioners.

All these recommendations for action have achieved a strengthening of the protection of the patient receiving a blood transfusion: there is an impressive increase of the cases reported over the years and, at the same time, a decrease in the percentage of deaths. However, fatalities remain, as IBCT could not be eradicated despite the frequency and the accuracy of the recommendations. The errors (that may result in IBCT) occur in any part of the transfusion chain, which makes it difficult to control.

To avoid/decrease acute- and delayed-transfusion reactions (ATR/DTR):

- 1996/97:
  - national requirements for samples and investigation following acute- or delayed-transfusion reactions should be reviewed;
  - guidelines for pre-transfusion compatibility testing should be followed.
- 1997/98:
  - all serious adverse reactions should be reported;
  - previous transfusion records should be accessible in order to check for historical clinically significant antibodies that are undetectable at the time of crossmatch.
- 1998/99:
  - transfusion services should re-examine the screening methods for hemolytic titers of iso-hemagglutinins.
- 1999/2000:
  - unnecessary transfusions should be avoided;
  - additional panels and techniques for antibody screening should be used.
- 2000/01:
  - patients receiving blood components should be monitored;
  - anaphylaxis should be investigated with more details;
  - a guideline for investigation and management of ATR is needed;
  - it is essential to perform a crossmatch, if clinical significant red blood cell (RBC) antibodies are found.

- 2001/02:
  - patients with severe allergic reaction should be investigated for IgA deficiency;
  - attention must be paid to patients with autoimmune hemolytic anemia (AIHA) or with recent positive Direct Antiglobulin Tests after transfusion;
  - patients with sickle cell disease should be transfused with Rh/Kell identical phenotype RBCs;
  - automated systems and changes to technology should be validated.
- 2003:
  - appropriate use of blood components is recommended;
  - internal audits are encouraged.
- 2004:
  - a toolkit with minimum standards to investigate of cases of ATR/DTR should be developed.
- 2005:
  - blood should not be transfused outside of core hours, unless clinically essential;
  - inconclusive antibody screens should be investigated prior to transfusion;
  - professionals are encouraged to publish case reports of Delayed Hemolytic Transfusion Reaction;
  - antibody cards should be issued to all patients with RBC antibodies;
  - period to keep the pre-transfusion sample should be reviewed.
- 2008:
  - as the mechanism of ATR is still not clear, the role of unselected testing for HLA, HPA, or HNA antibodies appears very limited;
  - a national register of patients with antibodies should be considered, linking up the red cell reference laboratories.
- 2009:
  - IgA should be measured in all patients who experience severe allergic or anaphylactic reactions.

Acute- and delayed-transfusion reactions are responsible for a few deaths and include a great variety of situations. On the other hand, they are essentially important because they act as a sentinel for reporting: the increased number of reports demonstrates also that the professionals have adhered to the notification of adverse reactions/events.

To avoid/decrease TTIs:

- 1996/97:
  - people are encouraged to report TTIs to allow a complete picture of the extent of infectious complications;
  - guidelines for bacteriological investigation should be followed;
  - donors should be excluded from blood donation if they have been resident as a child in a malaria area, unless they are shown to be negative for malaria antibodies;
  - methods and criteria should be introduced to exclude individuals with risk factors.
- 1997/98:
  - blood components that appear unusual should not be transfused and should be returned to the hospital blood bank/blood establishment.
- 1999/2000:
  - strategies to prevent transfusion transmitted bacterial infections should be given priority.
- 2000/01:
  - strategies to prevent transfusion of bacterially contaminated products (especially platelets) should be developed, such as disinfection of donor arm and diversion of the first 20–30 ml of blood collected;
  - blood services should review the residual risk of transfusion-transmitted HBV infection.
- 2001/02:
  - methods for testing platelets for bacterial contamination should be evaluated;
  - the residual risk of transmission of HBV is to be reviewed to assess the need for HBV RNA testing.
- 2008:
  - staff should maintain a high index of suspicion for bacterial causes when managing acute transfusion reactions;
  - cleaning protocols for cold rooms as well as processing and storage areas should be reviewed regularly and audited.

The main cause of TTIs is bacterial origin. In the 2009 report, only three cases were reported, all of them fatal. It is hypothesized that under-diagnosis of the bacterial contamination happens, because it can be confused with symptoms of the underlying disease, and that the recommendations to report these infections are probably not strictly followed. If this is the case, it may be concluded that the recommended actions have not achieved their objective and that further initiatives are needed.

More recommendations were made in the SHOT reports. Nevertheless, we believe that the list of recommendations we present is sufficient to demonstrate the achievements of SHOT in the transfusion safety, with a decrease of the number of deaths and a concomitant increase of reactions reported (see Figure 24.4).

It becomes obvious that in the UK the risks of transfusion are much better known than elsewhere; the efficacy of the recommendations have been demonstrated and will continue to be apparent in the future.

Results

The following material is a compilation of data gathered through the questionnaire mentioned above and retrieved from the annual reports of the different national hemovigilance systems.

In order to approach this information in a logical way, the three questions posted to the different countries (detailed in the earlier 'Methods' section on page 283) are covered consecutively. Each one is projected onto the blood chain and broken down into the "production" and "usage" segments of this chain. In order to make it as useful as possible, information is grouped into specific and general areas, starting with a few original answers, continuing with an overview in the form of a graph, describing the situation in the different countries (including a global view), and ending with a summary of the information received.

Problems and risks identified by hemovigilance

As an example Box 24.1 contains the original response from New Zealand.[6]

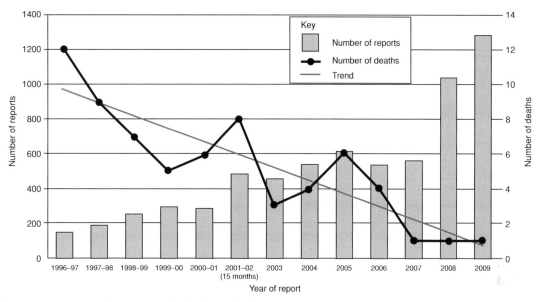

Figure 24.4 Number of reports and deaths definitely due to transfusion between 1996 to 2009 in the UK.

Box 24.1 New Zealand Hemovigilance: Original response

The New Zealand National Haemovigilance Programme was established just five years ago. Data acquired through this voluntary reporting scheme has enabled us to estimate the incidence of transfusion-related adverse events. Specific problems that have been identified to date include the following:

- There are inconsistencies in reporting between various hospitals.
- Platelet components are more frequently associated with reactions than other blood components; overall apheresis platelet units are more frequently associated with events compared to pooled platelets ($p = 0.01$); the rationale for this is not known (both types are suspended in donor plasma).
- TRALI reports have decreased since the implementation of male-donor FFP, however there is a residual risk associated with platelets collected from HLA alloimmunized female donors.
- Over 50% of IBCT involved errors originating in the laboratory.
- 64% of near-miss events occurred in the laboratory (blood bank or blood processing laboratory). These errors involve storage, labeling, irradiation, and expiry of blood components.
- Vasovagal reactions are the most common donor complication and occur more frequently in donors <20 years of age (odds ratio 2.2).

- 20% of errors relating to pre-transfusion samples/request forms involve a sticky label on the sample, although the hand-labeling policy was introduced in 2004 (prior to the Hemovigilance Programme).
- The rate of "wrong blood in tube" is not reducing.
- Minor ABO-incompatible transfusion (i.e., group O platelets or whole blood to nongroup O recipient) can cause severe hemolytic transfusion reactions in small (pediatric) recipients, despite hemolysin testing.

Specific risks and problems

Production segment (in the BE)

Figure 24.5 shows the different key processes in a blood establishment. Each of these processes is prone to deviations, errors, and weaknesses, possibly resulting into a more or less severe risk.

Although structured, systematic, and national donor-vigilance is quite new in nearly all the countries, it should not be forgotten that in many BEs all kinds of reactions, incidents, and accidents have been documented and analyzed in a local fashion for many years.

Nowadays, all are recorded and documented and form a solid basis for the following observations:

- adverse reactions experienced by donors are not rare;

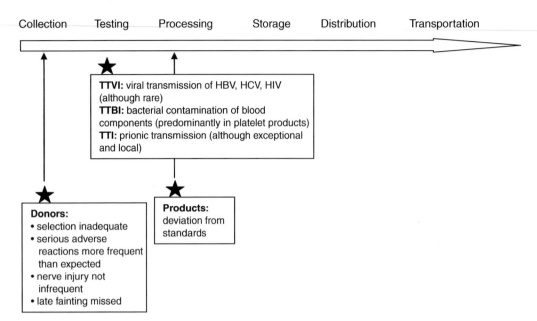

Figure 24.5 Risks and problems in the different key processes in a blood establishment from the collection of whole blood, plasma, or cells through testing of donor blood, preparation of blood components, storage, distribution, and transportation of finished blood products (TTVI = transfusion-transmissible viral infection, TTBI = transfusion-transmissible bacterial infection, TTI = transfusion-transmissible infection, HBV = Hepatitis B Virus, HCV = Hepatitis C Virus, HIV = Human Immunodeficiency Virus).

• vasovagal reactions are the most common donor reaction or complication (>90%);

• serious adverse reactions are more frequent than expected;

• hematoma and direct puncture can cause nerve injury/damage and need more intensive medical care and follow-up;

• late fainting of the donor (outside of the collection site) is recognized as a risky situation and needs to be tackled by better and individualized observation and guidance of bled donors before leaving the site.

It comes out of the HV reports and responses to the questionnaire that inadequate donor selection is a major cause for destruction/recall of blood components issued from donations where the donor acceptance was wrong due to noncompliance or imprecision of donor eligibility criteria.

Concerning products/processes in the BE, TTI agents are generally under control. Viral TTIs are rare, very rare even, but HBV, HCV, or HIV transmissions have not been completely eradicated. Bacterial TTIs continue to exist, but have drastically diminished since measures were taken: it is considered as a rare, but significant, occurrence (less now in PLT concentrates; relatively more in RBC concentrates). Prionic TTI also exists, but basically it is an exceptional and local (UK and France) problem. Product deviations from the preset standards leading to destruction of scarce resources have been qualified and quantified through HV and been identified as an area with significant potential for improvement.

Usage segment in the healthcare institution

Figure 24.6 illustrates the different key processes in the context of a blood transfusion in a hospital. Each of these processes is prone to deviations and errors possibly resulting into a risk.

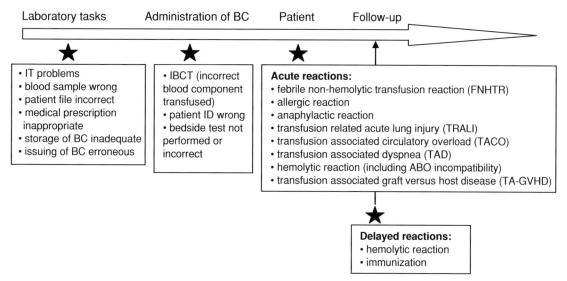

Figure 24.6 Risks and problems in the different key processes in the context of a blood transfusion in a hospital, from the collection of a blood sample from a patient through testing, administration of the transfusion, and follow-up of the transfused patient (BC = blood components, such as red cells, platelets, or plasma; ID = identity).

Traditionally, hemovigilance has focused on "side effects" in the recipient, during and after transfusion. Therefore, the longest experience and the largest datasets are in this area of the clinical segment of the blood chain:

- *acute reactions:* Hemolytic (it was recognized that it was mainly due to ABO-incompatibility), febrile non-hemolytic (HV has helped to quantify these), allergic, anaphylactic (HV has helped to identify patients at risk);
- *delayed reactions* (HV helped to capture these previously not recognized incidents);
- *respiratory complications* (TRALI was "discovered" by HV or made visible by HV; with TACO and TAD it was very similar);
- *TA-GVHD* (HV helped to prioritize this very serious disease in recipients);
- *immunization* (HV facilitated the quantification of formation of alloantibodies in transfused patients);
- *hypotensive reactions* (detected through HV).

HV also showed that many problems and risks can exist in a hospital: from receipt and storage of BCs, blood grouping of potential recipients, com-

patibility tests, issuing of BCs, and pre-transfusion measures to administration.

HV has helped to identify areas of risk and weakness where in the past there was little or no awareness:

- patient identification;
- medical prescription;
- pre-analytic steps (drawing of blood sample, labeling it);
- handling of BC (storage, distribution, warming, filtering);
- link to patient ("wrong blood to wrong patient"—IBCT—with or without clinical signs);
- pre-transfusion measures (clerical checks and bedside test).

Specific problems were recognized through HV in one single country related to a significant number of anaphylactic reactions in recipients (due to haptoglobin deficiency) and of TA-GVHD in transfused patients (unexplained at this moment, but fortunately eradicated by systematic irradiation of BC). These findings could not be confirmed to the same extent by other countries, which shows the diversity of situations and also the importance that each and every country establishes and maintains national HV.

General risks and problems

Right from the beginning it should be said that several countries responded that have not identified "special" problems or risks through HV. This can be explained in the way that these countries have learned from other HV systems; deficiencies identified elsewhere are not recognized as such by the latter because they were not "new" to them.

From the Netherlands,[7] Box 24.2 relates one interesting comment that illustrates this and shows that things that appear simple and easy in reality are not.

Box 24.2 The Netherlands Hemovigilance

The problems which we have seen had previously been detected by others. For this reason the question cannot be answered as currently phrased and the title of the questionnaire is over-optimistic (N.B. "Achievements through Hemovigilance").

Three important points have emerged from the work of the national hemovigilance office:
- risk of errors and under-reporting of errors;
- use of autologous blood not free of transfusion reactions and at least as prone to errors as allogeneic transfusion (use of peri-operative blood management techniques often escape the attention of the hospital blood transfusion committee)
- allergic and anaphylactic reactions poorly understood but numerically important.

The majority of countries found that HV was very valuable in revealing the following:
- errors and near-misses quite common;
- clinical blood use often inappropriate (sometimes irrational habits were detected);
- medical prescription inadequate and communication weak between the hospital players;
- noncompliance recognized regularly as a major problem;
- nonconformities, complaints, and errors are a major issue in many BEs (probably also due to the fact that most of the BEs have established QMS and reporting is part of it);

- IT problems unexpectedly frequent (most were due to inadequate validation, frequently in the context of installation of software updates).

One problem that was mentioned again and again in HV reports was that of wrong patient ID and of incorrect/omitted bedside test.

More general comments in this context focus on: organizational problems in the HV system itself, diversity in the use of definitions, in reporting (especially when a national system is built up from regional modules), and in training of transfusion practice (insufficient and/or inadequate including the problem that certain groups/professions dealing with transfusion are not reached by any educational activity).

As can be seen from the above, HV has been very successful in detecting and identifying problems and risks existing all along the blood/transfusion chain.

Actions and measures triggered by hemovigilance

We turn now to actions and measures triggered by HV, and it will become apparent that there are some important challenges ahead.

Once sufficient data are collected and analyzed, it may become obvious that a risk or a problem exists and that it is necessary to eliminate or reduce it. Such measures or actions (corrective or preventive in nature, CAPA) are taken at national, regional, local, or institutional level (reaching down to departments, processes, and subprocesses, including specific routine activities and steps of them).

Box 24.3 contains the response from New Zealand on this aspect.

Box 24.3 New Zealand Hemovigilance: Actions and measures

In February 2008, the New Zealand Blood Service began to produce FFP (for transfusion) from male donors with no history of transfusion, by apheresis procedures. This led to a dramatic reduction in the number of TRALI cases reported per year (despite small numbers overall). In the past year, a project assessing HLA and HNA

---

alloimmunization in plateletpheresis donors, has commenced. Further strategies to reduce the residual risk of TRALI are under consideration.

Platelet additive solution, replacing 2/3 of the plasma from a pooled platelet unit, has been introduced at two of the four blood processing sites in New Zealand. These units (PAS platelets) will be used for transfusion in the near future; we will monitor closely for any trends in adverse events. Replacement of plasma with platelet additive solution may reduce the reports of allergic reaction and TRALI.

Bacterial monitoring of platelet concentrates commenced prior to the hemovigilance scheme. The New Zealand Blood Service has implemented BacTalert bacterial detection systems and aims to test as many platelet units as possible, on Day 2 and on Day 8 if not transfused. During 2009, over 80% platelet components were tested. The frequency of confirmed positives was 1:6,000 (Day 2) and 1:1,800 (Day 8).

Specific actions

Production segment (in the BE)

Figure 24.7 shows the different key processes in a blood establishment. In order to reduce or eliminate the risks possibly affecting these processes, specific actions (corrective or preventive in nature) may be suggested.

As can be seen, the measures taken rely upon the following:

• *New analytic technologies:* Nucleic Acid Testing (NAT) as a diagnostic amplification technique has been used for quite a while, but its adaptation as a large-scale laboratory tool is much more recent and the demand from the BEs has been one of the driving forces. Different approaches are used, proprietary solutions as well as "in-house" developments, screening and quantification, pool testing

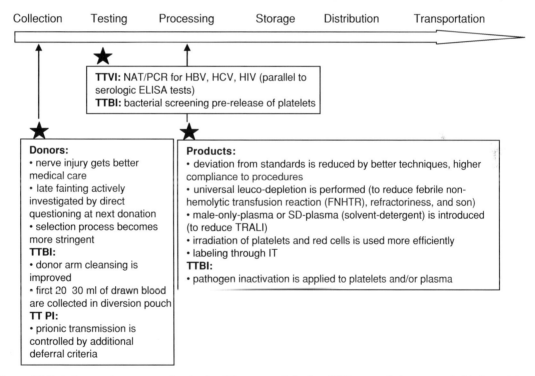

Figure 24.7 Actions and measures taken in the different key processes in a blood establishment from the collection of whole blood, plasma, or cells through testing of donor blood, preparation of blood components, storage, distribution, and transportation of finished blood products (TTVI = transfusion-transmissible viral infection, TTBI = transfusion-transmissible bacterial infection, HBV = Hepatitis B Virus, HCV = Hepatitis C Virus, HIV = Human Immunodeficiency Virus, NAT/PCR = Nucleic Acid Testing/Polymerase Chain Reaction, ELISA = Enzyme Linked Immunosorbent Assay).

(up to 96 samples at the same time), single sample testing, and so on. In all cases, NAT (in the majority as Polymerase Chain Reaction (PCR)) is added to the classical serological testing and performed in parallel to Enzyme Linked Immunosorbent Assay (ELISA) tests. Regardless of its high cost, this supplement was introduced and started predominantly in countries where the prevalence for HIV, HCV, (and HBV) in the general population and in the donor pool is already very low, whereas in countries with high prevalence it could not yet be started because of the tremendous expenditure although in the latter countries the benefit in terms of patient protection and of public health would be much more pronounced.

• Existing analytic technologies: Bacterial culturing is an "old" laboratory tool, but it was not very popular in BEs until TTBI was recognized as a major problem in blood transfusion. It is nowadays accepted as a standard for screening platelet concentrates (of whatever type): the most common strategy is that of pre-release bacterial culture of the platelets (which are stored up to five days between 20 and 24°C (68–75°F), in other words, at optimal growth conditions for most microbial organisms). A sample of the product content is drawn from the bag after 24 hours and cultivated at predefined conditions until the product is needed. Before release and distribution of the product, the result of bacterial culture is checked: if it is negative, the platelet concentrate is sent to the ordering hospital. In many BEs, bacterial culturing is continued until transfusion or outdating of the product.

• *New processing technologies:* Pathogen inactivation (p.i.) eliminates or attenuates a large spectrum of microorganisms: viruses, bacteria, parasites. Only prions and some spore forms are resistant to this innovative technology. p.i. has been developed and marketed (for PLT and FFP: Intercept®, Mirasol®; for plasma only: MB, SD). This additional processing step has been implemented in several BEs, although its usage remains limited at this point because of very high costs, complex activity, additional QC, and some drawbacks such as loss of platelets during the processing. There is no doubt that in the future p.i. will gain more markets and can contribute to increased safety in the recipient.

For the moment the technology is confined to the treatment of PLT products and FFP, it cannot yet be applied to RBCs, which represent the large majority of transfused blood components (up to 80%).

• *Existing processing technologies:* Filtration of blood is an "old" technique used in the past at the bedside in selected patients. With the recognition and ranking of Febrile Non-Hemolytic Transfusion Reaction (FNHTR) as the most common adverse reaction in recipients, research concluded that the leucocytes and the subsequent cytokine production during storage of the BC were the major cause. Pre-storage universal leuco-depletion (u-LD) through large-scale filtration of whole blood (or of resulting BCs) was introduced in many countries. Again, this is a very costly and complex action. For many decades, irradiation has been well known for its preventive effect in the context of TA-GVHD. In several countries, this adverse reaction was given a high priority, due to its very high mortality rate. Different approaches were chosen in different countries, from issuing special cards for those patients at risk in the UK[8] to systematic irradiation of cellular BCs in Japan.[9]

• *Organizational changes:* Probably the most striking measure was and is the introduction of quality management (QM) in BEs and hospitals. Since the mid-1990s, QMS were put in place by many BEs (in the EU, according to the Blood Directives, worldwide more and more responding to ISO9001 requirements), by many laboratories (some according to ISO17025 or ISO15128), and by hospitals. Without doubt, this has led to significant improvement of products and activities, in the production as well as the usage segment of the blood chain.

Beside the changes mentioned above, it is quite remarkable how many additional safety steps have been introduced in relation to the donors (for the protection of the donor and the recipient). Whereas in the past, BEs had local, isolated documentation and registries of donor complication, networking revealed the necessity to focus more on donors. And the more data were collected, the more obvious it became that donor complications were probably underestimated and that especially serious and very serious ones were not captured as it could be. So came into life donor-HV, inspired directly by recipient-HV and relying on similar, if not the same, tools.

Usage segment in the healthcare institution

Figure 24.8 illustrates the different key processes in a hospital in the context of blood transfusion. In order to reduce or eliminate the risks possibly affecting these processes specific actions (corrective or preventive in nature) may be suggested.

In the hospitals several specific actions have been taken, mostly related to clinical practice:

• improvement of medical prescription (unambiguous ID, clear instructions on transfusion therapy, use of guidelines, and so on);
• adequate choice of blood components (to avoid TA-GVHD: ordering exclusively irradiated BCs; to reduce TACO: giving clear and detailed instructions on transfusion rate and volume in patients at risk; to decrease anaphylactic shock: identifying patients with haptoglobin or IgA deficiency).

Additional actions include the following:

• correct ID of patient (making sure that procedure is followed and that wrist bands used) and product

to be transfused (performing clerical checks without exceptions);
• bedside test (performing it systematically as well as technically correct, with the right interpretation of the results).

General actions

One must be aware that many different actions have been taken in the hospitals, but at the same time it should be recognized that most of these measures relate to simple and general elements of QM:

• procedures and SOPs;
• training and education;
• compliance enforcement;
• reporting of abnormalities;
• audits and reviews (through HTCs).

In addition, new standards and guidelines have been enacted in many of the responding countries, relating to BEs and healthcare institutions.

In the BEs, donor-HV has received a much higher attention and is intensified at a broader range.

In hospitals, governance in transfusion matters has been strengthened (mainly through the

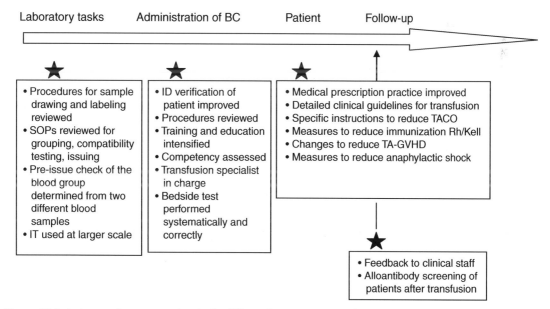

Figure 24.8 Actions and measures taken in the different key processes in a hospital in the context of blood transfusion from the collection of a blood sample from a patient, through testing, administration of the transfusion and the follow-up of the transfused patient (BC = blood component, SOPs = Standard Operating Procedures).

establishment of HTCs). Clinical audits on blood usage have been initiated here and there.

At national/regional levels, the curriculum of the different professional bodies have been revised, updated, and completed to cover more extensively issues related to blood transfusion. Special postgraduate training programs have been introduced and online material is largely available for e-learning by different professional groups and disciplines.

In an effort to boost impact, some countries have started joint ventures. These are alliances of patient groups, blood services, hospitals, authorities, professional and scientific societies, and so on cooperating with the aim of improving quality and safety in blood transfusion.

Finally, reporting and analysis of information collected through HV have become more convenient, secure, and efficient through the use of common definitions, introduction of IT tools, and regular feedback.

Outcomes and achievements through hemovigilance

As already mentioned the conclusions on outcomes call for prudence because one single change may have several impacts and one single improvement may be due to different interventions and, of course, combinations of both make things even more complex.

Box 24.4 shows the original response from New Zealand.

Box 24.4 New Zealand hemovigilance: Outcomes and achievements

The only measurable outcome since the establishment of a hemovigilance system has been the reduction in TRALI cases following the implementation of male-donor FFP. However it is possibly too early to detect outcomes, given the relative youth of our Hemovigilance Programme and the small population in New Zealand.

International data from other hemovigilance schemes have influenced blood safety in New Zealand. Universal pre-storage leuco-depletion was implemented in 2001. The major hospitals in New Zealand have a local Transfusion Nurse Specialist who is regularly involved in education relating to blood safety. These specialist nurses collaborate regularly and undertake transfusion audits. Results and recommendations from the multicenter audits are relayed back to HTCs. We suspect that improvements prompted by these initiatives occurred prior to the establishment of the Hemovigilance Programme.

Specific outcomes and achievements

Production segment (in the BE)

Figure 24.9 summarizes the achievements recorded for the different key processes in a blood establishment. Deviations, errors, and weaknesses are not excluded and may generate risks, requiring corrective or preventive actions that should lead to measurable outcomes.

The highlights in terms of outcome through measures triggered by HV and put in place by BEs are developed together with the reflections relating to the hospitals: it would be somewhat arbitrary to make a distinction between the two segments of the blood chain when it comes to outcome.

Usage segment in the healthcare institution

Figure 24.10 demonstrates the achievements recorded for the different key processes in a hospital in the context of a blood transfusion. Deviations, errors, and weaknesses are not excluded and may generate risks, requiring corrective or preventive actions that should lead to measurable outcomes.

Specifics and general outcomes and achievements

As discussed, both BEs and hospitals have taken numerous actions to correct and prevent incidents and errors/near-misses. As a result of these measures and changes, there is without any doubt improvement along the blood chain to the benefit of donors, patients, and society in general.

Listed below are the outcomes as they are seen in the reporting countries (one or more) along the blood chain:

• The number of recalls of donations and BCs (prepared from index donations) has decreased in several countries for different reasons:

  ○ the medical questionnaire to assess donor eligibility has been reviewed and updated,

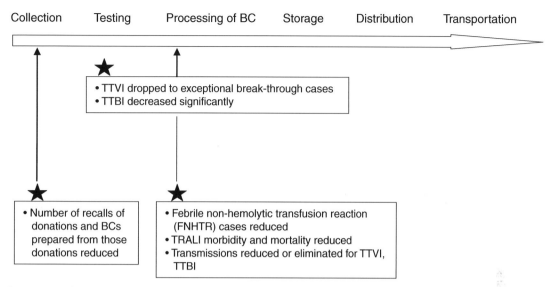

Figure 24.9 The achievements recorded for the different key processes in a blood establishment from the collection of whole blood, plasma, or cells through testing of donor blood, preparation of blood components, storage, distribution, and transportation of finished blood products (BC = blood components, TTVI = transfusion-transmissible viral infection, TTBI = transfusion-transmissible bacterial infection).

(rendering the questions clearer and adding more precise questions on risk behavior);

  ○ the process of medical selection of donors has been strengthened (increasing compliance to the acceptance criteria after training and re-training of staff in charge).

• The number of transfusion-transmitted viral infections (TTVIs) has decreased, especially in countries with a higher prevalence of relevant viruses in the general population. This is due to the introduction of systematic NAT testing, parallel to the classical serological screening. Nevertheless exceptional break-through cases continue to exist, transgressing all safety barriers including testing (negative results in ELISA as well as in PCR for donors coming to donate blood, very shortly after viral contamination).

• The number of transfusion-transmitted bacterial contaminations (TTBIs) has dropped significantly in those countries where specific measures have been taken: because platelet concentrates are most at risk, they are subject to bacterial pre-release testing

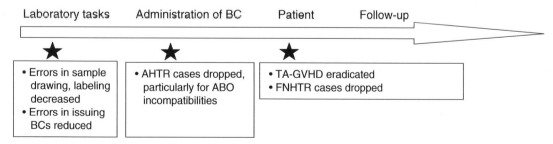

Figure 24.10 The achievements recorded for the different key processes in a hospital in the context of a blood transfusion, from the collection of a blood sample from a patient through laboratory testing, administration of blood, and follow-up of the transfused patient (BC = blood components).

(culturing in the BE's laboratory of samples from the finished product until the product is distributed upon negative test result).

• TRALI morbidity and mortality have been significantly reduced or even eradicated in a majority of countries since the introduction of new plasma components for transfusion:

  ○ male-only plasma (prepared from donations by nontransfused male donors) eliminates passive transfer of leucocyte-antibodies from donor to recipient, a prerequisite for the development of TRALI;

  ○ in SD-plasma (prepared from a pool of multiple plasmas and subject to treatment by solvent-detergent), leucocyte-antibodies (if present) are diluted during pooling probably to a point where they can no longer trigger the pathomechanism for TRALI.

• Despite this positive impact one should not forget that TRALI still happens, at a much lower rate and linked to transfusion of RBCs and PLTs.

• This beneficial TRALI outcome is one of the most visible and dramatic achievements of HV and it is observed consistently in the countries where the new policies for FFP transfusion are adopted.

• FNHTR is greatly reduced due to universal pre-storage leuco-depletion of RBCs and PLTs. Filtration of the intermediate products during processing lowers the number of residual leucocytes to a level that no longer allows sufficient production of cytokines (of different kinds) during the following storage, thus decreasing the incidence of the typical symptoms of FNHTR.

• Besides new testing strategies (see above), transmission of infectious agents through transfusion can be eliminated by pathogen inactivation of PLTs and/or FFP, but not for RBCs. The effect is less visible for viral transmissions because these have already become exceptional after the introduction of NAT. In eliminating bacterial contaminations through transfusion of certain BCs, p.i. has had a positive outcome without doubt.

• Eradication of TA-GVHD has been achieved in one country through routine irradiation of cellular BCs (elimination of the transfer through transfusion of viable T-lymphocytes from the donor to a patient). In other countries it has become very

rare because the medical prescription practice has improved and its execution is more disciplined.

• HV has uncovered sample drawing and tube labeling as one of the most critical and vulnerable steps of the blood chain. A marked reduction of errors and near-misses at these steps has been shown year after year based on HV data. This is not due to a single corrective intervention but to several: better procedures, clearer SOPs, intensified training, re-training, and increased compliance after education have all had their input on the "output" (in terms of outcome). Again, this achievement through HV is one of the most important and spectacular ones.

• A similar trend has been observed in different countries when it comes to issuing of BCs from the hospital blood bank to the requesting ward. Improved procedures in the laboratory in charge, better SOPs, more training, but also the support by IT during this important step have led to a drop in errors and near-misses when BCs move from the laboratory to the site of transfusion.

• Another impressive achievement is the drop in acute hemolytic transfusion reactions (AHTRs), particularly in the frequency of ABO-incompatible transfusions. It is not surprising that more stringent ID checks of the patients as well as clerical controls of the issued BC have reduced mix-ups. In those countries were the bedside test was already mandatory and in those where it was rendered compulsory, these dramatic accidents are rare if the bedside test is performed systematically (good compliance), with good *lege artis* (good material and good technique) and the correct interpretation of the results (good personnel).

• In a more general way, HV has certainly had a significant impact on the mentality of those involved in blood transfusion and has greatly increased awareness of the real transfusion risks. This is reflected in increased demand for consultation from experts by hospital staff, increased reporting of ARs/AEs, errors, and near-misses in hospitals, better risk management, rationalization of transfusion practice, better clinical use, and decrease in the number of blood transfusions. Now, the latter may be demand-driven (related to decreasing donation and collection in many countries), motivated by costs of blood components, or impacted by optimal use of blood. Whatever the cause (mono-causal or multi-factorial), the endpoint one can see is a decrease in mortality attributable to blood transfusion.

- HV has been finally integrated into the QMS (especially in BEs): nonconformities of blood components, complaints of customers in the hospital, and errors in the processes are much better managed and followed-up and the result is a drop of the former, indicating improvement in the blood chain.

If we speak about achievements in the context of HV, we should not forget that improvements are not always measurable, for different reasons, and that specific outcomes may not yet be assessable, if actions have only been taken only recently. So, the benefit of HV may be even higher than we can assess today.

Conclusions

Through HV, numerous different risks and problems have been detected and reported.

Adverse reactions, adverse events, incidents, accidents, side effects, errors, near-misses, deviations, and so on have been observed all along the blood chain from the donor to the recipient, including the processes, subprocesses, and activity steps.

The first global achievement of HV is the correct and wide documentation of these and particularly their quantification (or at least an order of magnitude). This is of special interest in the context of TTIs with viruses (HIV in the first place, but also for HBV, HCV, HTLV, and so on) and with bacteria. In the first category it became evident that the risk was overestimated; in the second that it was underestimated.

The second global achievement of HV is the discovery and re-discovery of important entities (infection, disease, situation, and so on) before, during, and after transfusion, but also in the context of donation. Most of these risks and problems were known before structured, organized HV started, but others were recognized as "new" dona-

tion, respectively, transfusion-associated entities, such as on one side "painful arm" and on the other TRALI. Some have a wide range of expression characteristics: IBCT is certainly a good example—from the absence of symptoms after transfusion of the wrong blood component to lethal outcome after massive hemolysis of an ABO-incompatible red cell unit. Other pathologies had also been described before HV started, but for others the link to blood transfusion was less obvious or less direct: one might cite here TACO, TA-GVHD, undertransfusion, and so on.

The third important achievement of HV is that it has triggered the closure of a gap in the quality cycle of "Plan, Do, Check, Act" with significant improvements in different activities.

Many different actions and measures were taken to reduce or eliminate these risks and problems. HV is considered to be a quality tool and as such is integrated into QA, QM, and QMS. In general this was easier in BEs than hospitals, which was not really surprising because BEs operating as production sites under GMPs had an overall higher level of quality culture level. Nevertheless it should not be forgotten that the hospitals (and especially their blood banks) have caught up very rapidly in this field.

Important changes may come from errors and near-misses that happened all along the blood chain: it is nowadays accepted as a principle that these are a valuable source for learning (and improving). The invisible becomes a trigger for change and this is another step from "reactive" to "proactive" (or preventive).

If we concentrate now on the last 20 years of institutionalized HV, it cannot be denied that significant, objective, and measurable achievements have occurred in the context of blood transfusion.

As already mentioned HV has brought general and specific achievements in relation to recipients, donors, products, and processes/systems. But HV also has had other impacts:

- politics (blood transfusion has gained in attention, interest, and priority);
- legislation (the core of legal requirements has grown at breath-taking speed, at national and international level);

• media (blood has been again and again the object of a "story", although in the last few years it is usually treated in a more objective and positive way);

• mentality, sensitivity, and awareness (all influenced by data and information generated by HV);

• approach (blood transfusion has seen a more evidence-based orientation).

Looking into the experiences of the last 20 years of HV and taking into account the achievements (directly measurable and those indirectly tangible), it can be concluded beyond reasonable doubt that HV has been very successful and efficacious.

This is particularly true in the context of the protection of patients with transfusion needs. At this moment in time, the most obvious and striking "negative" side effects of transfusion in recipients have nearly disappeared (or at least they have been dramatically reduced). To improve this segment of the blood chain in the future will become increasingly difficult. In other words, the "easiest" things have been done first. But new challenges are ahead to improve further the safety for patients through the quality tool named HV: effects of transfusion on the immune system and its biological valence; effects of undertransfusion of patients in need for a blood transfusion (no transfusion or not enough transfusion); and so on—many challenges remain.

This applies even more to the donor segment. In general, donor-HV has just started (or is about to do so) in a structured, organized, and scientific way, reaching beyond observational value. Many questions await an answer: What is the impact of frequent apheresis procedures on the organism of regular blood, plasma, platelet, and multicomponent donors? What is the effect (positive or negative) on depleting partially the iron stores of donors (especially of menstruating females)? What is the psychological influence on donors of deferred (temporarily or permanently) donation? There is also a direct interface with Human Ethics and Medical Deontology. A lot remains to be done.

When it comes to products, the pharmaceutical principle of "highest purity" has become a leitmotiv for the BE. Recipient-HV has clearly shown that some of the adverse reactions (serious and less serious) are due to blood constituents that are not needed by the patient. Specific blood components

contain less and less residual "contaminating" elements that should not part of the product (for example, less leucocytes in RBC or PLT, less plasma in RBC or PLT, less cells in plasma). Additional screening tests and/or pathogen inactivation have been introduced or are about to be implemented to increase safety of the products. In any case, availability (of donations and products) will probably become the biggest challenge in the future.

In relation to processes/systems, QM is indicating the future direction: efficacious, comprehensive QMS help keep the processes under control and give them the necessary stability. HV systems, which encompass errors and near-misses, detect weaknesses and deviations that subsequently are the target of CAPA. Processes and activities in the BE are more and more approaching pharmaceutical principles and standards, and so achieving higher safety and quality levels.

What we have said above is within the domain of hemovigilance (labile blood components: allogeneic and autologous; for transfusion/administration, collection, testing, processing, storage, and distribution). In several countries, there is a new trend to enlarge the scope to "biovigilance"[10] to embrace also organs, tissues, and cells. It is still too early to speak about solid data proving achievements in these new areas, but it can be anticipated without too much speculation that similar success can be expected in biovigilance because many similarities exist with blood, at all levels. But at the same time, organs, tissues, and cells present their specific risks, problems and challenges, and particularities.

Finally, after 20 years of structured, organized HV in some countries and its achievements, it is difficult to imagine a world of transfusion without HV, because it has significantly increased safety and quality of transfusion for the recipient and donation for the donor.

Acknowledgements

The following representatives of countries contributed to this chapter and the authors want to express their sincere thanks and deep gratitude to them. Without their valuable contributions this chapter could not have been a colorful and multi-faceted look:

Australia (Erica Wood and Chris Hogan), Belgium (Ludo Muylle and Micheline Lambermont), Canada/Québec (Pierre Robillard), Croatia (Dorotea Sarlija), Denmark (Jan Jorgensen), Finland (Mirja Korkolainen), France (Philippe Renaudier), Greece (Constantina Politis), Italy (Giuliano Grazzini), Ireland (Emer Lawlor), Japan (Hitoshi Okazaki), Luxembourg (Jean-Claude Faber), The Netherlands (Jo Wiersum and Martin Schipperus), New Zealand (Dorothy Dinesh and Peter Flanagan), Norway (Oystein Flesland), Portugal (Jorge Condeco and Fatima Nascimento), Singapore (Ramir Alcantara and Mickey Koh), Slovenia (Marjeta Potocnik), South Africa (Francis Ledwaba and Heide Schmalberger), Spain (Magdalena Perez Jimenez and Elena Moro), Sweden (Miodrag Palfi), Switzerland (Morven Rüesch), United Kingdom (Clare Taylor) and many more.

References

1 European Union, 2003, Directive of the European Parliament and of the Council setting standards of quality and safety for the collection, testing, processing, storage and distribution of human blood and blood components and amending Directive 2001/83/EC. *Official Journal of the European Communities* L33/30–L33/40.

2 Faber JC, 2004, The European Blood Directive: A new era of regulation has begun. *Transfusion Medicine TME* **14**: 257–73.

3 Faber JC, 2002, Haemovigilance around the world. *Vox Sang* **83**(Suppl 1): 71–6.

4 European Centre for Disease Prevention and Control, 2009, Annual epidemiological report on communicable diseases in Europe, revised edition. http://ecdc.europa.eu/en/publications/publications/0910_sur_annual_epidemiological_report_on_communicable_diseases_in_europe.pdf [accessed February 28, 2012].

5 Serious Hazards of Transfusion (SHOT) Office, Hazards of Transfusion, Annual Reports 1996/97 through 2009. Manchester Blood Centre, Manchester, UK.

6 Dinesh D, and Flanagan P (New Zealand), personal communication.

7 Schipperus M, and Wiersum J (the Netherlands), personal communication.

8 Taylor C (UK), personal communication.

9 Okazaki H (Japan), personal communication.

10 de Vries RRP, Faber JC, Strengers P, 2011, Haemovigilance: An effective tool for improving transfusion practice. *Vox Sang* **100**: 60–7.

PART 6
Developments

CHAPTER 25

Vigilance of Alternatives for Blood Components

Dafydd Thomas

Abertawe Bro Morgannwg University Health Board, Morriston Hospital, Swansea, UK

Introduction

The development of hemovigilance has occurred at the same time as a number of blood conservation and blood avoidance programs. The realization that blood transfusion can cause transmission of blood-borne diseases has been well documented since the initial development of blood transfusion services. However, it was only from the 1980s that there seemed to be an explosion of transfusion transmitted infections (TTIs) that suddenly required a coordinated scientific and organizational approach to minimize the harm that could result from the transmission of infection through blood transfusion.

Attempts at minimizing transmission of infection have been concentrated on viral and bacterial testing of donated blood, but the avoidance of allogeneic transfusion can also avoid such transmission. Use of autologous transfusion techniques, the use of other strategies that withhold transfusion, use pharmacological agents to stimulate erythropoiesis, or reduce blood loss during surgery, have been used with positive effect.

As one might expect, the introduction of novel and alternative processes are usually welcomed by some practitioners with a degree of enthusiasm but with cynicism from others.

It is true to say that even the most promising developments in medicine are often accompanied by problems or risks. They may be well recognized risks that apply to the old as well as the new process or indeed reveal new previously unknown risks that may be specifically associated with the new treatment.

Throughout this chapter these themes will be repeated as we explore the risks and problems identified by hemovigilance, a process that has to be applied to old and new transfusion therapies and the alternatives to allogeneic transfusion. The chapter describes the alternatives that may be used, each description providing a short summary of the alternative therapy and how it can be used either individually or in combination with others to minimize or prevent the use of allogeneic blood and/or component therapy, followed by examples of problems that have been recognized and would need to be incorporated in any hemovigilance program of alternative therapies.

It needs to be stated at this stage that all other measures to minimize blood loss occurring at the time of surgery need to be taken. This includes fastidious surgical attention to stop bleeding and to prevent unnecessary blood loss and complementary anesthetic techniques to reduce venous engorgement and arterial hypertension, which can also lead to increased bleeding. The details of such interventions will not be discussed further in this chapter as they are not likely to be recorded or considered under hemovigilance schemes. The withholding of transfusion as an intervention to allow a lower hemoglobin in the patient and therefore lead to a decrease in transfusion rates does need to be monitored, but is dealt with in Chapter 26.

Before we embark on a detailed description of the individual techniques, however, it must be emphasized that the generic headings into which we divide hemovigilance for allogeneic products still apply to autologous and pharmacological alternatives to allogeneic transfusion. The assumption that any alternative therapy that we employ to avoid the use of allogenic blood is ultimately beneficial to patients needs to be challenged and the same rigorous standards that we employ to the collection, storage, and ultimate transfusion to patients applied to the alternative therapy. Data on the safety of cell savers and the antifibrinolytics are lacking.[1] Although the RCT evidence is sparse, many of these techniques are in common use and it may be that data from hemovigilance schemes can provide an objective opinion of the safety and effectiveness of these alternate techniques.

Autologous blood transfusion techniques

There are three main categories of autotransfusion that can be used to provide autologous blood:
- preoperative autologous deposit/predeposit;
- acute normovolemic hemodilution and acute hypervolemic hemodilution;
- red cell salvage, which can be undertaken intra-operatively, post-operatively, or during both, when it is referred to as *peri-operative cell salvage* (POCS).

Predeposit

The use of preoperative collection of autologous blood (PAD), where the patient acts as donor in the preceding weeks prior to surgery, became very popular in the initial years following the discovery of the HIV problem and subsequent AIDS crisis. The use of PAD increased dramatically, more than 17-fold, in the United States.[2] The collection, storage, and re-transfusion during surgery associated with major blood loss was shown to reduce allogeneic transfusion during such procedures as cardiac, orthopedic, and pediatric surgeries.

The use of PAD can be considered when blood would usually be typed and crossmatched, for example, all procedures with an anticipated blood loss in excess of 1000 ml.

Apart from the obvious difficulty and possible distress in persuading pediatric patients to pre-donate, there are few contraindications to using PAD because anyone scheduled for elective surgery with expected major blood loss is probably able to predonate providing the hematocrit is above 33%. Contraindications to PAD include recent myocardial infarction, chronic heart failure, aortic stenosis, transitory ischemic events, arrhythmias, hypertension, and unstable angina pectoris. Patients with an obvious bacteremia are excluded as are patients with poor venous access, which may include some children.

The collection of the blood needs to occur no longer than four weeks prior to the date of surgery, otherwise the shelf life of the first donated unit runs out. If this happens there needs to be a reinfusion of the first collected blood to allow further donation to occur. This is known as "leap-frog" donation but is not advisable and every effort needs to be made to ensure that collection of blood and surgical intervention are carefully coordinated. Prior to taking blood from a patient for this procedure, informed consent needs to be obtained and the risks associated with donation explained such as hematoma, infection, fainting, nausea, and so on. As will be explained later, despite the assumption that this sort of procedure is safe inherent risks need to be discussed as well as the logistical and storage problems that may arise. In addition, patients will need to give consent for their blood to be tested for all the known infections to which allogeneic blood is currently subjected. More importantly, if any of these tests are positive further investigation and treatment may be required. These tests include HIV, HBV, HCV, syphilis, ABO, and Rh type.

The collection of 3–4 units in the month before surgery is the norm with the last unit being collected not later than 72 hours prior to surgery to allow equilibration of the blood volume of the patient. More aggressive donations may be considered but have to be organized carefully to provide the best risk–benefit ratio for the patient. In these instances it may be necessary to supplement the process with the use of erythropoietin and iron supplementation, which may help stimulate the patient's response to the induced anemia and help minimize the hematocrit drop as a consequence of the PAD. These interventions bring increased cost and complexity to the procedure, adding further potential for risk to the patient.

When it comes to the reinfusion of PAD blood, the perception that it is without risk itself may lead to complications as the physician and patient expect reinfusion to take place. If such a transfusion is physiologically unnecessary at the time, this may bring its own problems such as circulatory overload. Equally if the collected blood is not reinfused, considerable waste occurs as the blood then runs out of date, is not retransfused to the patient, and not able to be used for any other patient. The cost of collecting, testing, and storing the blood, as well as the inconvenience and administrative cost, leads to a very uneconomic process.

The initial promise of this technique has subsequently been tainted by problems involved with collection of blood from patients, unpredicted adverse costs and efficacy, and most recently within Europe by the European Blood Directive.[3] The use of PAD therefore is rather heterogeneous across the world with pockets of enthusiasm among some institutions while others rarely offer it to their patients.

Potential pitfalls and problems that may serve as a template for hemovigilance are described in the later section "Hemovigilance of alternatives" starting on page 314.

Hemodilution

There are different types of hemodilution: hypervolemic and normovolemic. This latter technique is best described as *acute predeposit* or more correctly as *acute normovolemic hemodilution* (ANH), and is where blood is removed from the patient immediately prior to the surgical intervention and blood volume maintained with plasma expanders. The patient's blood is therefore diluted with either crystalloid or colloid to reduce the overall hematocrit. These techniques were first described and advocated by

Konrad Messmer in the early 1960s, explaining the deliberate dilution to make the patient anemic.[4,5] Further developments including the technique of hyperoxic hemodilution have been described by Oliver Habler.[6]

Acute hypervolemic hemodilution (AHH)

This technique is performed by infusing large amounts of crystalloids or colloids. It dilutes the patient's red cells so that a temporary expansion of the blood volume is achieved, therefore increasing the allowable blood loss of a more dilute blood. A target hematocrit of 25% is aimed for. The eventual result is that less red cells per milliliter are lost.

AHH requires a patient who can tolerate hypervolemia. Although one could assume that Transfusion Associated Circulatory Overload (TACO) may be a side effect of this technique while the patient remains anesthetized an excessive increase in blood pressure is avoided by the use of the vasodilatory effect of anesthetic drugs. Care is obviously needed particularly in the immediate post-operative period when patients with cardiac and autonomic nervous disorders will not be able to make the necessary adjustments to the excessive volume and display symptoms of TACO. Selected patients will require intact renal function to allow excretion of the excess blood volume. Providing appropriate patient selection, AHH can be a simple and safe method of reducing allogenic blood use.[7]

Acute normovolemic hemodilution

Unlike the acute hypervolemic hemodilution technique, with ANH blood is removed and then immediately replaced with crystalloid or colloid to ensure that normovolemia is maintained. In this way the problems of volume overload is avoided and the technique can be used in a wider selection of patients. To ensure that the quality of the blood is as high as possible, it is advised to avoid excessive intravenous fluid administration prior to the venesection of the blood to be stored. The avoidance of general anesthesia until ANH is well underway may help in this regard as there will not be a need to compensate for the vasodilation induced to maintain blood pressure, because unlike AHH the aim is to maintain normovolemia. There is still a need, of course, to calculate how low to allow the hematocrit to drop and this will often depend on the cardio-respiratory status of the patient.

To calculate the amount of blood that can be safely removed from a patient the following calculation can be used:

$$ABV = EBV \times (H_O - H_T)/(H_O + H_T)/2$$

where ABV is the autologous blood volume withdrawn; H_O is the pre-hemodilution hematocrit; H_T is the target hematocrit; and EBV is estimated blood volume of the patient.

The use of ANH is contraindicated in patients with severe coronary artery stenosis, congestive heart failure, severe COPD, hemoglobinopathies, coagulation disorders, poor renal function, severe aortic stenosis, unstable angina pectoris, and major organ dysfunction.

Blood collection is usually started after the induction of anesthesia, but some practitioners feel it is safer to monitor the patient fully and to keep the patient awake during the blood collection and compensation of blood volume to ensure any symptoms of cardiac or cerebral ischemia can be immediately diagnosed. The blood is usually stored in identical blood bags to those used for routine donor blood collection and needs to be labeled with the patient's name and time of withdrawal. The blood is kept at room temperature after collection, stays with the patient, and is re-infused later in the procedure. Six (to eight hours) is accepted as a reasonable time to store at room temperature. The principle is to isovolemically hemodilute the patient to a lower hematocrit and then at the time of surgery a more dilute lower hematocrit blood is lost due to surgical trauma and bleeding. At the end of the procedure the patient's own blood is re-infused to boost the low hemoglobin at a time when surgical blood loss is low or has stopped. The blood has the added value of being relatively warm and containing normal levels of clotting factors and platelets to aid coagulation.

If the lowest acceptable hematocrit is reached earlier than the end of surgery then blood is returned in reverse order to the initial harvest so that the blood unit with the highest hematocrit and highest concentration of coagulation factors is infused last.

The principles and the potential advantage of ANH were elaborately discussed in a paper by Brecher.[8] The mathematical model explained that the saving of 1 equivalent unit of red cells would require the removal of 4 units of blood from the patient at the beginning of the procedure.

Peri-operative cell salvage (POCS)

Peri-operative cell salvage can be divided into intra-operative cell salvage (ICS) and post-operative cell salvage.

ICS is usually understood to be a process where spilt blood is collected from a body cavity during a surgical procedure. The method of collection requires specific equipment, comprising a double lumen suction tubing that usually delivers anticoagulant (either citrate or heparinized saline) to a point close to the suction tip where it prevents clotting in the collected blood and allows the salvaged blood to be stored for a period of time prior to processing. Processing consists of filtration and washing, producing a red cell concentrate resuspended in 0.9% saline for reinfusion into the patient. Some systems have been marketed in the past that required systemic anticoagulation of the patient (as occurs in most cardiac and vascular procedures) but no washing process, simply filtration. More recently this form of the unwashed system has recently been advocated for intra-operative use once more.

Post-operative cell salvage, although used historically to collect and re-infuse blood collected from intercostal chest drains following cardiothoracic procedures, is most commonly used these days in orthopedic joint-replacement procedures. The wound drainage collected during the post-operative period is re-infused following a washing procedure or unwashed with a device that simply filters large aggregates and fat particles prior to re-infusion. There are advocates and critics of both techniques, but hitherto reports of harm to patients receiving unwashed blood are small in number and do not seem to reflect any significant problem when considering the prevalence of these procedures using unwashed blood following ortho-pedic operations.

Use of ICS during obstetric interventional procedures

In 2005, after extensive consultation, the National Institute for Clinical Excellence (NICE) in the UK accepted[9] that in situations of massive hemorrhage it would be considered appropriate that ICS be used to salvage the autologous blood being lost at the time of interventional delivery and often re-laporotomy for bleeding in parturient women and during the postpartum period. The evidence was accepted that much of the fetal contamination would be removed with the washing procedure and that the remaining contamination could be removed by the use of a leucoreduction filter, which had been shown by a large number of researchers to reduce the fetal contaminants.

As a result, the use of cell salvage in obstetrics showed a significant increase across the UK.

The use of ICS in parturient women had been introduced as routine practice in some institutions in the US, championed by Jonathan Waters who has a database of such use in over 7000 women. Since its introduction in the UK and expansion of use there have been some reports of adverse events reported to Serious Hazards of Transfusion's (SHOT's) new category of autologous transfusion.[10] These incidents do not seem to be related to problems envisaged such as amniotic fluid embolism but rather to the leucoreduction filters used to try and minimize fetal contamination in the woman receiving the re-infused blood.

Use of ICS during cancer surgery

As with the use of ICS in obstetrics, NICE consulted about its use in urological procedures such as radical prostatectomy[11] and again came to the conclusion that such use seemed to be safe and recommended use in these cases within the context of current evidence.

Possible problems with autologous blood collection

Popovsky and co-workers reported an increase in adverse events among those patients present-ing to predonate when compared with healthy donors.[12,13] This led to a more cautious approach and remains relevant today as the risk of viral transmission currently is lowering for the pathogens we know about. Goodnough and colleagues also contributed to this debate by showing that the true cost of predeposit in terms of quality added life years (QALY) was extremely expensive.[14,15]

When this is added to the effect that the European directive had on predeposit, its slow development within the UK has been completely arrested due to the need for local blood banks (where the predeposited blood was stored) to become blood establishments and inspected as such under the Medicines and Healthcare products Regulatory Agency (MHRA) umbrella.

It is not surprising that the problems that might occur in using alternative therapies to allogeneic transfusion will have the same generic errors that are associated with allogeneic transfusion, namely

- procedural errors such as patient mis-identification and blood sampling errors, and transfusing the wrong blood component;
- reactions such as acute transfusion reactions (for example, fever and chills) and bacterial infections.

There is always the potential that blood removed from a patient can be re-infused to the incorrect patient, particularly if rigorous labeling of the blood bag is not undertaken. If we take as our first example any form of autologous blood that can be collected whether pre-operative donated blood (PAD), blood collected during acute normovolemic hemodilution (ANH), or peri-operative cell salvaged red cells (POCS), they all have a short and finite time after they are removed from the patient. Depending on the technique, this time may be anything from a period of 15 minutes to 42 days but during this period the blood needs to be labeled and stored correctly. PAD blood will need to be stored at 4°C (39.2°F) and may need to be leucoreduced or divided into separate components depending on the individual requirements. ANH collected blood or peri-operatively salvaged red cells may be stored at room temperature for up to 6 hours depending on locally agreed protocols and standard operating procedures (SOPs).

Equally, labeling of these samples needs to be consistent and clear so that when re-infusion is required, similar forms of administrative checks to those applied to allogeneic components can be employed. Certainly prolonged storage of blood or red cells collected using ANH or POCS is not advisable and can lead to significant problems and potential confusion among clinical staff. Personal communications and reports to some hemovigilance schemes have reported inappropriate storage and re-infusion of such collected components. Despite the fact that this is autologous blood, the possibility of an incompatible blood component being transfused remains and similar checking procedures to identify the recipient and the component being transfused to ensure compatibility is essential.

The storage of blood collected using either ANH or POCS is at room temperature and storage for a longer period is not used. In these instances, as the blood is not stored for long periods bacterial contamination is rarely a problem. However quality assurance programs are advised to document the frequently encountered pathogens that may be isolated in the collected blood so that a locally registered inventory can be kept together with antibiotic sensitivities for these bacteria. In the case of PAD, blood storage criteria need to be exactly the same as for allogeneic blood with all the same pathogen testing.

Similarly, it is foolish to think that the storage lesion will not affect autologous blood. The lesion will be exactly the same as with allogeneic blood depending on length of storage and storage medium used. It can be assumed therefore that similar problems will occur, albeit less frequently because of the lower frequency of autologous blood use. If as is anticipated there is a promotion of such autologous alternatives it is very important that we monitor the adverse events that will occur so that we can continue to deliver best care and respond to developing patterns of adverse events.

As ANH is not routinely practiced in some institutions, it is important that SOPs are in place. A number of personal communications outside a hemovigilance process have been received. One related to the placement of the patient's unlabeled blood in a blood refrigerator because it was not immediately infused at the end of the procedure. This blood was wasted, meaning it was an unnecessary procedure for the patient that left the person with lower hemoglobin than would have been the case if ANH had not been undertaken. Of course in institutions that conduct ANH regularly, these problems rarely occur, but they remain a potential hazard in less-experienced arenas.

Poor patient selection will lead to clinical problems. Including any of the patients who are normally excluded from the process will reveal clinical symptoms earlier than in those patients correctly included; however, reports still arise in the literature showing how even in the most compromised patients the technique can be undertaken safely.[16,17]

The most obvious potential problem is the accelerated way in which a patient will reach a target hematcrit or hemoglobin level following removal of blood than if left untouched to reach this level in the course of the surgery. This may lead to a decompensation within the patient resulting in organ ischemia. The most obvious and easiest type to monitor is myocardial ishemia.

The signs of ECG-documented ischemia have been described.[18] In this case report, the potential to cause unintended harm was displayed in a fully monitored patient who was in the anesthetic room awaiting surgery. The patient was being invasively monitored with CVP, arterial line, ECG, and pulse oximetry. During the ANH procedure, the venesection of a unit of blood caused some ECG changes indicating myocardial ischemia. This was noticed by the anesthetist and the procedure altered. The blood was re-infused to the patient. As soon as this blood was re-infused there was a reversal of the ischemic changes shown on the electrocardiogram.[18]

Other authors have shown that this degree of organ hypoxia can be simply treated using hyperoxic ventilation using 100% oxygen. This enhances the amount of dissolved oxygen and also ensures as high an hemoglobin saturation as possible.[6,19]

Iron

The use of iron to treat anemia is fraught with difficulties because it is difficult to establish whether a lack of response is due to poor compliance, due to forgetfulness, or due to the unpleasant side effects that some patients experience with this therapy: G/I upsets, odd metallic taste symptoms, and rashes are the most common.

IV iron is a way of preventing some of these problems but there is a legacy of concern by older clinicians because they were experienced in using the iron dextran preparations that had a high incidence of anaphylaxis. Some of the earlier intravenous preparations were associated with very severe anaphylactoid reactions. These reactions prompted the FDA to require resuscitation equipment to be available when IV iron was given. The preparation used was an iron dextran preparation, which indeed did have a significant record of anaphylaxis.

These days there are safer products available and there are a number of different preparations, which all have specific problems with their use that could be included in a proforma for collecting adverse incidents related to its use.

The role of iron has long been accepted as an essential and simple therapy to correct iron-deficiency anemia. It is important that pre-operative iron deficiency anemia is appropriately investigated and corrected to prevent the unnecessary transfusion of allergenic blood, but more importantly that a diagnosis of the etiology of the anemia is defined and the appropriate treatment given. The well-known use and problems with oral iron therapy, however, have provided an opportunity for the development of very safe alternative intravenous iron preparations, which are now widely marketed.

Hemostatic fibrin sealants

The majority of hemostatic and adhesive surgical sealants invariably combine fibrinogen and thrombin. Their role in facilitating hemostasis has become part of the patient blood-management program with the aim of aiding surgical hemostasis and reducing total blood loss for the patient undergoing the procedure. The contribution to total blood loss may be minimal, but the minimizing of surgical ooze or troublesome bleeding from surgical intervention may allow quicker closure and shorter surgical procedures.

These products may contain human or bovine thrombin and fibrinogen and so use of them needs to be monitored by hemovigilance. Currently many such products are ordered by surgical teams and stored within a theater pharmacy for immediate use when troublesome bleeding occurs. The traceability of such products may not be to the standard considered necessary by a hemovigilance scheme and is not usually under the control of the hospital blood bank. It is important to remember that the available fibrin sealants both in Europe and the US tend to be of the new generation virally inactivated or virus removed fibrin sealants. However, prior to these products, which have been available since 1998 and 2003 respectively, there were reports describing a number of "homemade formulations."[20–24]

The use of plasma-derived products to facilitate hemostasis was first described in 1909.[25] Concern over the transmission of hepatitis with the use of human thrombin led to the substitution with bovine thrombin. Commercial concentrates containing clotable human fibrinogen plus fibrin stabilizing factor (Factor XIII) together with bovine thrombin were available in Europe in the late 1970s. All of these products contained an antifibrinolytic agent. The viral risk was reduced through donor selection followed by heat treatment of the human fibrinogen component. In addition, human thrombin (virally inactivated) has now replaced bovine thrombin.[20]

Despite these advances in viral safety, a few cases have been reported with the use of fibrin glues that relate more to the mode of use of these products. Although it has to be stated that the use of generic "fibrin glue" appears to be safe in the majority of cases, one report of a fatality when a syringe was used to administer the glue to a deep hepatic wound, the fatal hypotension, was thought to be related to a reaction to bovine thrombin.[26] Another recently reported case highlighted significant morbidity after using a pressurized fibrin glue aerosol, again in liver surgery, resulting in air embolism and intravascular thrombus. The air was identified with transoesophageal echocardiography in the right ventricle, with some air even finding a passage through to the left ventricle leading to cardiovascular collapse.[27]

In conclusion, the use of all types of fibrin glues appears to be increasing but the current practice seems to have little standardization of use with too little attention being paid to the traceability of the product used. This is of course very important when human thrombin, albeit treated and virally inactivated, is being used. A better system needs to be employed and a registry of patients who receive such products needs to be kept by the institution. In addition to the documentation, placement of a sticky label in the patient's notes identifying the product precisely needs to become a standard of care.

Erythopoietin (EPO)

Erythopoietin is a hormone produced by the kidney that promotes the formation of red blood cells in the bone marrow. EPO is a glycoprotein (a protein with a sugar attached to it). Human EPO has a molecular weight of 34,000. Using recombinant DNA technology, EPO has been synthetically produced for use in persons with certain types of anemia, such as the type due to kidney failure, that secondary to AZT treatment of AIDS, and that associated with cancer.

The kidney cells that make EPO are specialized and are sensitive to low oxygen levels in the blood. These cells release EPO when the oxygen level is low in the kidney. EPO then stimulates the bone marrow to produce more red cells and thereby increase the oxygen-carrying capacity of the blood. EPO is the prime regulator of red blood cell production. Its major functions are to promote the differentiation and development of red blood cells and to initiate the production of hemoglobin.

The theoretically obvious use of erythropoietin to boost low hemoglobin levels has been the topic of many research projects over the last 20 years. As

with many of the alternatives to allogeneic transfusion, it has not been the subject of hemovigilance.

It has been used to promote hemoglobin levels in those anemic patients awaiting elective surgery or in those undergoing PAD. The process of PAD will result in a decrease in the patient's hemoglobin level and therefore many patients will undergo surgery with a lower hematocrit and hemoglobin than they would have done if no PAD had been performed. To avoid this, and in an attempt to promote erythropoiesis, recombinant EPO has been used sometimes combined with oral or intravenous iron.[28–30]

EPO is thought to be especially dangerous if not closely monitored when being used in this way because an increase in the viscosity of the blood may increase the risk for heart attacks and strokes. The use of EPO is not recommended when a patient's hemoglobin is within the normal range, and even when used in patients with low levels of hemoglobin thrombo-embolic events can occur.

It is recognized that critical-care patients become anemic due to a number of factors including daily venesection for investigations, surgical interventions, and disordered erythropoiesis.[31,32] The use of recombinant erythropoietin to help stimulate the bone marrow has not proved to be as beneficial as expected with only minor increases in hemoglobin levels and small changes in transfusion incidences. Numerous studies show that there is very little benefit in terms of increased Hb levels when used in populations of ICU patients.[33] However, there do seem to be advantages in some patient groups due to the presence of erythropoietin receptors in other areas of the body and the experimental evidence that cell apoptosis can be reduced when EPO is administered.[34]

One of the findings again in critically-ill patients was increased mortality from vTE especially when these patients were not on thrombo-prophylaxis. Surprising in the same study was the dramatic decreased mortality in trauma victims (adjusted hazard ratio, 0.37; 99% CI 0.19–0.72).[35]

In addition there is emerging evidence that these events are more common when EPO is used to treat anemia associated with cancer. In addition, the stimulatory effect of EPO may be detrimental in this subgroup of patients because tumor growth may be promoted.

The European Medicines Agency and FDA have warned against the use of EPO in cancer patients to treat anemia, stating that blood transfusion should be the preferred method of correcting anemia. The advice followed further evidence showing an increased risk of tumor progression, venous thrombo-embolism, and shorter overall survival in cancer patients who received epoetins than those who did not.

Perhaps if the use of erythropoietin had been associated with an ongoing registry of use, a number of the resulting problems with its use would have been more apparent, with patterns of adverse events being recognized sooner. Likewise the benefits, such as its effect on cell apoptosis, may have been revealed earlier.

Aprotonin

Aprotonin was used extensively as an agent that prevented clot breakdown by its anti-fibrinolytic properties. Cochrane systematic reviews and meta-analyses suggested how effective this drug was in reducing the need for red cell transfusion particularly in cardiothoracic surgery.[36,37] A study published in 2006 by Mangano concluded that the association between aprotonin and serious end organ damage indicated that continued use of aprotonin to minimize operative blood loss in cardiac surgery was not prudent, advocating the use of cheaper and apparently safer anti-fibrinolytics such as the less-expensive generic preparations of tranexamic acid and aminocaproic acid.[38]

A subsequent multicenter, blinded study came to a similar conclusion, It was stated that despite a modest reduction in the risk of massive bleeding the strong and consistent negative mortality trend associated with aprotonin, as compared with other lysine analogues, precluded its use in high-risk cardiac surgery.[39] The identification of these significant long-term problems with the use of the drug eventually led the FDA to advise against its use in cardiac surgery and this led to withdrawal

of the drugs license in the US and subsequently in many other countries.

Tranexamic acid

The successful CRASH 2 study[40] suggested that the use of 1 g of tranexamic acid immediately to blunt trauma victims, followed by 1 g over 8 hours by infusion, did not lead to an increase in mortality due to thrombo-embolic problems and in fact led to improved survival in these patients. It is likely that use of this drug will increase as a result, in the hope that it will have an impact on the amount of blood transfusion required in this group of patients.

It is very important therefore that adverse events are reported. The precise way of achieving this is not certain at the current time and often these patients may have multiple co-morbidities, making it difficult to establish causality when problems develop in the post-trauma phase of treatment.

Recombinant VIIa

The rather widespread and enthusiastic "off licence" use of this drug to help control bleeding in patients who had received massive transfusion, followed initial experience in severely traumatized young patients. The drug, which is highly effective in patients with antibodies to factor VIII, was used often as a last resort in patients who had developed a secondary coagulopathy following large volume blood transfusion. Its compassionate use was monitored closely, not least because of its cost, but outcome in the cases it was used for was difficult to assess. The drug seemed to be helpful in reducing bleeding but the longer-term effects were often difficult to assess.[41,42]

There has been no convincing level one evidence to support its use. In Australia and New Zealand where a registry of use was established data collected provided valuable insight in clinical areas where it may have been beneficial. Subsequent RCTs have failed to show a benefit in terms of long-term survival despite the obvious immediate benefit of usually slowing or stopping bleeding from an acquired coagulation problem. It seems that as alterations have been made to the datasheet guidance, its use in massive hemorrhage may well decline. However, the capture of data on its use and any outcome data remain of interest.

Hemovigilance of alternatives

As mentioned previously, hemovigilance is a system of epidemiological surveillance of the undesirable effects associated with the use of blood products and their substitutes. It contributes to ensuring the optimal safety of the blood supply system.

It requires continuous and standardized data collection and analysis as well as dissemination of results. Therefore, it makes it possible to estimate the frequency of undesirable events, determine their causes, and prevent their appearance in recipients. It also ensures the traceability of blood products, that is, enables them to be monitored from donor to recipient. Moreover, the purpose of the hemovigilance system is the early detection of the appearance or resurgence of problems related to blood products and their substitutes.

It would be useful to explain how such a hemovigilance system can be applied to a specific area of practice aimed at replacing or minimizing red blood cell transfusion, namely red cell salvage. As an example, this section describes how within the UK's SHOT hemovigilance process a section on autologous transfusion was commenced as a pilot in 2007 and subsequently led to the establishment of a permanent section within the reporting system.

In the 2009 report there were 14 cases reported to SHOT concerning autologous transfusion. There were six related to intra-operative cell salvage and eight to post-operative cell salvage. There were five reports related to adverse reactions connected to post-operatively collected, unwashed autologous transfusion, including pyrexia, rigors, and bradycardia. Of the six intra-operative cell salvage cases, there were three hypotensive incidents, one machine error, and two operator errors. The mechanical failure of a laboratory machine may or may not lead to a clinically significant event. However, in the near-patient situation where there

may be less time to allow for machine failure, such an event may lead to a decreased quality of care. In this incident, there was only wastage of the blood collected and no clinical harm came to the patient. In these situations a clinical need may result in allogeneic blood transfusion, which may be regarded as routine care in some institutions.

There were no deaths either directly or associated with autologous use and no significant morbidity.

Clearly this reporting is in its early stages and it is highly likely to be an underestimation of the adverse events that may be occurring. It will take some time to reach a situation where reporting of these incidents becomes widespread and so we anticipate year-on-year increases to the number of reports submitted related to this section. SHOT will continue to collect these reports and is working in close collaboration with the UK Cell Salvage Action Group (UKCSAG) to promote best practice in this area and encourage adverse-event reporting when it occurs.

At the same time it has been impossible to gauge how many procedures were being undertaken. Unlike the situation for allogeneic transfusion, it is difficult to judge the incidence of adverse events because the denominator is unknown. The UKCSAG is a subcommittee of the appropriate Use of Blood Group, which itself reports to the National Blood Transfusion Committee. The UKCSAG has attempted to set up a UK database for the registration of all cell salvage procedures undertaken by developing and then using a network of cell salvage users throughout the UK. This followed the successful establishment of an All Wales Cell Salvage Database situated within the Better Blood Transfusion Team based at the Welsh Blood Service. Procedures were documented on a standardized form (see Figure 25.1) and returned to a data collector who placed them on a database for further analysis.

The success of the scheme was dependent on a financial incentive to the hospitals, where a proportion of the cost of the cell salvage disposables was reimbursed to the hospitals on the return of a completed audit form.

This scheme worked on a number of levels. As blood is issued to hospitals based on historical

All Wales Intra-Operative Cell Salvage Data Collection Form

This form should be completed for every surgical case where blood has been collected with
the intention of intra-operative call salvage EVEN if the blood collected is not processed.

1. Trust	Hospital	For BBT use only

2. Patient Details		3. Procedure Details	
Hospital number		Name of procedure	
Surname			
Forename		Date of operation	/ /
D.O.B		In hours	Emergency
Address		Out of hours	Elective
		Malignancy	Infected fields
		Obstetrics	Trauma
		Jehovah's Witness	
		Surgeon	
		Anaesthetist	
		Cell Salvage Operator	
Age	Male	Female	Patient died	No	Yes

4. Cell Saver Equipment Used

BRAT	Electa	Cell Saver 5	Orthopat	CATS	Other
Anti-coag used	Heparin		Citrate		Other
Blood filter used	40µ filter		Leucodepletion filter		None

Collection reservoir	Lot No.
Harness set	Lot No.

5. Salvaged Blood Volume Details			6. Total No. allogeneic units transfused during hospital stay	
Processed	**Yes**	**No**		
Intra-op processed (ml)				
Volume of anticoagulant intra-op (ml)			Red cells	
Volume of irrigation used (ml)			FFP	
Volume of swab wash (ml)			Platelets (adult dose)	
Volume salvaged RBC intra-op (ml)			Cryoprecipitate	
Post-op processed (ml)			Other	
Volume of anticoagulant post-op (ml)				
Volume salvaged RBC intra-op (ml)				
Time collection started			Pre-Op Hb	
Time re-infusion started			Discharge Hb	

7. Reason of blood was not processed

Inadequate volume collection	Training purposes	Technical problem

8. Problems/Faults

Technical	Machine	Bowl	Harness	Software
	Other (Please state)			

Procedural (Operator/Surgeon/Patient)

	Operator error	Communication failure
	Training issue	Unforeseen circumstance

Top copy — Patient notes	2nd copy – Audit form – WBS

All Wales ICS Form Version 5   Revised September 2005

Figure 25.1 All Wales intra-operative cell salvage data collection form.

use, hospitals in Wales do not pay per unit of blood actually used and the contract payment is somewhat dissociated from blood used. It therefore becomes difficult to incentivize hospitals toward a more appropriate use of blood products. It was decided that the small financial incentive may help the spread of cell salvage use within Wales. Previous studies at Morriston hospital had shown a financial benefit to the finances of the hospital by the use of cell salvage autotransfusion resulting in a decrease in allogeneic use particularly in the surgical specialties. This reduced demand on Welsh Blood Service (WBS) supplies and made the supply of allogeneic red cells therefore more resilient.

An additional benefit was the collection of the audit of use-forms, because payment was not made unless these forms were received, resulting in a fairly accurate reporting system and allowing the collection of data on activity that can be used when combined with the adverse reports received—also outlined on the same forms if necessary (see Table 25.1).

Even more benefit can be realized because the data on specialty use can be collated and data on the amount of red cells and red cell volumes saved per case can be analyzed. The patterns of use, as well as patterns of salvaged volumes, can then be used as predictors of when it might be advisable to use cell salvage and when its use would be inappropriate.

Table 25.1 Summary of the All Wales database showing specialty use of the technique.

Procedure	Cases
Vascular	1252
Orthopedic	5277
Urology/Gyn.	1244
General	693
Obstetric	430
Cardiac	4691
Transplant	15
Other	103
Unknown	134
Training	25

The UKCSAG has received financial support to develop a UK database for cell salvage using an online reporting system, which it is hoped will encourage a more timely and less complicated reporting processes. This database, which is in its infancy at present, when combined with the SHOT initiative on autologous hemovigilance, will give the two essential components necessary to calculate the incidence of adverse events occurring in this area of transfusion practice (see Figures 25.2 and 25.3).

Specific problems that are unique to the alternative being used will also occur (see Figure 25.4).

It is worth commenting on the value of the monitoring of alternatives by describing an example of how a problem has been identified after only a handful of reports being received (see Figures 25.5 and 25.6). It is thought that the cause of the event can be explained theoretically and this is backed by some experimental data.[43]

Three cases of severe hypotension were reported during the 2008 reporting year to SHOT. These incidents have continued, it appears at a very low incidence, and to date there have been no fatalities or major morbidities. The exact cause of these events has not been identified although they all occur when cell salvaged washed blood is being re-infused via a leucodepletion filter (LDF). Profound but transient drops in blood pressure have occurred with recovery of blood pressure on stopping the infusion of the salvaged blood. It is postulated that this may be in response to cytokine release as the few remaining white cells in the washed blood degranulate when in contact with the filter. Although bedside reaction was reported with allogeneic blood infusion with LDP filters, the reaction may be more significant when using cell saved blood that is already warmer at the time of re-infusion than stored red cells. It is likely that in some of these incidents there was an attempt to pressurize the blood through the filter again, a process that may make white cell fragmentation worse. Offering a theoretical explanation for the hypotension, vasoactive substances created by this degranulation have a short half-life. If the blood is being re-infused quickly it will have a more significant effect

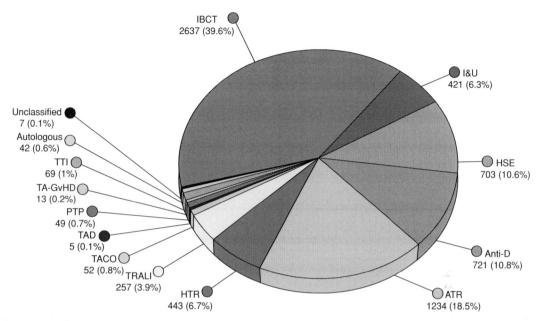

Figure 25.2 This graph shows the small percentage of reports arising from autologous blood transfusion. At this time it is anticipated there is significant under-reporting due to inadequate awareness and monitoring. A color version of this chart is available at the SHOT website www.shotuk.org (*source:* SHOT 2009).

	Total	IBCT	I&U	HSE	ANTI-D†	ATR	HTR	TRALI	TACO	TAD	PTP	TA-GvHD	TTI	AUTOL-OGOUS
Death in which transfusion reaction was causal or contributory	138	27	4	0	0	19	11	42	5	0	2	13	15	0
Major morbidity probably or definitely attributed to transfusion reaction (imputability 2/3)	495	116	3	0	25	58	48	165	18	1	13	0	48	0
Minor or no morbidity as a result of transfusion reaction	5998	3439	161	335	361	1154	383	50	29	4	34	0	6	42
Outcome unknown	15	11	0	0	0	3	1	0	0	0	0	0	0	0
TOTAL*	**6646**	**3593**	**168**	**335**	**386**	**1234**	**443**	**257**	**52**	**5**	**49**	**13**	**69**	**42**

*Total excludes 7 cases from 1998–1999 that were not classified
†Cases with potential for major morbidity included in the Anti-D data are excluded from this table

Figure 25.3 A summary and breakdown of autologous reports received (*source:* SHOT 2009).

Definition

Any adverse event or reaction associated with autologous transfusion including intraoperative and postoperative cell salvage (washed or unwashed), acute normovolaemic haemodilution or preoperative autologous donation.

DATA SUMMARY							
Total number of cases		14	**Implicated components**			**Mortality/morbidity**	
			Autologous Red cells	14		Deaths due to transfusion	0
			FFP			Deaths in which reaction was implicated	0
			Platelets			Major morbidity	0
Gender		**Age**		**Emergency vs. routine and core hours vs. out of core hours**		**Where transfusion took place**	
Male	5	18 years+	13	Emergency	2	ED	
Female	2	16 years+ to 18 years	1	Routine	11	Theatre + ITU/NNU/	
Unknown	7	1 year+ to 16 years	0	Not known	1	HDU/Recovery	6
		28 days+ to 1 year	0			Wards	8
		Birth to 28 days	0	In core hours	5	Community	
				Out of core hours	1	Other	
		Total	14	Not known/applicable	8	Not known	

Figure 25.4 Cumulative mortality/morbidity data 1999–2009 (TACO, TAD, and Autologous are new since 2008, and NSE and I&U were separated from IBCT in 2008).

on the recipient. The process of leucodepletion pre-storage for allogeneic blood means these vasoactive substances have disappeared by the time of re-infusion.

On the strength of these reports, the advice is to ensure that practitioners become aware of the problem and recognize it when it occurs. Treatment involves stopping the re-infusion and if need be treat with another less reactive fluid and the use of simple vasoconstrictors. The effect of the cytokines is short-lived and apparently easily reversible. If the need for red cells remains crucial, as in a massive hemorrhage situation, removal of the LDP altogether may be a justified step and commencement of the washed salvaged blood without the filter (see Figure 25.7).

This example serves to illustrate how the collection of adverse events via a hemovigilance process has great value for its qualitative reporting even if it is not possible to quantify the significance by producing a figure of true incidence of the event.

ICS incidents _n_ = 6

- Operator errors
  - Heparinized saline used in wrong bag, 1 case

- Machine errors
  - Faulty optic - red cells spilled into waste bag, 2 cases

- Clinical adverse events
  - Hypotension, 3 cases

Figure 25.5 Cell salvage incidents (_source:_ SHOT 2009).

PCS incidents _n_ = 8

- 1 system not assembled correctly

- 1 wrong infusion set used

- 5 pyrexia, rigor or bradycardia

- 1 excessive time to transfuse

Figure 25.6 Incidents reported with post-operative cell salvage (_source:_ SHOT 2009).

RECOMMENDATIONS

There are no new recommendations for this year.

Recommendations still relevant from last year

Year first made	Recommendation	Target	Progress
2008	All cell salvage operators must undertake initial and regular update training and be assessed as competent. There should be documented evidence of competence in the form of a training record. Competency-assessment workbooks are available for both ICS and PCS at www.transfusionguidelines.org.uk	**Cell salvage leads/HTT**	Online survey currently being undertaken by the UK Cell Salvage Action Group, asking about training and competency. Education workbook produced and available on the website.
2008	All ICS and PCS related adverse events should be reported to SHOT.	**Cell salvage leads/HTT**	There is a specially designed section of the new web-based SHOT reporting system to facilitate this.
2008	Monitoring of patients is as important for the reinfusion of red cells collected by ICS or PCS as it is for allogeneic red cells.	**Cell salvage leads/HTT**	
2008	Cell salvage machines are classified as Medical Devices, so all adverse events attributable to machine errors and failures should be reported to the MHRA as well as SHOT.	**Cell salvage leads/HTT**	

Figure 25.7 Recommendations highlighting areas of practice that need development and reminding of the need to report adverse events (*source:* SHOT 2009).

References

1 Vries RRP, Faber J-C, and Strengers PFW, 2011, Haemovigilance: An effective tool for improving transfusion practice. *Vox Sang* **100**(1): 60–7.

2 Popovsky M, *et al.*, 1997, Preoperative autologous blood donation. In Spiess BD, and Shander A (eds) *Perioperative Transfusion Medicine*. Williams and Wilkins, Baltimore, MD, USA.

3 European Union, 2003, Directive 2002/98/EC of the European Parliament and of the Council of 27 January 2003 setting standards of quality and safety for the collection, testing, processing, storage and distribution of human blood and blood components and amending Directive 2001/83/EC. *Official Journal of the European Union* L33/30–40.

4 Messmer K. *et al.*, 1967, Uberleban von Hunden bei acuter Verminderung der O2-Transportkapaziitat auf 2.8 g% Hamaglobin. *Pfugers Arch Physiol* **297**: R48.

5 Messmer K, 1975, Haemodilution. *Surg Clin North Am* **55**: 659.

6 Habler O, Kleen M, Kemming G, and Zwissler B, 2002, Hyperoxia in extreme hemodilution. *Eur Surg Res* **34**(12): 181–7.

7 Saricaoglu F, Akinci SB, Celiker V, and Aypar U, 2005, The effect of acute normovolaemic hemodilution and acute hypervolaemic hemodilution on coagulation and allogeneic transfusion. *Saudi Med J* **26**(5): 792–8.

8 Brecher ME, and Rosenfeld M, 1004, Mathematical and computer modelling of acute normovolaemic hemodilution. *Transfusion* **34**: 176–9.

9 National Institute for Heath and Clinical Excellence, 2005, Intraoperative blood cell salvage in obstetrics. Information about NICE Interventional Procedure Guidance No. 144. http://www.nice.org.uk/nicemedia/live/11038/30691/30691.pdf [accessed February 18, 2012].

10 SHOT, 2010, Annual Report 2009. http://www.shotuk.org/wp-content/uploads/2010/07/SHOT2009.pdf [accessed February 18, 2012].

11 National Institute for Heath and Clinical Excellence, 2008, Intraoperative red blood cell salvage during radical prostatectomy or radical cystectomy. Information about NICE Interventional Procedure Guidance No. 258. http://www.nice.org.uk/nicemedia/pdf/IPG258Guidance.pdf [accessed February 18, 2012].

12 AuBuchon JP, and Popovsky MA, 1991, The safety of preoperative autologous blood donation in the non-hospital setting. *Transfusion* **31**: 513–7.

13 Popovsky MA, Whitaker B, and Arnold NL, 1995, Severe outcomes of allogeneic and autologous blood donation: Frequency and characterization. *Transfusion* **35**: 734–7.

14 Goodnough LT, Grishaber JE, Birkmeyer JD, *et al.*, 1994, Efficacy and cost effectiveness of autologous blood predeposit in patients undergoing radical prostatectomy procedures *Urology* **44**(2): 226–31.

15 Birkmeyer JD, Goodnough LT, AuBuchon JP, *et al.*, 1993, The cost-effectiveness of preoperative autologous blood donation for total hip and knee replacement. *Transfusion* **33**: 544–51.

16 Spahn DR, Zollinger A, Schlumpf RB, Stöhr S, Seifert B, *et al.*, 1996, Hemodilution tolerance in elderly patients without known cardiac disease. *Anesth Analg* **82**: 681–6.

17 Spahn DR, Schmid ER Seifert B, and Pasch T, 1996, Hemodilution tolerance in patients with coronary artery disease who are receiving chronic beta-adrenergic blocker therapy. *Anesth Analg* **82**: 687–94.

18 Carvalho B, Ridler BM, Thompson JF, and Telford RJ, 2003, Myocardial ischemia precipitated by acute normovolaemic haemodilution. *Transfus Med* **13**: 165–8.

19 Meier J, Kemming G, Meisner F, Pape A, and Habler O, 2005, Hyperoxic ventilation enables hemodilution beyond the critical myocardial hemoglobin concentration. *R J Med Res* **10**(11): 462–8.

20 Jackson MR, MacPhee MJ, Drohan WN, Alving BM, 1996, Fibrin sealant: Current and potential clinical applications. *Blood Coagul Fibrinol* **7**: 737–46.

21 Cronkite EP, Lozner EL, and Deaver J, 1944, Use of thrombin and fibrinogen in skin grafting. *JAMA* **124**: 976–8.

22 Alving BM, Weinstein MJ, Finlayson JS, *et al.*, 1995, Fibrin sealant: Summary of a conference on characteristics and clinical uses. *Transfusion* **35**: 783–90.

23 Martinovitz U, and Saltz R, 1996, Fibrin sealant. *Curr Opin Hematol* **3**: 395–402.

24 Spotnitz WD, 1995, Fibrin sealant in the United States: Clinical use at the University of Virginia. *Thromb Haemost* **74**: 482–5.

25 Bergel S, 1909, Uber Wirkungen des Fibrins. *Drsch Med Wochenschr* **35**: 633.

26 Berguer R, Staerkel RL, Moore EE, *et al.*, 1991, Fatal reaction to the use of fibrin glue in deep hepatic wounds. *J Trauma* **31**: 408–11.

27 Ebner FM, Paul A, Peters J, *et al.*, 2011, Venous air embolism and intracardiac thrombus after pressurised fibrin glue during liver surgery. *BJ Anaes* **106**: 180–2.

28 de Pree C, Mermillod B, Hoffmeyer P, *et al.*, 1997, Recombinant human erythropoietin as adjuvant treatment for autologous blood donation in elective surgery with large blood needs (≥5units): a randomised study. *Transfusion* **37**: 708–14.

29 Mercurali F, Gualtieri G, Sanigaglia L, *et al.*, 1994, Use of recombinant human erythropoietin to assist autologous blood donation by anemic rheumatoid patients undergoing major orthopaedic surgery. *Transfusion* **34**: 501–6.

30 Price TH, Goodnough LT. Vogler WR, *et al.*, 1996, The effect of recombinant human erythropoietin on the efficacy of autologous blood donation in patients with low hematocrits: A multicentre, randomised, double blind, controlled trial. *Transfusion* **36**: 29–36.

31 Vincent JL, Baron JF, Reinhart K, *et al.*, 2002, Anemia and blood transfusion in critically ill patients. *JAMA* **288**: 1499–507.

32 Corwin HL, Gettinger A, Pearl RG, *et al.*, 2004, The CRIT study: Anaemia and blood transfusion in the critically ill-current clinical practice in the United States. *Crit Care Med* **32**: 39–52.

33 Corwin HL, Gettinger A, Pearl RG, *et al.*, 2002, Efficacy of recombinant human erythropoietin in critically ill patients: A randomized controlled trial. *JAMA* **288**: 2827–35.

34 van de Meer P, and Lipsic E 2006, Erythropoietin: Repair of the failing heart. *J. Am Coll Cardiol* **48**(1): 185–6.

35 Corwin HL, Gettinger A, Fabian TC, *et al.*, 2007, Efficacy and safety of epoetin alfa in critically ill patients. *N Eng J Med* **357**: 965–76.

36 Laupacis A, and Fergusson D, 1997, Drugs to minimize perioperative blood loss in cardiac surgery: Meta-analyses using perioperative blood transfusion as the outcome. *Anesth Analg* **85**: 1258–67.

37 Henry DA, Carless PA, Moxey AJ, *et al.*, 2007, Antifibrinolytic use for minimising perioperative allogeneic blood transfusion. *Cochrane Database Syst Rev* **4**: CD001886.

38 Mangano DT, Tudor JC, and Dietzel C, 2006, The risk associated with aprotonin in cardiac surgery. *N Eng J Med* **354**: 353–65.

39 Fergusson DA, Hebert PC, Mazer CD, *et al.*, 2008, A comparison of aprotonin and lysine analogues in high risk cardiac surgery. *N Eng J Med* **358**: 2319–31.

40 CRASH-2 trial collaborators, 2010, Effects of tranexamic acid on death, vascular occlusive events, and blood transfusion in trauma patients with significant haemorrhage (CRASH-2): A randomised, placebo-controlled trial. *Lancet* **376**(9734): 23–32.

41 Martinowitz U, Kenet G, Segal E, *et al.*, 2001, Recombinant activated factor VII for adjunctive hemorrhage control in trauma. *J Trauma* **51**: 431–38.

42 Martinowitz U, and Michaelson M, 2005, Guidelines for the use of recombinant activated factor VII (rFVIIa) in uncontrolled bleeding: A report by the Israeli Multidisciplinary rFVIIa Task Force. *J Thromb Haemost* **3**: 640–48.

43 Iwama H, 2001, Bradykinin-associated reactions in white cell-reduction filter. *Journal of Critical Care* **16**(2): 74–81.

CHAPTER 26

Surveillance of Clinical Effectiveness of Transfusion

Brian McClelland and Katherine Forrester
Scottish National Blood Transfusion Service, Edinburgh, UK

Introduction

In 1972, a distinguished predecessor in Edinburgh wrote a very far-sighted and characteristically modest statement that remains as relevant today as it was 40 years ago: "One of the factors of paramount importance in developing the range and quality of service which medicine will in future demand of us is the nature and extent of the requirement for the various components of blood. For this, collaborative clinical trials are essential."[1]

This might be casually dismissed as a statement of the obvious or, alternatively, could be taken as a text to guide our efforts to establish powerful surveillance data about the effectiveness of transfusion.

Why we transfuse blood components

Benefits

The only reason for giving a patient a treatment with as much potential for hazard as a blood transfusion is to make the person better. The patient may derive benefit in one of two ways. Transfusion may be used to replace some constituent of the blood that is believed to be defective or lacking in a way that affects the patient's health (for example, platelet transfusion for thrombocytopenic bleeding), or to provide support that makes it possible to subject the patient to another effective intervention such as surgery or chemotherapy (for example, platelet transfusion during a period of bone-marrow failure caused by chemotherapy).

We have chosen these examples because there is a clinical concensus, supported by a body of data from clinical trials, that both therapeutic and prophylactic platelet transfusion are clinically effective (although even with this example, there are some important reservations about prophylactic platelet transfusion).[2]

Risks

The patient and clinician need to know in advance the probability that the patient will have a net benefit from transfusion (more good than harm = effective treatment) and when the harms outweigh any benefit (more harm than good = bad medicine). It is important for all concerned in the healthcare process—patient, doctor, funder, or researcher into the effectiveness of care—to know in what circumstances a treatment such as transfusion is effective. Patients and their clinicians need to know, before the decision is taken to transfuse blood, that there is a strong probability that it will offer a net benefit. Funders, researchers, and policymakers—if they are to make rational decisions about the allocation of resources—need to know to what extent transfusion has benefited the health of the population for which they are responsible.

Hemovigilance: An Effective Tool for Improving Transfusion Safety, First Edition. Edited by René R.P. De Vries and Jean-Claude Faber.
© 2012 John Wiley & Sons, Ltd. Published 2012 by John Wiley & Sons, Ltd.

What is meant by hemovigilance

In this book hemovigilance has been defined as:

A set of surveillance procedures covering the whole transfusion chain (from the collection of blood and its components to the follow-up of recipients), intended to collect and assess information on unexpected or undesirable effects resulting from the therapeutic use of labile blood products, and to prevent their occurrence or recurrence.[3]

What hemovigilance can tell us

So defined, hemovigilance will provide us with information about effects of transfusion that cause harm (or that could predispose to a harmful effect). The value of this type of information is not in dispute, although it could be questioned whether there is high-quality evidence that would satisfy the health economist that expenditure on hemovigilance is justified by measurable improvements in outcome: "The risk of viral transmission has decreased by a factor greater than 1500 within the last 20 years. In comparison, the risk related to ABO error has decreased only by half."[4]

What hemovigilance does not tell us

Hemovigilance does not give us information about the health benefits of transfusion. Neither do current systems provide information about the adverse effects of failure to transfuse at a time when there is unarguable need (for example, insufficient or late ordering or slow provision of blood for obstetric hemorrhage).

The UK Confidential Enquiry into maternal deaths for the period 2000–2002, reported that 17 women died from hemorrhage; of these, 13 women sought obstetric care and were prepared to accept blood products. The following quote refers to these patients:

Most did have a transfusion, sometimes massive (range 7–82 units). Acknowledging the fact that death can occur very rapidly, it is nevertheless noteworthy that some women who died of haemorrhage seem to have received remarkably little blood. Despite repeated recommendations given in succes-

sive reports of this enquiry, some high-risk women are still being booked for delivery in hospitals with neither blood transfusion nor intensive care facilities on site and with poor lines of communication to the nearest of appropriate facilities. In one case, urgently needed blood had been withdrawn from the refrigerator by the blood transfusion service because it was out of date 30 minutes before it was required. One hospital reported malfunctioning of specimen transport systems, which led to delay in crossmatched blood being available.[5]

A further consideration is that the data collected by current hemovigilance systems may not identify possible influences of transfusion (or of higher hemoglobin levels) on all-cause mortality, such as the apparent negative effect of the liberal versus conservative transfusion regime observed in the TRICC study.[6]

A national study of anesthetic deaths in France revealed that some patients had died with profound anemia, in some cases with laboratory results documenting progressive falls in hemoglobin concentration over a number of days, and yet had not received any red cell transfusion.[7]

Information that would show how transfusion treatment influences the health of a population

Below is a suggested outline of the data required to describe the clinical use of blood components:
- Quantity of blood components *transfused.*
- Characteristics of the transfused patient population:
  - total population;
  - demography;
  - epidemiology.
- Clinical reasons for transfusion:
  - diseases;
  - interventions.
- Variations in use of blood for similar patient groups.
- Outcomes of transfusion: short and long-term:
  - health gain;
  - health loss;
  - net effectiveness.

Using these data, indicators of use of blood components would include the following:
- number of units transfused per 1000-population;
- proportion of the whole patient population transfused during a defined time period;
- proportion of patients with specified conditions and/or interventions transfused;
- rates of transfusion for patients with particular demographic features:
  - age;
  - gender;
  - socioeconomic or deprivation status.

Definitions and data quality

These broad outlines of the data conceal the need for rigorous attention to the precise definition of terms. Biggin et al.[8] reviewed blood utilization studies with the aim of describing methods that could be used for future comparative studies. They concluded that variability in methods precludes useful interpretation and understanding of comparisons of large, regional variations in blood use. The authors recommended that if blood utilization data is to be used for comparison or benchmarking of the factors associated with red cell transfusion, standardization and transparency of methods is essential. They proposed some basic standards for methodology in future studies:
- clear definitions of the source population and the means of appropriate selection of a representative study sample;
- clear definitions of data sources (specifically for transfusion events/records and records or episodes of clinical care) and clear definitions of record linkage processes;
- comparable methods for the classification of clinical data, the definition of clinical case groups, and the reporting of findings by case group;
- defined methods to associate transfusion events with clinical data including the definition of relevant time frames;
- use of a small number of standard metrics to facilitate comparison of findings.

A number of recent studies show how improvements in methods are leading to a point where data from different areas or countries could usefully be compared. For example, Madsen et al. analyzed data for the entire population of one county in Denmark and proposed that an age-standardized prevalence rate was necessary for meaningful comparisons between populations.[9] In the UK, the EASTR study[10,11] used a new approach to combine the ICD-10 codes with the surgical procedure codes to improve the assignment of clinical indication for transfusion. Bosch et al. collected data on transfused patients over four one-week periods in one year from every hospital in Catalonia, and used population and demographic data from the national statistics agency to estimate denominators.[12]

Transfusion and survival in a population

Kamper-Jørgensen et al. studied a population-based cohort of transfusion recipients in Denmark and Sweden, followed for up to 20 years after their first blood transfusion, and reported all-cause mortality among transfusion recipients as absolute rates and rates relative to the general population.[13]

Out of more than 1 million transfusion recipients, 62.0% were aged 65 years or older at the time of their first registered transfusion. Survival at 1, 5, and 20 years after transfusion was 73.7, 53.4, and 27.0%, respectively. The first three months after the first transfusion, the standardized mortality ratio (SMR) was 17.6 times higher in transfusion recipients than in the general population. One to four years after first transfusion, the SMR was 2.1 and even after 17 years the SMR remained significantly 1.3-fold increased. Prospective randomized controlled studies with long follow-up periods will be required to explore the extent to which transfusion itself—rather than factors that lead to transfusion—contributes to such excess mortality.

Hemovigilance in the future

One way in which hemovigilance programs might direct their resources in the future is to extend their scope to include the collection of data required for surveillance of the use of blood components and the associated outcomes. The availability of national or regional databases of population, demographic, healthcare, and mortality data can facilitate the assembly and analysis of data that should help us to understand better the variations in the use of blood components and the associated outcomes.

References

1 Cumming RA, 1972, Blood and blood products. *Proc Roy Soc Edinb B* **71**(Suppl 1): S3–6 [text slightly modified from the original].

2 Wandt H, Schäfer-Eckart K, Wendelin K, Rottmann M, Thalmeimer M, *et al.*, 2009, A therapeutic platelet transfusion strategy without routine prophylactic transfusion is feasible and safe and reduces platelet transfusion numbers significantly: Final analysis of a randomised study after high-dose chemotherapy and PBSCT. *Bone Marrow Transplantation* **43**(Suppl 1s): S23.

3 International Hemovigilance Network, 2011, Definition of hemovigilance. [cited February 1, 2011]. Available from www.ihn-org.com.

4 Auroy Y, Andreu G, Aullen JP, Benhamou D, Caldani C, *et al.*, 2010, Patient safety and root cause analysis. *Transfus Clin Biol* **17**(5–6): 386–9.

5 CEMACH (Confidential Enquiry into Maternal and Child Health), 2004, *Confidential Enquiry into Maternal and Child Health. Why Mothers Die 2000–2002: The Sixth Report of the Confidential Enquiries into Maternal Deaths in the United Kingdom*. RCOG Press: London.

6 Hébert PC, Wells G, Blajchman MA, Marshall J, Martin C, *et al.*, 1999, A multicenter, randomized, controlled clinical trial of transfusion requirements in critical care. Transfusion Requirements in Critical Care Investigators, Canadian Critical Care Trials Group. *N Engl J Med* **340**(6): 409–17.

7 Auroy Y, Lienhart A, Pequinot F, and Benhamou D, 2007, Complications related to blood transfusion in surgical patients: Data from the French national survey on anaesthesia-related deaths. *Transfusion* **47**(Suppl 2): 184S–9S.

8 Biggin K, Warner P, Prescott R, and McClelland B, 2007, A review of methods used in comprehensive, descriptive studies that relate red cell transfusion to clinical data. *Transfusion* **50**: 711–8.

9 Madsen JT, Kimper-Karl ML, Sprogøe U, Georgsen J, and Titlestad K, 2010, One year period prevalence of blood transfusion. *Transfus Med* **20**(3): 191–5.

10 Llewelyn CA, Wells AW, Amin M, Casbard A, Johnson AJ, *et al.*, 2009, The EASTR study: A new approach to determine the reasons for transfusion in epidemiological studies. *Transfus Med* **19**(2): 89–98.

11 Wells AW, Llewelyn CA, Casbard A, Johnson AJ, Amin M, *et al.*, 2009, The EASTR Study: Indications for transfusion and estimates of transfusion recipient numbers in hospitals supplied by the National Blood Service. *Transfus Med* **19**(6): 315–28.

12 Bosch MA, Contreras E, Madoz P, Ortiz P, Pereira A, and Pujol MM, on behalf of the Catalonian Blood Transfusion Epidemiology Study Group, 2011, The epidemiology of blood component transfusion in Catalonia, Northeastern Spain. *Transfusion* **51**(1): 105–16.

13 Kamper-Jørgensen M, Ahlgren M, Rostgaard K, Melbye M, Edgren G, *et al.*, 2008, Survival after blood transfusion. *Transfusion* **48**(12): 2577–84.

CHAPTER 27

Biovigilance

Jerry A. Holmberg[1], Matthew J. Kuehnert[2], and D. Michael Strong[3]

[1]Formerly of the US Department of Health and Human Services, currently Novartis Vaccines and Diagnostics, Inc., Emeryville, CA, USA

[2]Division of Healthcare Quality Promotion, Centers for Disease Control and Prevention (CDC), Atlanta, GA, USA

[3]Department of Orthopaedics and Sports Medicine, University of Washington School of Medicine, Seattle, WA, USA

Definition of biovigilance and surveillance

Hemovigilance systems have been implemented in most developed countries to monitor the adverse reactions and errors associated with the transfusion of blood products. In the early stages of hemovigilance, the concept was little more than coordination of existing data but over the years analysis and process improvement has led to enhanced patient safety and donor health.

Clearly the monitoring of blood and blood components adverse events is just one aspect of total biological product surveillance based on risk that is inherent in substances of human origin. Aspects of donor health and patient safety are shared concerns related to transfusion (e.g., blood, blood products, and fractionated plasma products) and transplantations (e.g., organs, human cells, tissues, and cellular- and tissue-based products).

Biovigilance extends the term hemovigilance beyond blood to incorporate monitoring of reactions/events associated with tissue, organs, and cellular components. The term biovigilance can be deconstructed to help understand the meaning of the word. First, the prefix "bio" comes from the Greek meaning "life". In the context of our discussion, this is referred to as the biological products that sustain life and includes blood, blood components, organs, human cells, tissues, and cellular and tissue-based products (HCT/Ps). "Vigilance" is, of course, the state of being attentive or watchful, which implies that vigilance is influenced by the attitude or motivation to be actively engaged.

Some experts have framed the basic elements of biovigilance as including: adverse event (AE) monitoring (for recipients and donors), product quality assurance (including processing controls and error management), and emerging threat assessment using epidemiologic and laboratory data (e.g., TTI bioinformatics, repositories). The World Health Organization (WHO) guideline on AE reporting emphasizes that the effectiveness of such systems should be measured not only by data reporting and analysis, but also by the use of such systems to improve patient safety.[1] In operational terms, this is Monitoring and Evaluation (M&E) for improved patient/donor safety.

There are two main types of surveillance approaches to these issues:

- utilizing aggregate data to analyze trends to reveal new concerns or the efficacy of interventions or policies; or
- utilizing a "sentinel network" to detect quickly singular events that may have public health impact.

The former has been described as "cold" or "passive" surveillance, while the latter has been described as "hot "or "active" surveillance.

When examining frameworks for the implementation of biovigilance systems, including the use of such systems for quality improvement, one must consider what types of events are captured in M&E.

For instance, in order to capture rare events that are of significant singular importance for patient safety, a sentinel system should be

- extremely sensitive, perhaps at the expense of specificity;
- operated in real time in order to allow immediate registry of events; and
- configured so that communication about the event allows critical response actions to take place.

On the other hand, surveillance of more common events of interest may be more comprehensive. Capture of more common events also may allow benchmarking through comparison of event rates among facilities, which are most helpful if they are adjusted for factors that are not the focus of comparison. Such risk-adjusted rates allow valid comparisons and analysis, so that a quality program can be implemented and continuously evaluated, before, during, or after an intervention takes place.

An effective biovigilance program should be operationally capable of providing the core tools, infrastructure, and logistics necessary to support timely communication of critical information to the right people, in order to make essential real-time interventions to avert clinical catastrophe and protect public health.

Background of need

Advances in science and healthcare technology have led to more biologic products being collected to sustain and improve the quality of human life. In the United States (US) in 2008, over 23 million units of blood or blood products, 28,000 organs, and 2 million tissue allografts were transfused or transplanted.[2] Despite these large numbers, demand often exceeds availability, particularly for organs. Challenges exist to monitor and ensure appropriate access to and availability of safe products, both in the domestic and global arenas. Also, efforts to increase the availability of these products may increase the opportunities for transmission of infectious pathogens, including viruses, bacteria, parasites, and prions. These risks are mul-

tiplied when there are multiple recipients from a common donor. Examples of diseases or organisms transmitted through blood, organs, or other tissues include: Human Immunodeficiency Virus (HIV), hepatitis B virus (HBV), hepatitis C virus (HCV), human T-cell lymphotrophic virus types I and II (HTLV-I/II), West Nile virus (WNV), rabies virus, lymphocytic choriomeningitis virus (LCMV), Group A Streptococcus, *Mycobacterium tuberculosis*, malaria, babesiosis, variant Creutzfeldt-Jakob Disease (vCJD), and *Trypanosoma cruzi* (the etiologic agent of Chagas disease). Transmitted malignancies have been reported primarily through organ transplantation.

Beyond disease transmission, other concerns include adverse immunologic response, reaction to toxins, or decrease in expected function. These noninfectious events may be due to deficiencies in the product, or a mismatch between the product and recipient immunologic profile, but consequences may be as severe as for infectious disease transmission events.

Biologic-based products or technologies are likely always to carry an inherent risk. Although solid organs cannot be altered to reduce infectivity, some tissues can be processed with chemicals or radiation, and blood can be modified, for example, through leukocyte filtration or irradiation. However, no process can completely eliminate the inherent risks of transfusion and transplantation. The role of patient-safety efforts is to drive that risk to the lowest level reasonably achievable without unduly decreasing the availability of these life-saving resources, so that the overall benefit outweighs risk.

In the US, a great example of success in vigilance has been in recognition of the magnitude of healthcare-associated infections (HAI). Although this surveillance for HAIs has been in place within local medical institutions for many years, the impact on patient safety and healthcare cost has been only recently realized. Patient safety and cost recovery data are only currently becoming available but indicate that huge cost savings can be made if proper vigilance systems are used as part of a total quality system. Only by starting to look at various processes within the healthcare setting can one become aware of the health burden and the impact on health economics. While many in the health professions would like to believe that healthcare changes are made for improved patient outcomes, in reality the cost of change and the mitigation strategies to avoid adverse outcomes ultimately is the driving force.

Coordinating public health and approach to risk

In an effective biovigilance program, there needs to be integration of surveillance into the quality system of blood, organs, and HCT/P into all aspects of public health. It is not just monitoring or surveillance but analysis of processes, products, and patient/donor outcome to prevent AEs and improve the process. Human errors, process errors including equipment, or supply defects can compromise donor health and the biologic outcome in patients. There can also be unknown causes of adverse outcomes, such as with emerging infectious diseases (EID). Being vigilance to monitor, detect, and analyze data as available is essential for an effective biovigilance program.

Risk of human errors, process errors, near-misses, quality of the product, and outcome to the patient should be detectable through various checkpoints in a quality process. As data are collected, they can be analyzed for cause through risk assessment. Once the risks are identified and assessed for probable cause, strategies for mitigation and appropriate risk management through process improvement, standards of practice, or regulations can implemented.

Throughout both the risk analysis and risk-management activities of biovigilance, risk needs to be communicated carefully and transparently to all stakeholders (see Figure 27.1). Although the level of communication must be messaged appropriately for the audience, risk and benefits of findings must be adequately communicated for appropriate informed consent from the patient, family members, and healthcare providers.

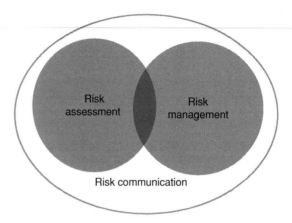

Figure 27.1 Public health biovigilance view to risk communication, once the risk has been analyzed and mitigation strategies have been identified for effective management.

Biovigilance in the United States: Efforts to bridge a critical gap in patient safety and donor health

In many developed or developing countries, the responsibility of public health lies with the Minister of Health. In the US, this is equivalent to the Secretary of Health and Human Services (HHS) who designates the Assistant Secretary of Health (ASH) to coordinate Public Health Services (PHS) and to ensure the safety of the US blood supply. This role was established as an outcome of an internal review of the Institute of Medicine's report in the mid-1990s. The ASH carefully considers public discussion of issues and recommendations from the Advisory Committee on Blood Safety and Availability (ACBSA). In addition, the ASH leads internal government discussions with the Blood, Organ, and Tissue Senior Executive Council (BOT-SEC), which provides input and recommendations on transfusion and transplantation safety matters.

Coordinated safety and public health efforts are shared among operating divisions of HHS, the Centers for Disease Control and Prevention (CDC), the Food and Drug Administration (FDA), the National Institutes of Health (NIH), the Health Resources and Services Administration (HRSA), and the Centers for Medicare and Medicaid Services (CMS).[3]

The FDA has regulatory responsibility for blood and blood products, and takes on most of the risk management. In the US, blood and plasma is collected, processed, and distributed by private industry that is regulated by the FDA primarily under the authority of two national laws.[4,5]

Blood collection and transfusion organizations also comply with state laws and voluntary standards developed by stakeholder organizations such as the AABB (formerly the American Association of Blood Banks) and the PPTA (Plasma Protein Therapeutics Association). Interstate distribution of biological products (including distribution outside of the US) is only permissible under FDA license. There are approximately 1090 FDA-licensed blood-collection establishments and 374 FDA-licensed plasma-collection establishments. Approximately 770 unlicensed but registered whole-blood facilities collect and manufacture blood components for intrastate distribution.

Reporting to the FDA is required for blood and blood components when a fatal AE occurs related to donation or transfusion.[6] Based on data collected in 2009, the top five leading transfusion-related fatality categories were: Transfusion Related Acute Lung Injury (TRALI) (30%); Transfusion Associated Circulatory volume Overload (TACO) (27%); non-ABO hemolytic transfusion reaction (18%), microbial infection (11%), and ABO blood group hemolytic transfusion reactions (9%). Collection of information from the currently required FDA fatality reports for disorders such as TRALI have led to increased understanding of the possible role of plasma and antibodies (anti-HLA and anti-leukocyte antibodies) in TRALI pathogenesis.

In addition, there is a requirement for licensed and registered blood establishments and transfusion services to file biological product deviation reports when a deviation from standards, such as a variation in current Good Manufacturing Practice (GMP), may affect the safety, purity, or potency of a blood product and the unit leaves the facility's or a contracted facility's control before the problem is identified and rectified. For nonfatal AEs, blood collection and transfusion facilities are required to conduct investigations and maintain records and reporting to the FDA is encouraged, but not required, and is uncommon.

Medical device manufacturers must submit AE reports to the FDA involving deaths and serious injuries or illnesses connected with medical devices used for the collection or administration of blood components for patient treatment or diagnosis.

For voluntary reporting related to any FDA-regulated product, patients, family members, physicians, pharmacists, and any other reporter can submit information to the FDA's AE Reporting System (AERS)/MedWatch.[7] This system gathers information on a variety of products including drugs, devices, and other medical and nutritional products.

Regulatory oversight of hospital transfusion services occurs through the CMS or accredited organizations granted deemed status under the Clinical Laboratory Improvement Amendment of 1988 (CLIA). Although transfusion services are subject to applicable FDA regulations, they are not required to register with the FDA unless they also manufacture blood or blood components and they are not routinely inspected by the FDA. However, hospital transfusion service laboratories are required to be certified by the CLIA program, and they are routinely surveyed for CLIA compliance. CLIA regulations require laboratories to report transfusion fatalities to the FDA, and the CMS and FDA routinely cooperate in the investigation of these fatalities. CLIA regulations directly reference certain FDA regulations that apply to transfusion services.

The CDC's mission is to collaborate with state and local health departments to create the expertise, information, and tools needed to protect public health through health promotion, disease prevention, and preparedness for new health threats. Areas of focus concerning blood, organ, and tissue safety at the CDC include public health investigation, surveillance, research, prevention, and risk communication. A CDC objective is to improve surveillance for AEs associated with the use of biologic products (e.g., blood, organs, and tissues), vaccines, drugs, or devices by coordinating HHS efforts to enhance rapid detection and implementation of novel prevention. Proposed measures and actions include implementation of transfusion and transplant AE surveillance. One CDC system for healthcare-related event surveillance is the National Healthcare Safety Network (NHSN). The NHSN is a secure internet-based surveillance system that collects data from voluntarily participating healthcare facilities in the US to permit benchmarking of AEs, including HAI, among patients and healthcare personnel.

The CDC has had in place since 1998 a blood-safety monitoring system in the bleeding disorder community, the Universal Data Collection program, managed by the Division of Blood Disorders, which provides annual testing for hepatitis and HIV and stores blood specimens in a serum bank for use in future blood-safety investigations.[8] The CDC works with local state health departments to investigate any seroconversions in bleeding disorder patients. A similar system has been established in several centers in the US that treat patients with thalassemia who depend on frequent blood transfusions for survival. Currently there are over 70,000 plasma specimens on patients with bleeding disorders (primarily hemophilia) and about 1000 specimens on patients with thalassemia in the CDC bleeding-disorder repository.

The National, Heart, Lung, and Blood Institute (NHLBI) of the NIH is responsible for funding basic, translational, and clinical research related to transfusion. Other than the National Institute for Diabetes and Digestive and Kidney Diseases, translational and clinical research for organ and HCT/P is limited.

The Division of Transplantation of the HRSA oversees the transplantation of human organs, including kidney, liver, heart, lung, pancreas, and intestine. The National Organ Transplant Act (NOTA) of 1984 established the Organ Procurement and Transplant Network (OPTN), resulting in a national computerized system to maintain a waiting list and allocate organs, including a 24-hour organ-recipient matching operations center. In 1986, the United Network for Organ Sharing (UNOS) was awarded the first contract to operate the OPTN, and has held the contract since then through a competitive award process. UNOS has developed an online database system, called UNet, for the collection, storage, analysis, and publication

of all OPTN data pertaining to the patient waiting list, organ matching, and transplants. The OPTN Final Rule became effective in March of 2000. This rule established a regulatory framework for operation of the OPTN, requirements for policy development, and member compliance with these policies, including policies consistent with the recommendations of the CDC for the testing of donors and follow-up of transplant recipients to prevent the spread of infectious diseases. The Division of Transplantation also administers the Scientific Registry for Transplant Recipients contract, as well as various grant programs and initiatives to increase organ donation and transplantation.

Through its oversight role, the HRSA monitors the activities of the OPTN to include member compliance with NOTA, the OPTN Final Rule, and other applicable federal law. The OPTN Final Rule requires the OPTN, with the assistance of the OPTN contractor, to review member compliance with federal law and regulations and the policies and bylaws of the OPTN. The OPTN contractor is also required to conduct periodic and special compliance reviews of OPTN members. Members found not to be in compliance are referred to the Membership and Professional Standards Committee (MPSC) for review. Unlike the on-site inspections conducted by the professional State Facility Surveyors under the CMS, much of the OPTN oversight is generally carried out through confidential peer reviews or on-site peer reviews by audit teams. The OPTN has the authority to take certain actions against OPTN members that are not in compliance, including issuing letters of warning, letters of admonition, letters of reprimand, placing the member on "Probation" and making the member a "Member Not in Good Standing." The two latter actions are public ones, which in the case of transplant programs may impact the program's ability to receive contracts from insurance companies. In addition to actions that may be taken by the OPTN, particularly egregious noncompliance issues may be referred by the OPTN Board of Directors to the Secretary of HHS for further action, including removing a transplant program's ability to receive donor organs and ability to participate in Medicare and Medicaid.

Solid organ transplant programs that participate in the Medicare program are required by the CMS to comply with the following Conditions of Participation (per 42 CFR Part 482.96) regarding AEs. The precise regulations, 42 CFR 482.69(b), are as follows:

> (b) *Standard: Adverse events.* A transplant center must establish and implement written policies to address and document AEs that occur during any phase of an organ transplantation case.
>
> **1** The policies must address, at a minimum, the process for the identification, reporting, analysis, and prevention of AEs.
>
> **2** The transplant center must conduct a thorough analysis of and document any AE and must utilize the analysis to effect changes in the transplant center's policies and practices to prevent repeat incidents.

The CMS has various options at its disposal to ensure transplant program compliance with these Conditions of Participation.

The FDA regulates HCT/Ps, which are defined as articles containing or consisting of human cells or tissues that are intended for implantation, transplantation, infusion, or transfer into a human recipient. Examples of HCT/Ps include bone, ligament, skin, dura mater, heart valves, cornea, tendon, oocytes, semen, and hematopoietic progenitor cells (HPCs) derived from peripheral and umbilical cord blood (UCB). Minimally manipulated bone marrow for homologous use and not combined with a drug or a device is not considered an HCT/P,

and is not regulated by the FDA. The HRSA has oversight of minimally manipulated bone marrow from unrelated donors. This oversight is executed through the Bone Marrow Coordinating Center, a component of the CW Bill Young Cell Transplantation Program, by contract with the National Marrow Donor Program (NMDP). Minimally manipulated bone marrow for homologous use that is not combined with another article and is for autologous or related use is not subject to federal oversight. For the most part, the collection and infusion of these products occurs in establishments that manufacture HPCs that are subject to oversight. Table 27.1 summarizes PHS agency responsibility for federal oversight/regulation of HPCs.

Together, these HHS agencies identify and respond to potential threats to blood, organ, and HCT/P safety, develop safety and technical standards, monitor supplies, and help industry provide an adequate supply. However, by their design, the existing systems focus primarily on reporting of sentinel events. The existing systems do not provide comprehensive baseline surveillance reporting of known events in relation to blood product exposures. Thus, in the US, currently it is not possible routinely to monitor AE rates outside of limited, specially designed studies.

AEs associated with HCT/P in the US

A major difference between blood, organs, and HCT/Ps is that many HCT/Ps undergo processing to disinfect; effectiveness of these methods varies

Table 27.1 US federal oversight/regulation of hematopoietic progenitor cells (minimally manipulated, for homologous use, and not combined with another article such as a drug or device).

Source	Marrow	Peripheral blood	Cord blood
Autologous	No federal regulation	FDA regulation as HCT/P	FDA regulation as HCT/P
Related allogeneic (first-degree or second-degree blood relative)	No federal regulation	FDA regulation as HCT/P	FDA regulation as HCT/P
Unrelated allogeneic	HRSA oversight of program*	HRSA oversight of program*; FDA regulation as HCT/P	HRSA oversight of program*; FDA regulation as HCT/P

*C.W. Bill Young Cell Transplantation Program

by processor, tissue type, and method employed. Although manufacturers validate their methods and have standard procedures, methods are not required to be FDA-reviewed before use, and the eventual risk of contamination of final products is not well-quantified, although it is understood to be quite low for many types of product and disinfection procedures. Better quantification of the potential risk based on the effectiveness of disinfection procedures will help investigators decide whether reported infections should be attributed to implanted tissues.

An adverse reaction, as defined by US federal regulation, means a noxious and unintended response to any HCT/P for which there is a reasonable possibility that the HCT/P caused the response. HCT/P manufacturers must investigate any adverse reaction involving a communicable disease related to an HCT/P they made available for distribution. Manufacturers must report to the FDA an adverse reaction involving a communicable disease if it is

- fatal;
- life-threatening;
- causes permanent impairment/damage; or
- necessitates medical or surgical intervention.

The current understanding of the risk of tissue-associated disease transmission largely is derived from what is learned from case reports because rates of transmission are unknown. For example, in 2001, the CDC investigated a case involving a musculoskeletal tissue allograft recipient who died as the result of *Clostridium* infection from a contaminated graft. In the course of its investigation, the CDC identified a total of 14 patients with *Clostridium* infections associated with musculoskeletal tissue allografts from this and other donors.[9] As a result of this case, the FDA published guidance for immediate implementation that emphasized existing regulatory requirements for the prevention of tissue contamination during processing.

In a 2005 article, investigators described transmission of HCV to several organ and tissue recipients from a donor who was antibody negative but later determined to be infected with HCV.[10] This case generated much publicity because of the numbers of organs and tissues (44 transplants into 40 recipients) produced from this single donor.

Through genetic comparison of isolates from donor and recipient serum, investigators determined that eight recipients (three organ recipients and five tissue recipients) were infected with HCV transmitted by the donor. Two of the tissue recipients and one organ recipient were diagnosed with HCV several months before many of the tissues were transplanted. Some of the subsequent tissue recipient infections would have been prevented if donor transmission had been recognized and communicated to the tissue establishments at the time of diagnosis of the three initial cases.

Another issue of significant concern is tracking of HCT/Ps to the level of the recipient. During 2005 and 2006, HHS became aware of two HCT/P recovery firms committing serious violations of federal regulations. An FDA investigation found that the firms were recovering tissues from donors in a manner that did not prevent the transmission of communicable disease. Other violations included creating and maintaining inaccurate and incomplete records related to: the medical/social history interview with next of kin; medical history, including place, time, and cause of death; and communicable disease screening and testing. These practices presented a danger to public health, and the FDA ordered the firms to cease manufacturing operations and retain tissues in inventory. In the first violation, tissue had been sent to a number of processors, then processed, distributed, and subdistributed. Tissues from over 1000 donors were recovered during a three-year period of time. An estimated 25,000 tissues were distributed to hospitals and other healthcare providers in the US and internationally for transplantation. The magnitude of distributions puts in perspective the current difficulties of timely tracking of HCT/Ps, something that is particularly important when there is concern about safety. A system such as the recently piloted Transplantation Transmission Sentinel Network (TTSN) is one such solution to these concerns.[11,12] Implementation of such a network may help to address issues related to tracking on a national level.

The lack of a uniform labeling standard as exists for blood and blood products may also contribute to the problems of tracking and traceability. The key to satisfying these requirements lies in standardization: globally unique identifiers for products, standardized terminology, and a means to convey information electronically that is recognized by computer systems throughout the world. Towards this end, *ISBT 128* coding has been developed and maintained by the International Council for Commonality in Blood Banking Automation (ICCBBA). The National Health Service Blood and Transplant, Tissue Services in the United Kingdom was the first to use *ISBT 128* for labeling tissues in 2003.[12,13] Since then, facilities in other countries have implemented the standard. In the US, the American Association of Tissue Banks (AATB) has been working with other organizations, and tissue banks, including the European Association of Tissue Banks (EATB), to establish common terminology for tissue products, the first step in the standardization process leading to universal coding.

Cell therapy organizations have moved toward universal acceptance of *ISBT 128*. In 2005 the Boards of Directors of AABB, American Society for Blood and Marrow Transplantation (ASBMT), American Society for Apheresis (ASFA), European Group for Blood and Marrow Transplantation (EBMT), Foundation for the Accreditation of Cellular Therapy (FACT), ICCBBA, International Society of Blood Transfusion (ISBT), International Society for Cellular Therapy (ISCT), ISCT Europe, Joint Accreditation Committee of ISCT and EBMT (JACIE), NMDP, and the World Marrow Donor Association (WMDA) released a Consensus Statement confirming their support for the international use of *ISBT 128* in the coding of hematopoietic progenitor cells and other therapeutic cell products and announcing the establishment of a cosponsored International Cellular Therapy Coding and Labelling Advisory Group.

This group began working to expand *ISBT 128* for use in the field of cellular therapy. Although a number of facilities had used *ISBT 128* for cellular therapy products since the late 1990s, this group greatly expanded the terms and definitions to meet evolving needs. Their work was published in a variety of journals.[14]

Beginning in 2008, *ISBT 128* terminology was required by FACT, JACIE, and AABB standards for labeling cellular therapy products. The requirement by these organizations for full *ISBT 128* labeling (bar codes and label design) is still a few years off to allow for enhancement of computer systems. However, some cellular therapy facilities that also handle blood are already in the process of implementing the full label and nearly 200 facilities in 36 countries are registered with the ICCBBA.

Representatives of the European Eye Bank Association, Eye Bank Association of America, Eye Bank Association of Australia and New Zealand, Eye Bank Association of India, and Pan-American Association of Eye Banks are working together to develop a global standard terminology to describe ocular tissue for transplant. The project is being coordinated by the ICCBBA.

Solid organ AE report in the US

Transmission of infectious agents, both known and unknown, from an organ donor represents a particular hazard to the transplant recipient because, unlike a recipient of blood transfusion, the immunosuppression regimen (required to prevent organ rejection) weakens the patient's host defense mechanisms against invading organisms. The resulting infection is thus more likely to result in devastating, and sometimes fatal, consequences. As such, biovigilance takes on added importance in the setting of solid organ transplantation. Although it is estimated that the risk of acquiring an infectious disease through organ transplantation is an infrequent occurrence, it is still higher than through blood or tissue transplantation. This risk is balanced against the life-saving indications for transplantable organs and the substantial number of patients who die each year due to the lack of organs.

There is a need to capture more complete data on the transmission of infectious diseases and malignancies of donor origin. Several factors make the task of identifying potential transmissible infections in deceased solid organ donors more problematic than for blood donors:

• Information about medical history and social/behavioral risk factors of deceased organ donors is often incomplete and suboptimal (usually obtained from family or acquaintances).

- Potential organ donors are typically admitted to the hospital emergently with catastrophic medical or traumatic events, and may receive multiple transfusion products with the small risk of transfusion-transmitted disease.
- Organ recovery often is done urgently (due to the donor's deteriorating clinical status) and the retrieved organs must be transplanted within hours of recovery, limiting the amount of time available to obtain the results of donor-screening tests or perform extensive confirmatory lab testing of any abnormal test results prior to the transplant of the organs.
- The number of patients waiting for organ transplants far exceeds the number of available organs, which makes it important that screening tests for infectious agents in a potential organ donor are accurate to avoid unnecessarily discarding useable organs.

In addition, because of the limited supply of organs, even individuals known to have risk factors for infectious diseases may be accepted as organ donors. Hence, the transplant community, including potential transplant patients, must balance the risk of acquiring an infection or other disease from a potential donor against the potential for death or morbidity if an organ from a particular donor is rejected.

Three recent changes in organ donor procurement practices and transplantation have heightened interest in an effective nationwide biovigilance system that includes solid organ transplantation.

First, due to the ever-expanding waiting list of patients in need of transplantable organs, deceased donors with various behavioral and social risks, which would categorized them as "high-risk" donors, are being accepted with the expectation that all available information will be provided to all involved. Although donors are screened and tested for infectious diseases, the inherent limitations of less-than-perfect screening tests for infectious agents have increased the potential for missing a potentially serious infection in such "high-risk" donors. Screening tests are not identical to those used in blood and tissue donors, in part because of concerns over timeliness and false positive results,

potentially impacting availability. A fully operational nationwide biovigilance system can improve the capabilities to detect and respond swiftly to such transmissible agents when these events occur thus minimizing the consequences in all recipients of organs from that affected donor.

Second, in an attempt to further increase the number of organs, especially kidneys, available from individuals with a demonstrated wish to donate, the transplant community is pursuing organ procurement following cardiac arrest and failed cardiopulmonary resuscitation in both the hospital and community settings. This has been termed Uncontrolled Donation after Circulatory Death (UDCD) or Donation after Cardiac Death (DCD). In these still infrequent situations, it may be difficult to procure suitable screening test specimens prior to death. How this might affect disease transmission from UDCD solid organ donors remains to be seen.

Third, a recent advance in the field is the transplantation of vascularized composite allografts (VCA), a variety of body parts composed of multiple types of tissues transplanted as an anatomical unit. The most notable types of VCAs to date have been hand and face transplants. Given the anticipated increase in VCA transplants, the HRSA published a Request for Information (RFI) on March 3, 2008, in the Federal Register for the purpose of soliciting feedback from stakeholders and the public as to whether VCAs should be included within the definition of organs covered by the OPTN Final Rule and/or added to the definition of human organs covered by section 301 of NOTA (73 Federal Register 11420).

Development of Vigilance and Surveillance (V&S) systems for HCT/P and organs

Development of vigilance and surveillance systems for tissues and cells used in transplantation is a recent undertaking in most of the world. Since biovigilance was established in France by a decree in 2003, annual reports now include AE reporting of cells, tissues, and organs.[15,16] The European

Union Standards and Training for the Inspection of Tissue Establishments (EUSTITE), co-funded by the European Commission, assisted member states by providing guidance documents and training in the areas of AE and reaction reporting for tissue and cells, as well as inspection training for compliance. The project developed V&S tools consistent with and complementary to existing ones, such as hemovigilance systems. Globally this is now being led by the Department of Essential Health Technologies at the WHO.

The EUSTITE project closed after three years at the end of 2009. The criteria for the reporting of serious AEs, the imputability scale for evaluating the link between a reaction and the tissues and cells applied, and the severity scale for a reaction have all been incorporated into the guidance provided by the European Commission to Member States. The project submitted Final Vigilance Recommendations to the Commission, which highlighted a number of areas for further work, particularly in relation to the need for investigation guidance and training, guidance for vigilance in assisted reproduction and the investigation of illegal and fraudulent activity, and for greater engagement of clinicians to ensure effective vigilance.

These issues are now being carried forward in a new EU-funded project: "Vigilance and Surveillance of Substances of Human Origin (SOHO V&S)," which started in March 2010 and is also led by Centro Nazionale Trapianti (CNT) in Italy in collaboration with WHO (www.sohovs.org). SOHO V&S is gathering essential information on EU Vigilance and Regulation of Tissues and Cells in cooperation with experts from around the world. A survey is currently being conducted to gather detailed information on the systems in place in EU member states for V&S in the field of tissues and cells for transplant and for assisted reproduction.

SOHO V&S and WHO's Project NOTIFY (Notifiable Organs, Tissues and Cells Incidents to be Flagged by You) have the broad goal to assist current global endeavors to improve V&S for the benefit of all countries, as a step toward building global vigilance and surveillance for substances of human origin.[17] The project will focus on the pivotal role of the clinician in the chain of vigilance, clearly for the identification of reportable situations but also for the elucidation of cause and consequence. The clinician will ultimately benefit from the improvements in patient care brought by vigilance and surveillance. The project will publish a reference didactic booklet on the notification of adverse reactions and events in organs, tissues, and cells. This booklet will be directed primarily at clinicians who use human organs, tissues, and cells and will provide detailed guidance on the detection and notification of appropriate corrective and preventive actions to be taken. Specific types of reactions and events, serious adverse reactions and events, as well as the steps that should be taken to elucidate and confirm the origins/causes will be considered by type of human substance.

In North America, the Public Health Agency of Canada (PHAC) has carried out a series of pilot projects to develop a national tissue and organ surveillance system (TOSS), which will be primarily focused on three types of adverse and severe reactions: transmission of infectious diseases; malignancy transfer; and graft failure.[18] Health Canada requires that source establishments investigate and submit reports of certain adverse reactions, errors, and accidents involving cells, tissues, and organs to the Canada Vigilance Program. Health professionals and consumers may submit voluntary reports to the Canada Vigilance Program as well.

Also in North America, the US FDA's Center for Devices and Radiological Health (CDRH) launched the Medical Product Safety Network (MedSun) in 2002 to identify and share information about problems with the use of medical devices. MedSun (www.medsun.net) is a targeted surveillance program that involves AE reporting from a sentinel network of around 350 healthcare facilities throughout the US. Currently the FDA is operating a sub-network involving a subset of MedSun sites, called TissueNet. TissueNet is the first enhanced surveillance program for HCT/P-related adverse reactions and boosts the numbers of voluntary reports submitted for these products. It is the goal that MedSun along with sub-networks like TissueNet will build relationships between the FDA and the front-line product users in specific "high-risk" clinical care areas. TissueNet enhances the Center for Biologics Evaluation and Research's understanding of the use of HCT/Ps and provides a resource for communication with the clinical tissue and cell transplant community. The objectives are to describe the frequency and types of reports following HCT/P transplants; identify potential causes or "near-misses"; and improve the safety of HCT/Ps. TissueNet sites use MedSun to report HCT/P-related AEs or product problems to the FDA via a secure Internet-based data entry portal.

Several professional organizations also perform tissue biovigilance activities. The Joint Commission (TJC) accredits and certifies more than 15,000 healthcare organizations and programs in the US. In 2005, TJC published standards related to tissue storage and issuance. These standards require the assignment of responsibility for handling tissue within a hospital to a single coordinating entity. The oversight responsibility includes: supplier certification; incoming inspection and logging in of tissue; traceability and recordkeeping; storage temperature monitoring; investigation of adverse outcomes; reporting tissue-related infections to the tissue supplier; sequestering tissue reported by the supplier as contaminated; the notification of surgeons and recipients if tissue donors are subsequently found to harbor infection; and compliance with federal and state regulations if supplying tissues to any other facility. The College of American Pathologists has adopted similar standards.

Many hospitals have turned to their blood bank where many of the capabilities for tissue management already exist. As a result, the AABB established a tissue task force to begin to develop guidance documents and assistance to hospital blood banks to prepare for managing tissue within their facilities. In an attempt to better understand how tissues were being managed within hospitals, the AABB Tissue Task Force later prepared and distributed a survey to hospital institutional members. The survey contained questions on tissue types handled, the breadth of responsibility, and facilities within hospitals responsible for tissue. Of the 904 institutional members invited to participate, 402 gave interpretable responses; 325 reported the use of allogeneic or autologous human tissue. The sur-

vey indicated that the department of surgery was the most likely hospital department to have any responsibility for tissue use, followed by the blood bank. Surgery departments were most frequently responsible for tissue handling, documenting use, and for AE reporting; for the latter category only 23% reported infection control responsibilities.[19]

The AABB survey was corroborated by the 2007 Nationwide Blood Collection and Utilization Survey (NBCUS) report that of hospitals reporting, 14% responded that blood banks had responsibility for tissue management and 80% responded that operating rooms did.[20] AEs were reported in this survey. Although limited to hospital transfusion service data on facility events, there were 43 AE reports, including bacterial and viral infections and graft failures, from 229,115 grafts implanted for a ratio of 1:5300. Since healthcare facilities do not have reporting requirements (unless they are performing a manufacturing step and subject to FDA reporting regulations), one is left to extrapolate the actual number of AEs occurring.

The AATB has been publishing standards since 1984. AATB Standards state that tissue banks establish policies and procedures regarding adverse outcomes and recalls, and have a process for sharing information with other tissue banks known to have recovered or received tissue from the same donor. Tissue banks must document and investigate all reported or suspected adverse outcomes potentially related to an allograft. Tissue banks must assure that tissue can be tracked to the consignee, and must notify the consignee of its responsibility to maintain records traceable to the recipient. Typically, tracking to the recipient is facilitated through graft implant cards that accompany each allograft that is distributed. These cards contain information about the graft, and space for recording information about graft use (such as facility, surgeon, and recipient). Manufacturers ask hospitals and healthcare providers to return these records following transplants, but there is no enforceable requirement for the return of the implant cards. Compliance with return of these cards varies considerably from bank to bank depending on the degree to which the tissue bank pursues their return. A recent AATB survey, to which only 15 of over 100 banks responded, reported an average return rate of just over 50% with a wide range from less than 10% to as high as 95%.[21] Information about graft disposition and adverse outcomes can provide context for assessing the potential risk of tissue allograft transplantation.

The Eye Bank Association of America (EBAA) implemented its Medical Advisory Board (MAB) in 1991 in response to a 1990 requirement for all eye banks to seek 3–12-month follow-ups of all patient outcomes. EBAA's Online Adverse Reaction Reporting System (OARRS) was redesigned in 2005. The MAB reviews results on a biannual basis. Eye banks provide institutions with self-addressed envelopes to complete and return follow-up forms. Persons who submit reports on OARRS must provide information on the adverse reaction, surgery, microbiology results, tissue mate status, donor, and method of transporting the tissue from the source eye bank.

The HRSA awarded the Center for International Blood and Marrow Transplant Research (CIBMTR) a contract to establish and maintain the Stem Cell Therapeutic Outcomes Database (SCTOD) component of the C.W. Bill Young Cell Transplantation Program. Transplant centers must submit data annually to CIBMTR on all allogeneic transplant recipients. Although most data are focused on outcomes, some data also relate to AEs such as early and late graft failures, risk factors for Graft Versus Host Disease (GVHD), prevalence of microbiologically contaminated hematopoietic stem cell products, antibodies to the graft, infections and second cancers.

The NMDP collects data on donor AEs and post-donation symptoms. Data collected include serious and minor complications following marrow and peripheral blood stem cell collections, such as mechanical injury to tissue, anesthesia reactions, infection, seizures, excessive pain, and delayed return to normal work functions. Minor side effects such as hypotension, syncope, and collection site pain are reported in 75% of marrow donors. Peripheral blood stem cell (PBSC) donors are also monitored for AEs specific to filgrastim administration and central intravenous catheter placement, such as more serious degrees of headache, fatigue, bone pain, hypotension, vomiting, cen-

tral line placement complications, or more serious cytopenias. HRSA personnel are informed of AEs that are serious and unexpected and the FDA is also notified if a serious and unexpected AE occurs in a PBSC donor.

Emerging threat assessment: Looking to the future and beyond known transfusion/transplantation-related events

There is a need to develop informatics and laboratory repository capabilities to meet the challenges presented by emerging infectious diseases (EIDs) and other threats. For example, the NHLBI has sponsored two multi-center Retrovirus Epidemiology Donor Studies (REDS-I and the current REDS-II) that carry out investigator-initiated investigations of transfusion-transmitted viral and nonviral infections, noninfectious complications of transfusion, and other aspects. Several targeted specimen repositories were established by REDS-I, including a matched donor-recipient cell and serum collection (REDS Allogeneic Donor and Recipient—RADAR) that included seven blood centers and eight hospitals. The use of these repositories has been reported in peer-reviewed journals.[22] REDS-II has initiated targeted studies of TRALI and other important transfusion-related outcomes. In 2011, the NHLBI awarded a seven-year contract for Recipient Epidemiology and Donor Evaluation Study (REDS) III. As the name implies, the objectives of the contract differs from the first two contracts.

Rapid worldwide information exchange is also needed to assess the potential impact on means of transmission regarding new or re-emerging agents. Repositories, such as those maintained by funded NHLBI studies and CDC's Universal Data Collection bleeding disorder community repository, may be very useful in defining the onset of human infection with a new EID and learning about its epidemiology and natural history, but vital epidemiologic data must be gathered from global sources before such studies can be put into place. More sophisticated real-time informatics methods are needed for timely detection of potential threats to transfusion and transplant recipients.

Mandates for a Comprehensive Biovigilance Program and Future Challenges

The rapid growth and evolution in the scientific and technical fields of transfusion and transplantation call for a comprehensive biovigilance program. Specifically, AE monitoring for recipients and donors, quality assurance, and emerging threat assessment are critical components in a comprehensive system. The current biovigilance patchwork system environment is complex and nonintegrated. As part of a national biovigilance effort, it must be integrated meaningfully with other systems that are under development. Since the broadest interpretation of biovigilance represents an umbrella for multiple public and private surveillance and reporting mechanisms, one could imagine a common portal through which systems could be accessed depending on either interest or requirement. As electronic health records (EHR) and information exchange become more widely adopted,

electronic exchange of information directly from EHR systems for biovigilance reporting should be integrated. It will, in part, be the role of government to identify and address these challenges and create a sustainable biovigilance effort of the highest quality to support the public health needs of donors and blood recipients.

Governance of the system including its sustainability is critical. There are many forms of governance throughout the world (see Figure 27.2). One form of governance unique to the US is a proposed public–private partnership (PPP). A PPP has the unique opportunity to bring together stakeholders such as industry (e.g., healthcare facilities, payers, pharmacology, biomedical technologies, and information technologies), public (e.g., patients, public advocates, universities, and foundations), professional (e.g., professional organizations and providers), and government. Although there are many opportunities created by a public–private venture, there also need to be clear pathways for long-term governance, funding for sustainability, and clarity on data collection, analysis, and dissemination to improve practice.

Government and nongovernment partners have made substantial progress on national biovigilance

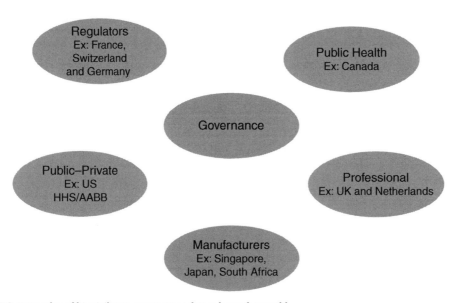

Figure 27.2 Examples of biovigilance governance throughout the world.

collaborations based upon voluntary reporting. This design offers many opportunities for improvements in national biovigilance capability, including time-trending based upon highly refined definitions and imputations, availability of benchmarking data to allow comparative assessment of errors and AEs at the institutional level, and establishment of national data for comparisons with other hemovigilance systems worldwide. Similarly, biovigilance efforts must also be designed to complement reporting with government safety reporting regulations.

For blood and blood products, there is a robust regulatory structure from collection to transfusion and accrediting organizations active in emphasizing patient safety, but coordinated surveillance for AE policy on reporting, particularly for nonfatal events, is lacking, both in donors and in recipients. For other tissues (i.e., HCT/Ps), regulation is narrower in scope, being limited to control of communicable diseases, but with no government regulation extending to the end-user in the clinical setting.

Common processes for data collection, analysis, and evaluation are either lacking or underdeveloped in both the private and public health communities. Compounding the lack of common processes is the lack of understanding of transfusion and transplant safety risks across the spectrum of products.

Surveillance for a wider array of AEs is needed for blood and blood products. Voluntary reporting of AEs may increase reporting if there are no punitive consequences to the facility, but such systems must be implemented widely to have an impact.

Mandatory reporting for HCT/P manufacturers, excluding reproductive tissue establishments, consists of adverse reaction reports involving communicable disease transmission, and deviations in manufacturing that may introduce risks of communicable disease transmission or contamination. For HCT/Ps also regulated as licensed biologics, mandatory reporting requirements are more extensive.

Finally, for solid organs, for which transmission risks are highest, oversight mechanisms feature an excellent database infrastructure through the OPTN, but such systems currently are focused on patient outcome, not disease transmission or other AEs. Evolution of the concept of hemovigilance to biovigilance has also exposed the need to expand from transfusion recipient safety to donor health and transfusion transmitted infectious (TTI) marker rates, as well as transplantation safety. A system that strengthens connections between organ and tissue recovery organizations and healthcare providers to solve multiple problems simultaneously may be the best approach.

Conclusions

Blood products, organs, and HCT/Ps are obtained and managed by independent local blood collectors, organ procurement organizations, and tissue establishments. National oversight includes monitoring through facility inspections or accreditation by professional organizations. Industry generally supports safety efforts, but encourages the government to minimize requirements to reduce burden and duplication of efforts. Thus, voluntary reporting of AEs would be more palatable but may hinder implementation of biovigilance without adequate enforcement.

A uniform biovigilance system may not be possible in some countries, given differences in government, oversight, and regulation of different biological products, but these differences should not be an obstacle to a common coordinated national program. Therefore, a concerted effort is needed for coordination among public health in government and organizations in the private sector to assure safe and available transfusion and transplantation. Systems need to avoid overlap in order to minimize reporting burden. However, mandatory regulatory components alone will not be sufficient, because data cannot be shared from these sources, emphasizing the need for voluntary nonregulatory components in parallel. Uncoordinated efforts without a clear governance plan may be the greatest threat to patient safety related to biovigilance, because progress may cease.

A comprehensive biovigilance program should bridge both regulatory and organizational gaps to meet public health needs. Regular assessment and evaluation of current measures are needed to determine risks to patient safety. Disease transmission and other AEs associated with transfusion and transplantation constitute risks that are evident but unevenly quantified, depending on the biologic. Although patient safety is paramount, the need to assess availability also needs to be taken into consideration. Well-defined transparent governance of a public–private partnership for biovigilance is in the best interest of the public.

References

1 WHO, 2005, Draft guidelines for adverse event reporting and learning systems. World Health Organization, Geneva, Switzerland.

2 US Department of Health and Human Services, 2011, The 2009 nationwide blood collection and utilization survey report. Office of the Assistant Secretary for Health, Washington, DC, USA.

3 Busch M, Chamberland M, Epstein J, Kleinman S, Khabbaz R, Nemo G, 1999, Oversight and monitoring of blood safety in the United States. *Vox Sang* **77**: 67–76.

4 US Department of Health and Human Services, 1994, Public Health Service Act, 42 USC 201 et. seq., Sections 351 and 361.

5 US FDA, 2006, Federal Food, Drug, and Cosmetic Act, 21 USC 201 and what follows.

6 Office of the Federal Register, 2006, Code of Federal Regulations, Title 21, *Food and Drugs*, Pt. 800–1299, **606**: 170(b).

7 US FDA, 2012, MedWatch: The FDA Safety Information and Adverse Event Reporting Program, http://www.fda.gov/medwatch/index.html [accessed February 17, 2012].

8 Centers for Disease Control and Prevention, 2003, Report on the Universal Data Collection Program. Special report summarizing data on female with von Willebrand disease. Division of Hereditary Blood Disorders, National Center on Birth Defects and Developmental Disabilities, Atlanta, GA, USA.

9 Kainer MA, Linden JV, Whaley DN, *et al.*, 2004, Clostridium infections associated with musculoskeletal tissue allografts. *N Eng Med* **350**: 2564.

10 Tugwell BD, Patel PR, Williams IT, *et al.*, 2005, Transmission of Hepatitis C virus to several organ and tissue recipients from an antibody-negative donor. *Ann Int Med* **143**: 678.

11 Strong DM, Seem D, Taylor G, Parker JB, Stewart D, and Kuehnert MJ, 2010, Development of a Sentinel Network to Improve Safety and Traceability of Organ and Tissue Transplants: The Need for Common Identifiers. *Cell Tissue Bank* **11**: 335–43.

12 Fehily D, Ashford P, Poniatowshi S, 2004, Traceability of human tissues for transplantation: The development and implementation of a coding system using ISBT 128. *Organs and Tissues* **2**: 83–8.

13 Strong DM, and Shinozaki N, 2010, Coding and traceability for cells, tissues, and organs for transplantation. *Cell Tissue Bank* **11**(4): 305–23.

14 Ashford P, Distler P, Gee A, Lankester A, *et al.*, 2007, *ISBT 128* implementation plan for cellular therapy products. *J Clin Apher* **22**(5): 258–64.

15 Samuel D, and Chabannon C (eds), 2010, Le report annuel biovigilance 2009. Agence francaise de securite sanitaire des produits de santé, Saint-Denise, France.

16 Roche M, and Creusvaux H, 2010, Biomedicine Adl. Rapprot annuel de sythese de biovigilance, Agence de la biomedicine, Saint-Denise, France.

17 Nanni CA, Noel L, Strong M, and Fehily D, 2011, NOTIFY exploring vigilance notification for organs, tissues and cells. *Organs Tissues & Cells*, November 14, **3**: Supp.

18 Moulton D, and Kondro W, 2010, Pilot projects lay foundation for national tissue surveillance and traceabiltly system. *CMAJ* **182**(6): E259–60.

19 Kuehnert MJ, Yorita KL, Holman RC, *et al.*, 2007, Human tissue oversight in hospitals: A survey of 402 AABB institutional members. *Transfusion* **47**: 194–200.

20 US Department of Health and Human Services, 2008, The 2007 nationwide blood collection and utilization survey report. Office of the Assistant Secretary for Health, Washington, DC, USA.

21 Rigney PR, Jr, 2008, AATB annual survey—2007 preliminary results. AATB 32nd annual meeting, Chicago, IL, USA.

22 Kleinman SH, Glynn SA, Higgins MJ, *et al.*, 2005, The RADAR repository: A resource for studies of infectious agents and their transmissibility by transfusion. *Transfusion* **45**(7): 1073–83.

Appendices

APPENDIX A
Glossary

Blood transfusion

Blood, blood products, and blood components

Blood

Whole blood collected from a donor and processed either for transfusion or for further manufacturing (ref: Directive 2002/98/EC).

Whole Blood (WB)

Whole blood for transfusion is blood taken from a suitable donor using a sterile and pyrogen-free anti-coagulant and container. The main use of whole blood is as a source material for blood component preparation (ref: Guide of the Council of Europe, EDQM).

Blood Component (BC)

A therapeutic constituent of blood (red cells, white cells, platelets, plasma) that can be prepared by various methods (ref: Directive 2002/98/EC).

Red Blood Cell Concentrate (RBC)

A component obtained by removal of part of the plasma from whole blood (ref: Guide of the Council of Europe, EDQM).

Note: It may prepared from a whole blood donation of 450 ml or 500 ml and it may come with or without additive solution, buffy-coat removed, leucocyte-reduced, leucocyte-depleted or filtered, cryopreserved, washed, and so on. Numerous variants of RBC exist. Therefore it is important to specify the characteristics of the RBC, especially within the context of studies or comparisons.

Platelet Concentrate (PLT)

A component derived from fresh whole blood that contains the majority of the original platelet content in a therapeutically effective form (recovered PLT). Or a component obtained by platelet apheresis of a single donor using automated cell separation equipment (ref. Guide of the Council of Europe, EDQM).

Note: It may be prepared from a whole blood donation of 450 ml or 500 ml and it may come with plasma or with additive solution, buffy-coat removed, leucocyte-depleted or filtered, cryopreserved, washed, pooled from 4–6 whole blood donors, and so on. It may come from an apheresis donation (single or multiple dose etc.). Several variants of PLT exist, and so it is important to specify the characteristics of the PLT, especially within the context of studies or comparisons.

Plasma

The liquid portion of anticoagulated blood remaining after separation from the cellular components (ref: Guide of the Council of Europe, EDQM).

Fresh Frozen Plasma (FFP)

A component for transfusion or fractionation prepared either from whole blood or from plasma collected by apheresis, frozen within a period of time and to a temperature that will adequately maintain the labile coagulation factors in a functional state (ref: Guide of the Council of Europe, EDQM).

Note: It may prepared from a whole blood donation of 450 ml or 500 ml (it is then commonly referred to as *recovered plasma*) or by apheresis.

Hemovigilance: An Effective Tool for Improving Transfusion Safety, First Edition. Edited by René R.P. De Vries and Jean-Claude Faber.
© 2012 John Wiley & Sons, Ltd. Published 2012 by John Wiley & Sons, Ltd.

It may come from a single donation or be pooled. It may be quarantined for a certain period before release, or be treated with inactivation methods (solvent-detergent SD, methylene blue, psoralene or others). Several variants of FFP exist. Therefore it is important to specify the characteristics of the FFP, especially within the context of studies or comparisons.

Blood Product (BP)

Any therapeutic product derived from human blood or plasma (ref: Directive 2002/98/EC).

Apheresis

Method of obtaining one or more blood components by machine processing of whole blood in which the residual components of the blood are returned to the donor during or at the end of the process (ref: Guide of the Council of Europe, EDQM).

Blood establishment and hospital blood bank

Blood Establishment (BE)

Any structure or body responsible for any aspect of the collection and testing of human blood or blood components, whatever their intended purpose, and their processing, storage, and distribution when intended for transfusion. This does not include hospital blood banks (ref: Directive 2002/98/EC).

Hospital Blood Bank (hBB)

A hospital unit that stores and distributes and may perform compatibility tests on blood and blood components exclusively for use within hospital facilities, including hospital-based transfusion activities (ref: Directive 2002/98/EC).

Distribution

Delivery of blood and blood components to other blood establishments, hospital blood banks, and manufacturers of blood and plasma derived products. It does not include the issuing of blood or blood components for transfusion.

Issuing

The provision of blood or blood components by a blood establishment or a hospital blood bank for transfusion to a recipient.

Recipient and donor

Recipient

Someone who has been transfused with blood or blood components (ref: Commission Directive 2005/61/EC).

Donor

A person in normal health with a good medical history who (voluntarily) gives blood or plasma for therapeutic use (ref: Guide of the Council of Europe, EDQM).

Donor, voluntary and nonremunerated

An individual who is at the origin of a donation, which is considered voluntary and nonremunerated if the person gives blood, plasma, or cellular components of his/her own free will and receives no payment for it, either in the form of cash or in kind that could be considered a substitute for money. This includes time off work other than that reasonably needed for the donation and travel. Small tokens, refreshments, and reimbursement of direct travel costs are compatible with voluntary, nonremunerated donation (ref: modified from Council of Europe Recommendation No. R(95) 14).

Autologous transfusion

Transfusion, in which the donor and the recipient are the same person (ref: Guide of the Council of Europe, EDQM).

Hemovigilance

Particularly in Europe, also spelled as "haemovigilance." We use hemovigilance throughout this book.

General

Hemovigilance (HV)

A set of surveillance procedures covering the whole transfusion chain (from the collection of blood and its components to the follow-up of recipients), intended to collect and assess information on unexpected or undesirable effects resulting from the therapeutic use of labile blood products, and to prevent their occurrence or recurrence (ref: IHN website, www.ihn-org.com).

Or a set of surveillance procedures of the whole transfusion chain intended to minimize adverse events or reactions in donors and recipients and to promote safe and effective use of blood components.

Donor (hemo)vigilance

The systematic monitoring of adverse reactions and incidents in the whole chain of blood donor care, with a view to improving quality and safety for blood donors.

Look-back

A look-back procedure is aimed at the tracing of recipients of potentially infectious blood components and notification of these recipients by their treating physicians.

Traceability of blood components

The ability to trace each individual unit of blood or components derived thereof from the donor to its final destination, whether this is a patient, a manufacturer of medicinal products or disposal, and vice versa.

Adverse events

Adverse Event (AE)

An undesirable and unintended occurrence in the blood transfusion chain (the collection, testing, preparation, storage, distribution, ordering, issuing, and administration of blood and blood components). It may or may not be the result of an error or an incident and it may or may not result in an adverse reaction in a donor or recipient.

Incident

Case in which the patient is transfused with a blood component that did not meet all the requirements for a suitable transfusion for that patient, or that was intended for another patient. It thus comprises transfusion errors and deviations from standard operating procedures or hospital policies that have led to mis-transfusions. *It may or may not have led to an adverse reaction* (ref: IHN-ISBT WP HV definition).

Near-miss

An error or deviation from standard procedures or policies that is discovered before the start of the transfusion and that could have led to a wrongful transfusion or a reaction in a recipient (ref: IHN-ISBT WP HV definition).

Adverse Reaction (AR)

An undesirable response or effect in a patient or donor temporally associated with the collection or administration of blood or blood component. It may be the result of an incident or of interaction between a recipient and blood, a biologically active product (ref: IHN-ISBT WP HV definition). The term transfusion reaction (TR) is also commonly used. Even when TR is used, imputability should be separately assessed and reported as appropriate (see below).

Imputability

The likelihood that an adverse reaction in a recipient can be attributed to the blood or blood component transfused or that an adverse reaction in a donor can be attributed to the donation process (ref: modified from Commission Directive 2005/61/EC).

Severity

Degree of expression of symptoms and signs of an adverse reaction in a recipient (a transfusion reaction) or a donor.

Look-back procedure

The objective is to identify the recipients of any previous potentially infectious donations made by this donor, and notify them so that they can be tested and counseled.

Epidemiological terms

Numerator

Number of cases (of a type of adverse reaction, incident, and so on) to be divided by a denominator figure for the calculation of the rate.

Denominator

The number of units, transfusions, and so on among which the observed adverse events occurred; the divisor for the calculation of the rate.

Rate

Number of (new) cases divided by a denominator, for example, the number of blood components transfused; it indicates the frequency of occurrence per 1000 (or other figure).

Adverse events in a recipient

Adverse reactions

Non-infectious adverse reactions

- Hemolytic Transfusion Reaction
- Acute Hemolytic Transfusion Reaction (AHTR)
- Delayed Hemolytic Transfusion Reaction (DHTR)
- Delayed Serologic Transfusion Reaction (DSTR)
- Febrile Non-Hemolytic Transfusion Reaction (FNHTR)
- Allergic reaction
- Anaphylactic reaction
- Transfusion Associated Graft-Versus-Host Disease (TA-GVHD)
- Post-transfusion purpura (PTP)
- Transfusion Related Lung Injury (TRALI)
- Transfusion Associated Circulatory Overload (TACO)
- Transfusion Associated Dyspnea (TAD)
- Hypotensive transfusion reaction
- Hemosiderosis
- Hyperkalemia
- Unclassified Complication of Transfusion (UCT)

Transfusion-transmitted infections (TTIs)

Viral infection (TTVI)

Following investigation, the recipient has evidence of infection post-transfusion and no clinical or laboratory evidence of infection prior to transfusion and either, at least one component received by the infected recipient was donated by a donor who had evidence of the same infection, or at least one component received by the infected recipient was shown to have been contaminated with the virus.

Bacterial infection (TTBI)

A TTBI should be clinically suspected if fever >39°C (102.2°F) or there is a change of >2°C (5.6°F) from pre-transfusion value; and rigors; and tachycardia >120 beats/min or a change of >40 beats/min from pre-transfusion value or a rise or drop of 30 mm Hg in systolic blood pressure within 4 hours of transfusion are present.

Possible TTBI:

- detection of bacteria by approved techniques in the transfused blood component but not in the recipient's blood; or
- detection of bacteria in the recipient's blood following transfusion but not in the transfused blood component and no other reasons are ascertainable for the positive blood culture.

Confirmed TTBI:

- detection of the same bacterial strain in the recipient's blood and in the transfused blood product by approved techniques.

Parasite infection (TTPI)

Detection of the same parasite in the recipient's blood and parasite or specific antibodies in the donor's blood.

Grading of imputability

Once the investigation of the adverse event is completed, imputability is the assessment of the strength of relation to the transfusion of the AE as follows (ref: IHN-ISBT WP HV definition):

- *Definite (certain):* When there is conclusive evidence beyond reasonable doubt that the adverse event can be attributed to the transfusion.
- *Probable (likely):* When the evidence is clearly in favor of attributing the adverse event to the transfusion.
- *Possible:* When the evidence is indeterminate for attributing the adverse event to the transfusion or an alternate cause.

- *Unlikely (doubtful):* When the evidence is clearly in favor of attributing the adverse event to causes other than the transfusion.
- *Excluded:* When there is conclusive evidence beyond reasonable doubt that the adverse event can be attributed to causes other than the transfusion.

Grading of severity

- *Grade 1 (Non-Severe):* The recipient may have required medical intervention (e.g., symptomatic treatment) but lack of such would not have resulted in permanent damage or impairment of a body function.
- *Grade 2 (Severe):* The recipient required in-patient hospitalization or prolongation of hospitalization directly attributable to the event; and/or the adverse event resulted in persistent or significant disability or incapacity; or the adverse event necessitated medical or surgical intervention to preclude permanent damage or impairment of a body function.
- *Grade 3 (Life-threatening):* The recipient required major intervention following the transfusion (vasopressors, intubation, transfer to intensive care) to prevent death.
- *Grade 4 (Death):* The recipient died following an adverse transfusion reaction. *Grade 4 should be used only if death is possibly, probably, or definitely related to transfusion. If the patient died of another cause, the severity of the reaction should be graded as 1, 2, or 3* (ref: IHN-ISBT WP HV definition).

Incidents

Incorrect blood component transfused (IBCT)

All reported episodes where a patient was transfused with a blood component that did not meet the appropriate requirements or was intended for another patient, even if the component was ABO-compatible and/or even if only a small quantity of blood was transfused and/or there was no adverse reaction (ref: ISBT WP).

ABO-incompatible transfusion

All cases where a blood component was transfused that was (unintentionally) ABO-incompatible: Includes all such events even if only a small quan-tity of blood was transfused, and/or no adverse reaction occurred.

All cases are to be included, whether the first error occurred in the blood establishment, in the blood transfusion laboratory, or in clinical areas.

Note that these are a subgroup of the IBCT category (ref: ISBT WP).

Wrong name on tube (WNOT) or Wrong blood in tube (WBIT)

All cases where it was found (in the reporting year) that a blood sample submitted for blood-group determination, irregular antibody screen, and/or compatibility testing was labeled with the identification details of a different patient. This is a ubiquitous and serious problem: includes all such events even if the error was detected by routine checks, such as repeat blood group determination; even if the error did not lead to an incorrect transfusion (for whatever reason); and even if the patient sampled was not (imminently) scheduled for transfusion.

Note that there can be overlap between cases of WNOT and ABO-incompatible transfusion or other IBCT subgroups, as well as near-misses (ref: ISBT WP and SHOT Annual Report).

Inappropriate and unnecessary transfusion (I&U)

Any case in which the intended transfusion is carried out and the component is suitable for transfusion and for the patient, but where the decision-making is faulty (ref: SHOT Annual Report).

Handling and Storage Errors (HSE)

Transfusion of a correct component to an intended patient, in which, during the transfusion process, the handling and storage may have rendered the component less safe (ref: SHOT Annual Report).

Adverse events in a donor

Adverse reactions or complications

Hematoma

A hematoma is an accumulation of blood in the tissues outside the vessels. Symptoms are bruising, discoloration, swelling, and local pain.

Hematoma is the second most common acute complication that occurs related to blood donation.

The symptoms are caused by blood flowing out of damaged vessels and accumulating in the soft tissues. As the volume of the hematoma increases, swelling occurs. The swelling puts pressure on the surrounding tissues. The strength of the pressure depends on size of the swelling and softness of the surrounding tissue. Pressure on nerves results in neurologic symptoms such as pain radiating down in forearm and hand, and of peripheral tingling.

If blood accumulates in the frontal deep layers of the forearm between muscles and tendons, the swelling is hard to recognize, but the pressure increases very easily. Therefore, complications such as injury of a nerve and even Compartment Syndrome occur more often related to a hematoma with this localization.

Arterial puncture

Arterial puncture is a puncture of the brachial artery or of one of its branches by the needle used for bleeding of donor. Symptoms may include weak pain localized to the elbow region. Objectively, a lighter red color than usual of the collected blood can be seen and perhaps some movements of the needle caused by arterial pulsation; the bag fills very quickly. In uncomplicated cases there may be no hematoma.

Complications are the increased risk of a large hematoma and thereby risks such as Compartment Syndrome in the forearm, Brachial Artery Pseudo Aneurysm, and Arterio-Venous Fistula.

Delayed bleeding

Delayed bleeding is the spontaneous recommencement of bleeding from the venipuncture site, which occurs after donor has left the donation site.

Nerve irritation

This is irritation of a nerve by pressure from a hematoma. Symptoms are of a nerve type such as radiating pain and/or paresthesia in association with a hematoma. The hematoma may not always be apparent at the time. Symptoms do not occur immediately on insertion of the needle but start when the hematoma has reached a sufficient size, some time after insertion of the needle.

Nerve injury

The injury of a nerve by the needle at insertion or withdrawal. Symptoms are pain often associated with paresthesiae. The pain is severe and radiating. It arises immediately when the needle is inserted or withdrawn.

Tendon injury

The injury of a tendon by the needle. Symptoms are very severe local nonradiating pain initiating immediately when the needle is inserted.

Painful arm

Such cases are characterized mainly by severe local and radiating pain in the arm used for the donation, arising during or within hours following donation, but without further details to permit classification in one of the already more specific categories mentioned above.

Thrombophlebitis

The inflammation in a vein associated with a thrombus. Symptoms are warmth, tenderness, local pain, redness, and swelling. Thrombophlebitis in a superficial vein gives rise to a subcutaneous red, hard, and tender cord. Thrombophlebitis in a deep vein gives more severe symptoms and may be associated with fever.

Allergy (local)

An allergic-type skin reaction at the venipuncture site caused by allergens in solutions used for disinfection of the arm or allergens from the needle. Symptoms are rash, swelling, and itching at venipuncture site.

Vasovagal reaction

A vasovagal reaction is a general feeling of discomfort and weakness with anxiety, dizziness, and nausea, which may progress to loss of consciousness (faint). Most instances give only minor symptoms, but a few have a more severe course with symptoms such as loss of consciousness and convulsions or incontinence. Symptoms are discomfort, weakness, anxiety, dizziness, nausea, sweating, vomiting, pallor, hyperventilation, convulsions, and loss of consciousness.

The reaction is generated by the autonomic nervous system and further stimulated by psychological factors, and the volume of blood removed relative to the donor's total blood volume.

Vasovagal reaction is the most common acute complication related to blood donation. Some of the most severe complications seen in relation to blood donation are accidents in donors who lose consciousness after leaving the donation site. In order to register these properly, the vasovagal reactions have been grouped as follows:
- *Immediate vasovagal reaction:* Symptoms occur before donor leaves the donation site.
- *Immediate vasovagal reaction with injury:* Injury caused by falls or accidents in donors with a vasovagal reaction and unconsciousness before donor leaves the donation site.
- *Delayed vasovagal reaction:* Symptoms occur after donor leaves the donation site.
- *Delayed vasovagal reaction with injury:* Injury caused by falls or accidents in donors with a vasovagal reaction and unconsciousness after donor leaves the donation site.

Grading of imputability

The strength of relation between donation and complication is
- *Definite or certain:* When there is conclusive evidence beyond reasonable doubt for the relation.
- *Probable or likely:* When the evidence is clearly in favor of a relation.
- *Possible:* when the evidence is indeterminate for attributing the complication to the donation or an alternative cause.
- *Unlikely or doubtful:* When the evidence is clearly in favor of attributing the complication to other causes.
- *Excluded:* When there is conclusive evidence beyond reasonable doubt that the complication can be attributed to causes other than the donation.

For international comparison of data on complications related to blood donation, it is recommended that only cases with an imputability of possible, probable, or definite be captured.

Grading of severity

Severity is graded in two main levels, severe and nonsevere, based on requirements for treatment and on outcome, in a way that corresponds to other systems in use internationally (i.e., ISBT for grading of adverse reactions to blood transfusion, European Commission for grading of transfusion reactions, among others).

Severe complications

Conditions that define a case as severe are as follows:
- *Hospitalization* if it was attributable to the complication.
- *Intervention* to preclude permanent damage or impairment of a body function to prevent death (life-threatening).
- *Symptoms causing significant disability or incapacity* following a complication of blood donation and persisted for more than a year after the donation (long-term morbidity).
- *Death* if it follows a complication of blood donation and the death was possibly, probably, or definitely related to the donation.

Non-severe complications

The nonsevere complications are complications that do not satisfy any of the requirements for being severe. The nonsevere level may be subdivided into mild and moderate complications as for instance for the following categories:
- *Hematoma:*
  - Mild: Local discomfort during phlebotomy, only minor pain or functional impairment
  - Moderate: As mild but with major discomfort during normal activities
- *Arterial puncture:*
  - Mild: No symptoms or local discomfort during phlebotomy and/or hematoma
  - Moderate: Local discomfort continuing after collection was terminated
- *Painful arm (subcategory specified or not):*
  - Mild: Symptoms for less than two weeks
  - Moderate: Symptoms for more than two weeks but less than one year
- *Vasovagal reaction:*
  - Mild: Subjective symptoms only
  - Moderate: Objective symptoms

At the border between mild and no complication there will be a gradual transition of the severity of the symptoms. It is likely that this border will not be placed at the same level in different settings and the number of mild cases may vary considerably from region to region. It is hoped that international sharing of data will gradually lead to improved uniformity.

References

Commission Directive 2005/61/EC

Directive 2002/98/EC

Guide to the preparation, use and quality assurance of blood components, 15th edition. Council of Europe, January 2010

IHN-ISBT WP HV definitions: www.ihn-org.com

SHOT annual report: see www.shotuk.org

APPENDIX B

Proposed Standard Definitions for Surveillance of Non Infectious Adverse Transfusion Reactions

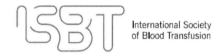

International Society
of Blood Transfusion

WORKING PARTY ON HAEMOVIGILANCE

**PROPOSED STANDARD DEFINITIONS FOR SURVEILLANCE OF
NON INFECTIOUS ADVERSE TRANSFUSION REACTIONS**

JULY 2011

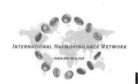

INTERNATIONAL HAEMOVIGILANCE NETWORK

Hemovigilance: An Effective Tool for Improving Transfusion Safety, First Edition. Edited by René R.P. De Vries and Jean-Claude Faber.
© 2012 John Wiley & Sons, Ltd. Published 2012 by John Wiley & Sons, Ltd.

INTRODUCTION

The definitions proposed in this document were prepared by a sub-group of members of the ISBT Working Party on Haemovigilance comprising:

Dr Mark Popovsky, USA
Dr Pierre Robillard, Canada
Dr Martin Schipperus, Netherlands
Dr Dorothy Stainsby, United Kingdom
Dr Jean-Daniel Tissot, Switzerland
Dr Johanna Wiersum-Osselton, Netherlands.

The definitions were inspired from a document written by Dr Juergen Bux on proposed definitions by the European Haemovigilance Network, from existing definitions in various haemovigilance systems and from published literature. The definitions were reviewed and adopted by the ISBT Working Party on Haemovigilance at its meeting in Capetown on September 2, 2006. Case scenarios from actual haemovigilance reports were developed and volunteers from various haemovigilance systems agreed to classify the cases using the standard definitions. Good agreement was obtained for the case definitions but a less good agreement was obtained for imputability grading. It was decided to keep imputability grading as developed because already in use in multiple haemovigilance systems.

These definitions are for the sole purpose of surveillance of adverse events related to the transfusion of blood components in haemovigilance systems. They are not intended as strict diagnostic criteria. Standard definitions are essential if comparisons from different haemovigilance systems are to be made. The purpose of this document is to provide such standard definitions that need to be simple yet precise enough to be able to classify most adverse transfusion events.

We first propose general definitions of adverse transfusion events, near misses, incidents and reactions. The non infectious reactions are then addressed with hemolytic and non hemolytic reactions followed by a proposed classification of severity and imputability (strength of association with transfusion) of adverse events.

This document does not provide categories and definitions for types of transfusion errors and near misses.

The proposed definitions of adverse reactions apply to the adult population of patients. Adaptations of the definitions will have to be made by institutions for the pediatric patient population and especially for neonates.

We hope this document will help the various haemovigilance systems to classify the adverse reactions reported to them in order to generate data that will be comparable at an international level.

Pierre Robillard, MD
Chair, ISBT Working Party on Haemovigilance

1 GENERAL DEFINITIONS OF ADVERSE EVENTS

An **adverse event** is an undesirable and unintended occurrence before, during or after transfusion of blood or blood component which may be related to the administration of the blood or component. It may be the result of an error or an incident and it may or not result in a reaction in a recipient.

An **incident** is a case where the patient is transfused with a blood component which did not meet all the requirements for a suitable transfusion for that patient, or that was intended for another patient. It thus comprises transfusion errors and deviations from standard operating procedures or hospital policies that have lead to mistransfusions. It may or may not lead to an adverse reaction.

A **near miss** is an error or deviation from standard procedures or policies that is discovered before the start of the transfusion and that could have led to a wrongful transfusion or to a reaction in a recipient.

An **adverse reaction** is an undesirable response or effect in a patient temporally associated with the administration of blood or blood component. It may, but need not, be the result of an incident.

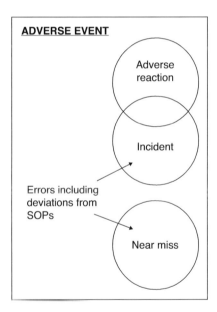

2 HEMOLYTIC TRANSFUSION REACTIONS

A hemolytic transfusion reaction is one in which symptoms and clinical or laboratory signs of increased red cell destruction are produced by transfusion. Hemolysis can occur intravascularly or extravascularly and can be immediate (acute) or delayed.

2.1   Acute hemolytic transfusion reaction (AHTR)

An AHTR has its onset within 24 hours of a transfusion. Clinical or laboratory features of hemolysis are present.

Common signs of AHTR are:
- Fever
- Chills/rigors
- Facial flushing
- Chest pain
- Abdominal pain
- Back/flank pain
- Nausea/vomiting
- Diarrhea
- Hypotension
- Pallor
- Jaundice
- Oligoanuria
- Diffuse bleeding
- Dark urine

Common laboratory features are:
- Hemoglobinemia
- Hemoglobinuria
- Decreased serum haptoglobin
- Unconjugated hyperbilirubinemia
- Increased LDH an AST levels
- Decreased hemoglobin levels

Not all clinical or laboratory features are present in cases of AHTR.

Blood group serology usually shows abnormal results but absence of immunological findings does not exclude AHTR. AHTR may also be due to erythrocyte auto-antibodies in the recipient or to non immunological factors like mechanical factors inducing hemolysis (malfunction of a pump, of a blood warmer, use of hypotonic solutions, etc.).

2.2   Delayed hemolytic transfusion reaction (DHTR)

A DHTR usually manifests between 24 hours and 28 days after a transfusion and clinical or laboratory features of hemolysis are present. Signs and symptoms are similar to AHTR but are usually less severe. DHTR may sometimes manifests as an inadequate rise of post-transfusion hemoglobin level or unexplained fall in hemoglobin after a transfusion. Blood group serology usually shows abnormal results.

2.3   Delayed serologic reaction (DSTR)

There is a DSTR when, after a transfusion, there is demonstration of clinically significant antibodies against red blood cells which were previously absent (as far as is known) and when there are no clinical or laboratory features of hemolysis. This term is synonymous with alloimmunization.

3   NON HEMOLYTIC TRANSFUSION REACTIONS

3.1   Febrile non hemolytic transfusion reaction (FNHTR)

There is a FNHTR in the presence of one or more of:

- fever ($\geq 38°C$ oral or equivalent and a change of $\geq 1°C$ from pretransfusion value),
- chills/rigors

This may be accompanied by headache and nausea.

occurring during or within four hours following transfusion without any other cause such as hemolytic transfusion reaction, bacterial contamination or underlying condition.

FNHTR could be present in absence of fever (if chills or rigors without fever).

FOR THE PURPOSE OF INTERNATIONAL COMPARISONS ONLY THE MOST SERIOUS CASES OF FNHTR SHOULD BE ACCOUNTED FOR:

- fever ($\geq 39°C$ oral or equivalent and a change of $\geq 2°C$ from pretransfusion value) and chills/rigors

3.2   Allergic reaction

An allergic reaction may present only with mucocutaneous signs and symptoms:

- Morbilliform rash with pruritus
- Urticaria (hives)
- Localized angioedema
- Edema of lips, tongue and uvula
- Periorbital pruritus, erythema and edema
- Conjunctival edema

occurring during or within 4 hours of transfusion. In this form it usually presents no immediate risk to life of patient and responds quickly to symptomatic treatment like anti-histamine or steroid medications. This type of allergic reaction is called 'minor allergic reaction' in many hemovigilance systems.

For the purpose of classification this type of allergic reaction would be graded as 1, i.e. non-severe.

An allergic reaction can also involve respiratory and/or cardiovascular systems and present like an anaphylactic reaction. There is anaphylaxis when, in addition to mucocutaneous systems there is airway compromise or severe hypotension requiring vasopressor treatment (or associated symptoms like hypotonia, syncope). The respiratory signs and symptoms may be laryngeal (tightness in the throat, dysphagia, dysphonia, hoarseness, stridor) or pulmonary (dyspnea, cough, wheezing/bronchospasm, hypoxemia). Such a reaction usually occurs occurring during or very shortly after transfusion.

For the purpose of classification this type of allergic reaction would be graded as 2 (severe), 3 (life-threatening) or 4 (death) depending on the course and outcome of the reaction.

An allergic reaction classically results from the interaction of an allergen and preformed antibodies. A rise of mast cell tryptase can support the diagnosis of an allergic reaction. IgA deficiency and/or anti-IgA in the recipient has been associated with severe allergic reactions but is only one infrequent cause out of many others.

3.8   Transfusion associated graft-versus-host disease (TA-GVHD)

TA-GVHD is a clinical syndrome characterised by symptoms of fever, rash, liver dysfunction, diarrhea, pancytopenia and findings of characteristic histological appearances on biopsy occurring 1-6 weeks following transfusion with no other apparent cause.

The diagnosis of TA-GVHD is further supported by the presence of chimerism.

3.7   Post transfusion purpura (PTP)

PTP is characterized by thrombocytopenia arising 5-12 days following transfusion of cellular blood components with findings of antibodies in the patient directed against the Human Platelet Antigen (HPA) system.

3.3   Transfusion-related acute lung injury (TRALI)

In patients with no evidence of acute lung injury (ALI) prior to transfusion, TRALI is diagnosed if a new ALI is present:
- Acute onset
- Hypoxemia
  - $PaO_2 / FiO_2 < 300$ mm Hg or
  - Oxygen saturation is < 90% on room air or
  - Other clinical evidence
- Bilateral infiltrates on frontal chest radiograph
- No evidence of left atrial hypertension (i.e. circulatory overload)
- No temporal relationship to an alternative risk factor for ALI

during or within 6 hours of completion of transfusion.

Alternate risk factors for ALI are:
- Direct Lung Injury
  - Aspiration
  - Pneumonia
  - Toxic inhalation
  - Lung contusion
  - Near drowning
- Indirect Lung Injury
  - Severe sepsis
  - Shock
  - Multiple trauma
  - Burn injury
  - Acute pancreatitis
  - Cardiopulmonary bypass
  - Drug overdose

It has been suggested by the Toronto TRALI Consensus Panel to add a category of *possible TRALI* that would have the same definition as TRALI except for the presence of a temporal relationship to an alternative risk factor for ALI (as described above). In such a circumstance TRALI should be indicated with a *possible* imputability to transfusion.

TRALI is therefore a clinical syndrome and presence of anti-HLA or anti-HNA antibodies in recipient nor confirmation of cognate antigens in donors are required for diagnosis.

3.6   Transfusion associated dyspnea (TAD)

TAD is characterized by respiratory distress within 24 hours of transfusion that does not meet the criteria of TRALI, TACO, or allergic reaction. Respiratory distress should be the most prominent clinical feature and should not be explained by the patient's underlying condition or any other known cause.

3.4   Transfusion associated circulatory overload (TACO)

TACO is characterized by any 4 of the following:
- Acute respiratory distress
- Tachycardia
- Increased blood pressure
- Acute or worsening pulmonary edema on frontal chest radiograph
- Evidence of positive fluid balance

occurring within 6 hours of completion of transfusion.

An elevated BNP is supportive of TACO.

3.5   Hypotensive transfusion reaction

This reaction is characterized by hypotension defined as a drop in systolic blood pressure of $\geq$ 30 mm Hg occurring during or within one hour of completing transfusion and a systolic blood pressure $\leq$ 80 mm Hg.

Most reactions do occur very rapidly after the start of the transfusion (within minutes). This reaction responds rapidly to cessation of transfusion and supportive treatment. This type of reaction appears to occur more frequently in patients on ACE inhibitors

Hypotension is usually the sole manifestation but facial flushing and gastrointestinal symptoms may occur.

All other categories of adverse reactions presenting with hypotension, especially allergic reactions, must have been excluded. The underlying condition of the patient must also have been excluded as a possible explanation for the hypotension.

3.6   Other transfusion reactions
a)   **Haemosiderosis**

Transfusion-associated haemosiderosis is being defined as a blood ferritin level of $\geq$ 1000 micrograms/l, with or without organ dysfunction in the setting of repeated RBC transfusions.

b)   **Hyperkalemia**

Any abnormally high potassium level ($>$ 5 mml/l, or $\geq$1.5 mml/l net increase) within an hour of transfusion can be classified as a transfusion-associated hyperkaliemia.

c)   Unclassifiable Complication of Transfusion (UCT)

Occurrence of an adverse effect or reaction temporally related to transfusion, which cannot be classified according to an already defined ATE and with no risk factor other than transfusion and no other explaining cause.

4 Severity

Grade 1 (Non-Severe):
  – the recipient may have required medical intervention (e.g. symptomatic treatment) but lack of such would not result in permanent damage or impairment of a body function.
Grade 2 (Severe):
  – the recipient required in-patient hospitalization or prolongation of hospitalization directly attributable to the event; and/or
  – the adverse event resulted in persistent or significant disability or incapacity; or
  – the adverse event necessitated medical or surgical intervention to preclude permanent damage or impairment of a body function.
Grade 3 (Life-threatening):
  – the recipient required major intervention following the transfusion (vasopressors, intubation, transfer to intensive care) to prevent death
Grade 4 (Death)
  – the recipient died following an adverse transfusion reaction

Grade 4 should be used only if death is possibly, probably or definitely related to transfusion. If the patient died of another cause, the severity of the reaction should be graded as 1, 2 or 3.

5 Imputability

This is, once the investigation of the adverse transfusion event is completed, the assessment of the strength of relation to the transfusion of the ATE.

Definite (certain):   when there is conclusive evidence beyond reasonable doubt that the adverse event can be attributed to the transfusion
Probable (likely):   when the evidence is clearly in favor of attributing the adverse event to the transfusion
Possible: when the evidence is indeterminate for attributing the adverse event to the transfusion or an alternate cause
Unlikely (doubtful): when the evidence is clearly in favor of attributing the adverse event to causes other than the transfusion
Excluded: when there is conclusive evidence beyond reasonable doubt that the adverse event can be attributed to causes other than the transfusion

Only possible, probable and definite cases should be used for international comparisons.

REFERENCES

Alyea EP, Anderson KC. Transfusion-associated graft-vs-host disease. In: Transfusion Reactions. Popovsky MA (editor). AABB Press, Bethesda, 2007: 229-250.

Ambruso DR. Acute hemolytic transfusion reactions. In: Blood Banking and Transfusion Medicine – Basic principles and Practice. Hillyer CD, Silberstein LE, Ness PM, Anderson KC (editors). Churchill Livingstone. Philadelphia, 2003: 391-5.

Arnold DM, Hume AH. Hypotensive transfusion reactions. In: Transfusion Reactions. Popovsky MA (editor). AABB Press, Bethesda, 2007: 251-273.

Brecher ME. Hemolytic transfusion reactions. In: Principles of Transfusion Medicine. Rossi EC, Simon TL, Moss GS, Gould SA (editors). Williams and Wilkins. Baltimore, 1996: 747-63.

Canadian Transfusion Adverse Event reporting Form – User's Manual. Health Canada. April 2004.

Corriveau P, Lapointe M, Robillard P. Rapport d'incident/accident transfusionnel : Guide d'utilisation du RIAT en ligne. Ministère de la santé et des services sociaux, Québec, Canada, 2001.

Davenport RD. Hemolytic transfusion reactions. In: Transfusion Reactions. Popovsky MA (editor). AABB Press, Bethesda, 2007: 1-55.

Haemolytic transfusion reactions. In: Mollison's Blood Transfusion in Clinical Medicine. Klein HG and Anstee DJ (editors). Blackwell Publishing, Oxford, 2005: 455-95.

Heddle NM, Kelton JG. Febrile nonhemolytic transfusion reactions. In: Transfusion Reactions. Popovsky MA (editor). AABB Press, Bethesda, 2001: 45-82.

Kleinman S, Caulfield T,. Chan P, et al. Towards an understanding of transfusion-related acute lung injury (TRALI): Statement of a Consensus Panel. Transfusion 2004; 44: 1774-89.

McFarland JG. Posttransfusion purpura. In: Transfusion Reactions. Popovsky MA (editor). AABB Press, Bethesda, 2007: 275-300.

Rigamonti Wermelinger V, Senn M. Hémovigilance – Rapport annuel 2004. Swissmedic, Switzerland, 2006.

Roush KS. Febrile, allergic and other non infectious transfusion reactions. In: Blood Banking and Transfusion Medicine – Basic principles and Practice. Hillyer CD, Silberstein LE, Ness PM, Anderson KC (editors). Churchill Livingstone. Philadelphia, 2003: 401-411.

Sampson HA, Munoz-Furlong A, Bock SA, et al. Symposium on the definition and management of anaphylaxis: summary report. J Allergy Clin Immunol 2005; 115: 584-91.

Serious Hazards of Transfusion. Annual report 2004. Serious Hazards of Transfusion Steering group. Royal College of Pathologists. United Kingdom. Nov. 2005.

Shirey RS, King KE, Ness PM. Delayed hemolytic transfusion reactions. In: Blood Banking and Transfusion Medicine – Basic principles and Practice. Hillyer CD, Silberstein LE, Ness PM, Anderson KC (editors). Churchill Livingstone. Philadelphia, 2003: 395-400.

Some unfavourable effects of transfusion. In: Mollison's Blood Transfusion in Clinical Medicine. Klein HG and Anstee DJ (editors). Blackwell Publishing, Oxford, 2005: 666-700.

Toy P, Popovsky MA, Abraham E, et al. Transfusion-related acute lung injury: definition and review. Crit Care Med 2005; 33: 721-6.

Transfusie Reacties in Patienten Rapport 2005. TRIP Foundation, Netherlands 2006.

Vamvakas EC. Allergic and anaphylactic reactions. In: Transfusion Reactions. Popovsky MA (editor). AABB Press, Bethesda, 2007: 105-156.

ISBT Working Party on Haemovigilance

Standard for Surveillance of Complications Related to Blood Donation

Working Group on Complications Related to Blood Donation

International Society of Blood Transfusion Working Party on Haemovigilance

European Haemovigilance Network

2008

Hemovigilance: An Effective Tool for Improving Transfusion Safety, First Edition. Edited by René R.P. De Vries and Jean-Claude Faber.
© 2012 John Wiley & Sons, Ltd. Published 2012 by John Wiley & Sons, Ltd.

Contents

Introduction

In 2004 the *International Society of Blood Transfusion* (ISBT) and the *European Haemovigilance Network* (EHN) set up a *Common Working Group on Complications Related to Blood Donation* (DOCO). The task was to create a set of definitions of issues in this new field, definitions which could be used internationally, and thereby facilitate international benchmarking. The aim is to contribute to efforts to increase safety of blood donors world wide.

The DOCO group has consisted of the following members: Elisabeth Caffrey (UK, 2004 -2007), Jo Wiersum (The Netherlands, TRIP, since 2007), Hitoshi Okazaki (Japan, Japanese Red Cross Blood Service, since 2008), Peter Tomasulo (US, Blood Systems, writing member since 2008) and Jan Jorgensen (Denmark, chair, since 2004).

The intention of this standard is to present an internationally accepted description of the complications, including severity and imputability grades, which can be used for benchmarking and international presentations. The present version results from critical review of the Madrid 2007 version by a large international panel. This led to regrouping of the categories and some adjustments to the descriptors of the severity levels.

A total of 18 categories have been defined. They are grouped according to the localization of the symptoms (local or general), complications especially related to apheresis and a final group of "others". A description of a complication category is only given for the most common complications (occurrence >1% of all complications) and not for the rare events associated with blood donation (<1% of all complications). Some of the rare complications are of a serious nature and will often be diagnosed by medical professionals outside the blood service. Medical terms used in categories are defined as indicated in common medical dictionaries. Severity and imputability are graded as shown in annex 2. Definitions of other issues used for the description of the categories are given in annex 3.

This Standard deals, as stated above, with common complications (adverse reactions or incidents) related in time to a blood donation (whole blood or apheresis). The complications related to apheresis are included as categories only, but definitions may be developed in the future. In the present version there are no categories or definitions for complications related to donation of more than one unit, long term effects following several donations or adverse events related to the donation process as such. If these prove necessary these will be addressed in a future edition of the Standard.

Jan Jorgensen, MD
Chair of Working Group

Description of Categories

A. Complications mainly with local symptoms.

These complications are directly caused by the insertion of the needle. Some of these are mainly characterized by occurrence of blood outside vessels, whereas others are mainly characterized by pain

A 1. Complications mainly characterized by the occurrence of blood out-side the vessels.

Haematoma
A haematoma is an accumulation of blood in the tissues outside the vessels.
Symptoms are bruising, discolouration, swelling and local pain.

Haematoma is the second most common acute complication which occur related to blood donation.
The symptoms are caused by blood flowing out of damaged vessels and accumulating in the soft tissues. As the volume of the haematoma increases, swelling will occur. The swelling will put pressure on the surrounding tissues.
The strength of the pressure will depend on size of the swelling and softness of the surrounding tissue. Pressure on nerves will result in neurologic symptoms like pain radiating down in forearm and hand, and of peripheral tingling.
If blood accumulates in the frontal deep layers of the forearm between muscles and tendons swelling is hard to recognize, but the pressure increases very easily. Therefore, complications like injury of a nerve and even a compartment syndrome occurs more often related to a haematoma with this localization.

Arterial puncture
Arterial puncture is a puncture of the brachial artery or of one of its branches by the needle used for bleeding of donor.
Symptoms: There may be weak pain localized to the elbow region. Objectively a lighter red colour than usual of the collected blood can be seen and perhaps some movements of the needle caused by arterial pulsation; the bag fills very quickly. In uncomplicated cases there may be no haematoma.
Complications: The risk of a large haematoma is increased and thereby risks such as Compartment Syndrome in the forearm, Brachial Artery Pseudo Aneurysm and arterio-venous Fistula.

Delayed bleeding
Delayed bleeding is spontaneous recommencement of bleeding from the venipuncture site, which occurs after donor has left the donation site.

A 2. Complications mainly characterized by pain

Nerve irritation
Irritation of a nerve by pressure from a haematoma.
Symptoms are nerve type as radiating pain and/or paraesthesiae in association with a haematoma. The haematoma may not always be apparent at the time. Symptoms do not occur immediately on insertion of the needle but start when the haematoma has reached a sufficient size, some time after insertion of the needle.

Nerve injury
Injury of a nerve by the needle at insertion or withdrawal.
Symptoms are pain often associated with paraesthesiae. The pain is severe and radiating. It arises immediately when the needle is inserted or withdrawn.

Tendon injury
Injury of a tendon by the needle.
Symptoms are very severe local non-radiating pain initiating immediately when the needle is inserted.

Painful arm
Cases characterized mainly by severe local and radiating pain in the arm used for the donation and arising during or within hours following donation, but without further details to permit classification in one of the already more specific categories mentioned above.

A 3. Other kinds of categories with local symptoms

Thrombophlebitis
Inflammation in a vein associated with a thrombus
Symptoms are warmth, tenderness, local pain, redness and swelling. Thrombophlebitis in a superficial vein gives rise to a subcutaneous red, hard and tender cord.
Thrombophlebitis in a deep vein gives more severe symptoms and may be associated with fever.

Allergy (local)
Allergic type skin reaction at the venipuncture site caused by allergens in solutions used for disinfection of the arm or allergens from the needle. Symptoms are rash, swelling and itching at venipuncture site

B. Complications mainly with generalized symptoms.

Vasovagal reaction
A vasovagal reaction is a general feeling of discomfort and weakness with anxiety, dizziness and nausea, which may progress to loss of consciousness (faint). Most give only minor symptoms, but a few have a more severe course with symptoms like loss of consciousness and convulsions or incontinence. Symptoms are discomfort, weakness, anxiety, dizziness, nausea, sweating, vomiting, pallor, hyperventilation, convulsions, and loss of consciousness. The reaction is generated by the autonomic nervous system and further stimulated by psychological factors, and the volume of blood removed relative to the donor's total blood volume.
It is the most common acute complication related to blood donation. Some of the most severe complications seen in relation to blood donation are accidents in donors who lose consciousness after leaving the donation site. In order to register these properly the vasovagal reactions have been grouped in

Immediate Vasovagal reaction
Symptoms occurred before donor has left the donation site

Immediate Vasovagal Reaction with injury
Injury caused by falls or accidents in donors with a vasovagal reaction and unconsciousness before donor has left the donation site

Delayed Vasovagal Reaction

Symptoms occurred after donor has left the donation site.

Delayed Vasovagal Reaction with injury

Injury caused by falls or accidents in donors with a vasovagal reaction and unconsciousness after donor has left the donation site.

C. Complications related to apheresis

Citrate reaction
Haemolysis
Generalised allergic reaction
Air embolism

D. Other complications related to blood donation

Annex 1. Categories of complications related to blood donation (overview)

Local symptoms	Blood outside vessels		Haematoma
			Arterial puncture
			Delayed bleeding
	Pain	Specified as	Nerve irritation
			Nerve injury
			Tendon injury
		or not specified	Painful arm
	Others		Thrombophlebitis
			Allergy (local)
Generalised symptoms	Vasovagal reaction		Immediate
			Immediate with injury
			Delayed
			Delayed with injury
Related to apheresis			Citrate reaction
			Haemolysis
			Generalised allergic reaction
			Air embolism
Other			

Annex 2 Grading of complication severity and imputability

Grading of severity

Severity is graded in two main levels severe and non-severe, based on requirements for treatment and on outcome, in a way which corresponds to other systems in use internationally (i.e. ISBT for grading of adverse reactions to blood transfusion, European Commission for grading of transfusion reactions, FDA for grading of drug adverse events).

Severe complications

Conditions which define a case as severe are:

Hospitalization:	If it was attributable to the complication.
Intervention:	To preclude permanent damage or impairment of a body function
	To prevent death (life- threatening)
Symptoms:	Causing significant disability or incapacity following a complication of blood donation and persisted for more than a year after the donation (Long term morbidity)
Death:	If it follows a complication of blood donation and the death was possibly, probably or definitely related to the donation.

Non-severe complications

The non-severe complications are complications which do not satisfy any of the requirements for being severe.

The non-severe level may be subdivided in mild and moderate complications as for instance for the following categories

Haematoma
Mild:	Local discomfort during phlebotomy only minor pain or functional Impairment
Moderate:	As mild but with major discomfort during normal activities

Arterial puncture
Mild:	No symptoms or local discomfort during phlebotomy and/or haematoma
Moderate:	Local discomfort continuing after the collection was terminated

Painful arm (subcategory specified or not)
Mild:	Symptoms for less than two weeks
Moderate:	Symptoms for more than two weeks but less than 1 year

Vasovagal reaction
Mild:	Subjective symptoms only
Moderate:	Objective symptoms

At the border between mild and no complication there will be a gradual transition of severity of the symptoms. It is likely that this border will not be placed at the same level in different settings and the number of mild cases may vary considerably from region to region. It is hoped that international sharing of data will gradually lead to improved uniformity.

Grading of imputability

The strength of relation between donation and complication is

Definite or certain:	when there is conclusive evidence beyond reasonable doubt for the relation
Probable or likely:	when the evidence is clearly in favor of a relation
Possible:	when the evidence is indeterminate for attributing the complication to the donation or an alternative cause
Unlikely or doubtful:	when the evidence is clearly in favor of attributing the complication to other causes
Excluded:	when there is conclusive evidence beyond reasonable doubt that the complication can be attributed to causes other than the donation.

It is recommended that for international comparison of data on complications related to blood donation only cases with imputability of possible, probable or definite be captured.

Annex 3. Definitions and remarks concerning issues used for the description of categories

Donation site is the area within which staff can observe donor and be responsible for care of donors with complications.

Complications related to blood donation are adverse reactions and adverse events with a temporal relation to a blood donation.

An immediate complication is a complication which occurs before donor has left the donation site.

A delayed complication is a complication which occurs after donor has left the donation site.

The relation of a delayed complication to the actual blood donation should be critically assessed (see grading of imputability).

Bruises and haematomas

Bruises can be very extensive but without any measurable swelling, whereas when the name a haematoma is used there would generally be swelling. However, as there is no physiological difference between bruises and haematomas except for the thickness, large skin discolouration can still be registered as a haematoma.

Annex 4. Scheme for registration of collected data

Category	Number of cases				
	Mild	Mode rate	Severe		Total
			Sympt >1 y	All severe	
Haematoma					
Arterial puncture					
Delayed bleeding					
Nerve irritation					
Nerve injury					
Tendon injury					
Painful arm					
Total number local sympt.					
VVR Immediate type					
VVR Immediate , accident					
VVR Delayed type					
VVR Delayed, accident					
Total number VV R					
Citrate reaction					
Haemolysis					
Generalised allergic reaction					
Air embolism					
Total					

Index

Note: page numbers in *italics* refer to figures; those in **bold** to tables or boxes.

Hemovigilance: An Effective Tool for Improving Transfusion Safety, First Edition. Edited by René R.P. De Vries and Jean-Claude Faber.
© 2012 John Wiley & Sons, Ltd. Published 2012 by John Wiley & Sons, Ltd.

Printed and bound by CPI Group (UK) Ltd, Croydon, CR0 4YY